Updates in Clinical Dermatology

Updates in Clinical Dermatology aims to promote the rapid and efficient transfer of medical research into clinical practice. It is published in four volumes per year. Covering new developments and innovations in all fields of clinical dermatology, it provides the clinician with a review and summary of recent research and its implications for clinical practice. Each volume is focused on a clinically relevant topic and explains how research results impact diagnostics, treatment options and procedures as well as patient management. The reader-friendly volumes are highly structured with core messages, summaries, tables, diagrams and illustrations and are written by internationally well-known experts in the field. A volume editor supervises the authors in his/her field of expertise in order to ensure that each volume provides cutting-edge information most relevant and useful for clinical dermatologists. Contributions to the series are peer reviewed by an editorial board.

Suzanne Wei Na Cheng
Chee Leok Goh
Editors

Updates on Lasers in Dermatology

Springer

Editors
Suzanne Wei Na Cheng
National Skin Centre
Singapore, Singapore

Chee Leok Goh
National Skin Centre
Singapore, Singapore

ISSN 2523-8884 ISSN 2523-8892 (electronic)
Updates in Clinical Dermatology
ISBN 978-3-031-71154-1 ISBN 978-3-031-71155-8 (eBook)
https://doi.org/10.1007/978-3-031-71155-8

This Springer imprint is published by the registered company Springer Nature Switzerland AG
The registered company address is: Gewerbestrasse 11, 6330 Cham, Switzerland

Foreword

The use of laser- and energy-based devices in dermatological application has gained much popularity in the last several decades. Asians' skin differs from that of Caucasians in many aspects, and photoaging among Asians tends to result in less wrinkles but more pigmentary conditions such as lentigo. Furthermore, Asians' skin tends to have more complications after laser treatment including post-inflammatory hyperpigmentation. For body contouring, Asians with a smaller physique tend to be less responsive to energy-based device treatment.

This book with authors from Asian countries is very special as it has gathered expert opinions regarding the use of lasers and energy-based devices in a wide range of dermatological applications from medical to cosmetic use among Asians. The editors and all the contributors have done an excellent work and are to be congratulated in providing such a scholarly and updated contribution to our current literature.

Henry H. L. Chan

Division of Dermatology
University of Hong Kong
Hong Kong, China

Wellman Center for Photomedicine
Massachusetts General Hospital
Boston, MA, USA

Preface

The therapeutic landscape of dermatology has been significantly enriched by the advent of laser technology, making it possible to address both medical and cosmetic skin conditions with precision and efficacy. This volume provides an up-to-date, illustrated synopsis of the therapeutic applications of lasers, shedding light on their efficacy and safety across a spectrum of dermatological conditions, from keloids, viral warts, skin malignancies, and infantile hemangioma to a wide range of cosmetic indications such as skin tightening, rejuvenation, resurfacing, and removal of birthmarks, pigmentation, and unwanted hair.

Authored by experts with years of clinical experience, this volume reflects the depth of knowledge and expertise that the field of dermatology has to offer. Each chapter meticulously focuses on newer advances and techniques, aiming not only to enlighten the reader but also to inspire innovation and a forward-thinking approach in their clinical practice. Since the 1960s, dermatologists have progressed from microsecond to nanosecond to picosecond pulse widths and from fully ablative lasers to fractional photothermolysis with diffractive handpieces. Laser removal of disfiguring facial birthmarks such as port-wine stain and nevus of Ota can now be successfully achieved with minimal scarring. We devote a chapter on special considerations of lasers in the pediatric population. This book serves as an essential guide to seasoned dermatologists seeking to refine their laser techniques and to novices eager to learn about the latest laser- and energy-based devices.

It is with great pride that we present this authoritative and comprehensive volume, "Updates on Lasers in Dermatology." As we turn the pages of this volume, let us embark on this journey of discovery and learning together. We would like to thank all the contributors who have worked hard to produce this volume.

Singapore, Singapore

Suzanne Wei Na Cheng
Chee Leok Goh

Contents

History of the Development of Lasers for Dermatological Applications

1

Woo Chiao Tay and Jun Khee Heng

Advent of Laser

German theoretical physicist Max Planck, in his effort to predict the spectral distribution of thermal radiation from a closed furnace ("black-body radiation"), introduced an accurate mathematical expression which is known today as Planck's law [1]. Planck presented the relationship between energy and frequency of radiation, with the conclusion that energy could only be emitted or absorbed in discrete "quanta."

Inspired by the theory of his mentor and professional colleague, physicist Albert Einstein in 1916 introduced the concept of stimulated emission, where excited photons (discrete quantum particle energy chunks delivered by light) could stimulate emission of new photons in the same phase, frequency, polarization, and direction of the original photon [2].

However, it was only four decades later in 1953 and 1954 when American and Russian physicists independently reported a device using ammonia molecules as active species to generate microwave, creating the acronym MASER, which stands for "microwave amplification by stimulated emission of radiation" [3–5]. Many experimental studies quickly followed. Arthur L. Schawlow and his brother-in-law Charles H. Townes showed that masers could be made theoretically to operate in the optical and infrared region in 1958 [6].

At that time, Theodore H. Maiman was an American physicist at Hughes Research Laboratories in Malibu. Then on 16 May 1960, Maiman constructed and fired the first functional optical maser, using synthetic chromium in corundum (ruby) excited by a photographic xenon flash lamp [7]. Maiman's work led to the development of multiple other optical masers, and the term LASER ("light amplification by stimulated emission of radiation") was coined by Gordon Gould, another American physicist.

Q-switch, or "quality-switching," was a technique to shorten pulse length to nanoseconds using an electro-optical shutter introduced in 1961 and 1962 by Fred J. McClung and Robert W. Hellwarth [8, 9]. Q-switch allowed for storage and release of gigawatts of energy.

Light and Laser in Dermatology

The use of light in dermatological treatment is hardly a novel concept. The ancient Egyptians treated vitiligo by using sunlight (bestowed upon them by the sun god Amun-Ra) to activate the naturally occurring photosensitizer psoralen in parsley. Physicians were also increasingly using light therapy to treat many diseases in the 1700s and 1800s—tuberculosis being the most well-

W. C. Tay (✉) · J. K. Heng
National Skin Centre, Singapore, Singapore
e-mail: woochiao.tay@mohh.com.sg; hengjk@nsc.com.sg

S. W. N. Cheng, C. L. Goh (eds.), *Updates on Lasers in Dermatology*, Updates in Clinical Dermatology, https://doi.org/10.1007/978-3-031-71155-8_1

known example. In dermatology, Finsen lamp was used to treat lupus vulgaris in 1899, and artificial UV light sources were used to promote wound healing and treat rickets after 1901 [10]. Finally, no discussion on phototherapy would be complete without mentioning William H. Goeckerman of Mayo Clinic and his first reported successful use of broad-spectrum UV radiation and topical crude coal tar in the treatment of severe psoriasis [11]. Given their familiarity with using light as a therapeutic option, it was not surprising that dermatologists quickly explored laser as an option to treat other skin conditions. An overview is summarized in Table 1.1.

1960s

Leon Goldman was an American dermatologist at the University of Cincinnati General Hospital (now the University of Cincinnati Medical Center) from 1945 until 1980 [12]. He had learnt of Theodore Maiman's invention of ruby laser in 1960, and Goldman started exploring using lasers as a tool to treat dermatological conditions. He founded the first biomedical laser research laboratory in 1961 at the university [10]. In his first studies in 1963, Goldman reported the effects of a ruby laser beam on the skin, selectively destroying pigmented cutaneous structures, including hair follicles with the beam of the ruby laser [13]. Pigmented structures (black hair follicles) were selectively destroyed with no change to the underlying white skin. Goldman also introduced Q-switch ruby laser treatment of tattoos, initially using 0.001-s pulses (1 ms) in 1965 and then improving the treatment specificity by using the shorter 10–30 ns pulses in 1967 [14, 15]. For all his contributions to the field of laser dermatology, Dr. "Golden Lion Man" was officially honored with the title "Father of Laser Medicine" 1979 at the Opto-Electronic Conference in Munich, Germany [12]. He also co-founded, with Ellet Drake, the American Society for Laser Medicine and Surgery in 1981 in San Diego, California [16].

1970s

Since 1960s, Goldman has been investigating the effects of different lasers in the treatment of dermatological conditions [17]. Although the first report of neodymium:yttrium-aluminum-garnet (Nd:YAG) laser was by Johnson in 1961 [18], it was only in 1973 that Goldman introduced its use to treat vascular lesions [10].

The basis of photodynamic therapy (PDT) started in 1900 by Oscar Raab, a medical student collaborating with Professor Hermann von Tappeiner in Munich, Germany. While exploring the impact of acridine dyes on protozoa, Raab uncovered during a thunderstorm that the fusion of acridine red and light proved lethal to infusoria, a type of paramecium.

However, it was Thomas J. Dougherty who initially investigated the photoactivated fluorescein in PDT as a potential anticancer treatment [19]. He was studying the use of lasers to activate photosensitive substances to preferentially destroy cancer cells. In 1975, Dougherty and his team at the Roswell Park Cancer Institute in Buffalo announced the first successful complete tumor cures using HpD and red light activation in the PDT treatment of experimental tumors in mice [20].

1980s

The next breakthrough in the field of lasers in dermatology came in 1983, thanks to the revolutionary selective photothermolysis principle introduced by R. Rox Anderson and John Parrish [21]. By utilizing specific wavelengths, this selective photothermolysis approach allowed for the targeted destruction of particular chromophores. Consequently, destructive thermal energy could be localized more accurately, minimizing damage to the surrounding tissue. The flashlamp-pumped pulsed dye laser (using an organic dye to produce yellow laser light at a wavelength of either 577 or 585 nm) was the first laser specifically developed for the treatment of vascular lesions.

Table 1.1 Summary of major historical milestones in laser in dermatological surgery

Before 1960s	**1916–1917** Stimulated emission concept (Einstein)	**1955** Maser (Townes/Gordon)							
1960s	**1960** Ruby laser (Maiman)	**1960–1961** HeNe laser (Javan)	**1961** Nd:YAG solid state lasers (Johnson)	**1961** QS technique	**1962** Semiconductor diode lasers	**1962** Argon laser (Bennett)	**1964** CO_2 laser (Patel)	**1965** Ruby laser on tattoo (Goldman)	
1970s	**1970** Excimer laser	**1972** Quantum well laser	**1973** Nd:YAG in vascular lesions	**1975** PDT and activated dyes as antitumour agents (Dougherty)	**1976** Free-electron laser				
1980s	**1981** Argon dye laser (Scheibner)	**1981** Flashlamp-pumped PDL	**1983** Selective thermolysis (Anderson, Parrish)	**1984** Laser light for PDT	**1985** CO_2 resurfacing on mucous membrane for actinic cheilitis	**1987** Laser-Assisted Drug Delivery (LADD) first described	**1989** FDA approval Q-switched ruby laser approved for tattoo removal		
1990s	**1991** High-energy pulsed CO_2 laser resurfacing	**1994** Semiconductor laser (simultaneously emission of widely separated wavelengths)	**Mid-1990s** IPL	**1996** Er:YAG laser resurfacing	**1996** PDL for acne scar	**1997** Pulsed alexandrite and pulsed diode hair removal laser 308-nm Excimer laser	**1999** Topical ALA and blue light for actinic keratoses	**1999** Nd:YAG—dermal remodelling (Tanzi)	**1999** Long-pulsed Nd:YAG for leg veins

(continued)

Table 1.1 (continued)

2000s	**2001**	**2002**	**2002**	**2003**	**2004**	**2004–2005**	**2007**	**2009**
	Long-Pulsed Nd:YAG Laser-Assisted Hair Removal	Long-pulsed PDL with dynamic cooling	Picosecond laser in tattoo removal	Long-pulsed PDL and PDT for acne vulgaris	Fractional photothermolysis or Fraxel (Manstein)	Light-emitting diode photomodulation	Xenon chloride excimer	Femtosecond pulsed laser
2010s	**2010s**	Fractional picosecond Nd:YAG laser technique for skin rejuvenation	Continuous evolution of current techniques for better efficacy and safety					
	Expansion of LADD (actinic keratoses, actinic cheilitis, squamous cell carcinoma in situ, and even hypertrophic scars and keloids)	Combination with optical elements e.g., DOE, MLA, holographic optical arrays						

HeNe Helium-neon, *Nd:YAG* neodymium-doped yttrium aluminium garnet, *QS* quality switch, CO_2 carbon dioxide, *PDL* pulsed dye laser, *PDT* photodynamic therapy, *IPL* intense pulsed light, *Er:YAG* erbium-doped yttrium aluminium garnet, *ALA* aminolevulonic acid

1990s

In the 1990s, we saw the rise of both ablative and non-ablative laser systems. There was an increased use of lasers in surface resurfacing, laser hair removal, and laser rejuvenation, particularly the use of pulsed, high-energy CO_2 and erbium:YAG lasers from the mid-1990s. Selective photothermolysis principle also led to the development of photoepilation, and in 1996, the American Food and Drug Administration approved the first ruby laser device for hair removal.

In 1997, Bonis et al. introduced 308 nm excimer laser for the treatment of refractory psoriasis [22]. The excimer laser uses xenon and chloride gases to create unstable "excited dimers." The dissociation of these dimers emits a 308 nm monochromatic coherent wavelength in the UVB spectrum.

Laser and PDT also saw an increase in its usage in this decade. In 1990, actinic keratoses and skin cancers were treated using a combination of topical 5-aminolevulinic acid (ALA) and noncoherent red light emitted from a slide projector equipped with a 600 nm red filter [23]. Subsequent to that, various other sources of red light (tungsten, xenon arc, halogen light) were utilized in combination with topical ALA. However, it was discovered that the combination of topical ALA with noncoherent blue light was the most effective in treating extensive areas of photodamaged skin and received FDA approval in 1999 for the treatment of actinic keratoses [24, 25].

Gold et al. first introduced the use of intense pulsed light (IPL) technology with the EpiLight Hair Removal System where they reported a 60% reduction in hair growth after a single treatment session, marking the initial published application of IPL for hair removal [26]. And since mid-1990s, there was a rise of IPL utilization in the dermatological field [27–29]. The IPL source emits noncoherent light in the 500–1200 nm range and has been successfully used to treat various vascular lesions like facial telangiectasias, port-wine stains, and hemangiomas. IPL can target both superficial and deep vessels effectively, particularly in patients with fair complexions, while minimizing the risk of adverse effects such as purpura and hyperpigmentation.

Although it was invented in 1962, the semiconductor diode laser only gained popularity in dermatology for use in late 1990s to 2000s [22–24]. The longer wavelength (800–810 nm) is absorbed sufficiently by melanin for laser hair removal, but at the same time lesser than that of ruby or alexandrite. This made the semiconductor diode laser a safer option for patients with darker skin phototypes.

2000s

Compared to other chromophores, tattoo pigments have very short thermal relaxation time of 10 ns. While Q-switched nanosecond lasers had been the laser of choice in the removal of tattoo pigments up till then, there was a demand for another method to delivery energy within even shorter pulse durations and hopefully enhance the efficacy of lasers in tattoo removal.

In the late 1990s and 2000s, the picosecond laser fulfilled this clinical need. Using a 1064 nm wavelength and graphite as pigment particle, Ho et al. used computer simulations of picosecond lasers to demonstrate that a predominantly photomechanical effect, as opposed to photothermal, resulted in successful removal of pigment tattoo particles. The quick increase in temperature generated a pressure wave that surpassed the tensile strength of pigment particles, causing them to fracture into smaller fragments. Using the optimal range of 10–100 ps, there was effective pigment clearance with little collateral damage [30].

From mid-1990s, ablative laser systems continued to expand its use to include atrophic scars, photodamaged facial skin, dyschromias, and photoinduced facial rhytides [31]. Fractional photothermolysis was introduced by Dieter Manstein as a new concept for cutaneous remodeling after microscopy thermal injury in 2004 [32]. It received FDA approval in 2004 for skin resurfacing and in 2005 for the treatment of melasma [33]. Using midinfrared laser light, the fractional photothermolysis laser creates numerous microscopic columns of dermal damage (microthermal zones) extending into the dermis. This "pixilated" treatment area initiates a wound repair phase with skin regeneration and remodeling. Fractional lasers can be categorized as ablative or non-ablative based on their effect on the stratum corneum. Ablative lasers cause complete skin destruction using longer wavelengths (2940–10,600 nm), while non-ablative lasers (1320–1927 nm) preserve the stratum corneum.

In the field of PDT, the combination of laser and photosensitizer also expanded. Different types of red light lasers, including copper vapor dye, Nd:YAG, and argon-ion dye lasers, were utilized in combination with topical ALA, resulting in varying rates of clearance. The 595 nm long-pulsed pulsed dye laser (PDL) was also employed with topical ALA to treat various forms of actinic disease, such as actinic keratoses, actinic cheilitis, and photoaging [34].

2010s to Now

Finally, in the past decade, developments in laser revolved more about improving the efficacy and safety of existing laser modalities and expanding its clinical indications. Fractional photothermolysis brought new spotlight onto laser-assisted drug delivery (LADD). Although first reported in 1987, the rapid evolution of LADD occurred in 2010s [35, 36]. LADD is considered a safe and improved drug delivery option in adults and adolescents, across all Fitzpatrick skin types and also in patients with immunosuppressants. Its use has been described in the treatment of actinic keratoses, actinic cheilitis, squamous cell carcinoma in situ, and even hypertrophic scars and keloids [37].

Existing technology continues to be enhanced. Fractional picosecond Nd:YAG laser technique has been combined with optical elements such as diffractive optical element (DOE), microlens array (MLA), holographic optical arrays to improve the effectiveness of skin treatment of pigmented lesions, and skin rejuvenation [38–41]. These special arrangements enable the energy to be focused within laser 2010s to now microbeams, leaving the surrounding tissue between these microspots unaffected [42]. Wat et al. first demonstrated in a prospective study the use of a 755 nm picosecond laser with diffractive lens array (DLA) in treating photoaging in Chinese individuals, with substantial enhancement observed in skin texture and reduction of skin discoloration after six sessions [43].

Nd:YAG laser has been reported to be used in the treatment of onychomycosis [44].

As what we have seen repeatedly in the history of laser development, small new technological advancements may need time to refine its clinical application before becoming the next groundbreaking advancement.

The Future

In conclusion, the field of dermatology has experienced significant advancements in laser technology over the years, with numerous historical milestones marking its transformative journey. From the earliest discoveries to the present day, researchers have persistently refined and expanded the application of lasers for the treatment of various skin conditions. As a result, today's laser technology offers highly accurate, effective, and minimally invasive solutions for a wide range of dermatological concerns. Moving forward, it is essential to appraise and embrace new laser technologies as they emerge, as the continuous evolution of this field promises to bring about even more innovations, further revolutionizing the way we approach skin care and treatment.

References

1. Klein MJ. Max Planck and the beginnings of the quantum theory. Arch Hist Exact Sci. 1975;1(5):459–79.
2. Einstein A. Zur Quantentheorie der Strahlung (On the quantum theory of radiation). Phys Z. 1917;18:121–8.
3. Gordon JP, Zeiger HJ, Townes CH. The maser-new type of microwave amplifier, frequency standard, and spectrometer. Phys Rev. 1955;99(4):1264–74.
4. Weber J. Amplification of microwave radiation by substances not in thermal equilibrium. Trans IRE Prof Gr Electron Devices. 1953;PGED-3(3):1–4.

5. Townes CH. Early history of quantum electronics. J Mod Opt. 2005;52(12):1637–45.
6. Schawlow AL, Townes CH. Infrared and optical masers. Phys Rev. 1958;112(6):1940–9.
7. Maiman T. Stimulated optical radiation in ruby. Nature. 1960;187(4736):493–4.
8. Hellwarth RW. Theory of the pulsation of fluorescent light from ruby. Phys Rev Lett. 1961;6(1):9–12. https://doi.org/10.1103/PhysRevLett.6.9.
9. McClung FJ, Hellwarth RW. Giant optical pulsations from ruby. J Appl Phys. 1962;33(3):828–9.
10. Geiges ML. History of lasers in dermatology. Curr Problems Dermatol. 2011;42:1–6.
11. Orseth ML, Cropley TG. What's in a name? JAMA Dermatol. 2013;149(12):1409. https://doi.org/10.1001/jamadermatol.2013.7477.
12. Ohshiro T. A tribute to the "Golden Lion Man"; Leon Goldman, MD, Father of laser surgery. Laser Ther. 2008;17(3):125–8.
13. Goldman L, Blaney DJ, Kindel DJ, Franke EK. Effect of the laser beam on the skin. Preliminary report. J Invest Dermatol. 1963;40:121–2.
14. Goldman L, Wilson RG, Hornby P, Meyer RG. Radiation from a Q-switched ruby laser. Effect of repeated impacts of power output of 10 megawatts on a tattoo of man. J Invest Dermatol. 1965;44(1):69–71. https://doi.org/10.1038/jid.1965.14.
15. Goldman L, Rockwell RJ, Meyer R, Otten R, Wilson RG, Kitzmiller KW. Laser treatment of tattoos. A preliminary survey of three year's clinical experience. JAMA. 1967;201(11):841–4.
16. ASLMS history. American Society for Laser Medicine and Surgery Inc. 2022. https://www.aslms.org/about-aslms/history.
17. Goldman L. Biomedical aspects of the laser. Heidelberg: Springer Berlin; 1967. https://doi.org/10.1007/978-3-642-85797-3.
18. Johnson LF. Optical maser characteristics of rare-earth ions in crystals. J Appl Phys. 1963;34(4):897–909.
19. Dougherty TJ. Activated dyes as antitumor agents. J Natl Cancer Inst. 1974;52(4):1333–6. https://doi.org/10.1093/jnci/52.4.1333.
20. Dougherty TJ, Grindey GB, Fiel R, Weishaupt KR, Boyle DG. Photoradiation therapy. II. Cure of animal tumors with hematoporphyrin and light. J Natl Cancer Inst. 1975;55(1):115–21. https://doi.org/10.1093/jnci/55.1.115.
21. Anderson RR, Parrish JA. Selective photothermolysis: precise microsurgery by selective absorption of pulsed radiation. Science. 1983;220(4596):524–7. https://doi.org/10.1126/science.6836297.
22. Bónis B, Kemény L, Dobozy A, Bor Z, Szabó G, Ignácz F. 308 nm UVB excimer laser for psoriasis. Lancet. 1997;350(9090):1522.
23. Kennedy JC, Pottier RH, Pross DC. Photodynamic therapy with endogenous protoporphyrin. J Photochem Photobiol B Biol. 1990;6(1–2):143–8.
24. Jeffes E. Levulan®: the first approved topical photosensitizer for the treatment of actinic keratosis. J Dermatol Treatment. 2002;13(Suppl 1):S19–23. https://doi.org/10.1080/095466302317414663.
25. Karrer S, Szeimies R-M, Hohenleutner U, Landthaler M. Role of lasers and photodynamic therapy in the treatment of cutaneous malignancy. Am J Clin Dermatol. 2001;2(4):229–37. https://doi.org/10.2165/00128071-200102040-00004.
26. Gold MH, Bell MW, Foster TD, Street S. Long-term epilation using the EpiLight broad band, intense pulsed light hair removal system. Dermatol Surg. 1997;23(10):909–13.
27. Tanzi EL, Lupton JR, Alster TS. Lasers in dermatology: four decades of progress. J Am Acad Dermatol. 2003;49(1):1–34.
28. Raulin C, Werner S. Treatment of venous malformations with an intense pulsed light source (IPLS) technology: a retrospective study. Lasers Surg Med. 1999;25(2):170–7. https://doi.org/10.1002/(sici)1096-9101(1999)25:2<170::aid-lsm11>3.0.co;2-v.
29. Raulin C, Schroeter CA, Weiss RA, Keiner M, Werner S. Treatment of port-wine stains with a noncoherent pulsed light source. Arch Dermatol. 1999;135(6):679. https://doi.org/10.1001/archderm.135.6.679.
30. Ho DD-M, London R, Zimmerman GB, Young DA. Laser-tattoo removal—a study of the mechanism and the optimal treatment strategy via computer simulations. Lasers Surg Med. 2002;30(5):389–97. https://doi.org/10.1002/lsm.10065.
31. Fitzpatrick RE. Maximizing benefits and minimizing risk with CO_2 laser resurfacing. Dermatol Clin. 2002;20(1):77–86.
32. Manstein D, Herron GS, Sink RK, Tanner H, Anderson RR. Fractional photothermolysis: a new concept for cutaneous remodeling using microscopic patterns of thermal injury. Lasers Surg Med. 2004;34(5):426–38. https://doi.org/10.1002/lsm.20048.
33. Houk LD, Humphreys T. Masers to magic bullets: an updated history of lasers in dermatology. Clin Dermatol. 2007;25(5):434–42.
34. Alexiades-Armenakas M. Laser-mediated photodynamic therapy. Clin Dermatol. 2006;24(1):16–25.
35. Jacques SL, McAuliffe DJ, Blank IH, Parrish JA. Controlled removal of human stratum corneum by pulsed laser. J Invest Dermatol. 1987;88(1):88–93.
36. Ng WHS, Smith SD. Laser-assisted drug delivery: a systematic review of safety and adverse events. Pharmaceutics. 2022;14(12):1–24.
37. Labadie JG, Ibrahim SA, Worley B, Kang BY, Rakita U, Rigali S, et al. Evidence-based clinical practice guidelines for laser-assisted drug delivery. JAMA Dermatol. 2022;158(10):1193–201.
38. Wong THS. Picosecond laser treatment for acquired bilateral nevus of Ota–like macules. JAMA Dermatol. 2018;154(10):1226. https://doi.org/10.1001/jamadermatol.2018.2671.
39. Lee CH, Jin EM, Seo HS, Ryu T-U, Hong SP. Efficacy and safety of treatment with fractional 1,064-nm picosecond laser with diffractive optic element for wrinkles and acne scars: a clinical study. Ann

Dermatol. 2021;33(3):254. https://doi.org/10.5021/ad.2021.33.3.254.

40. Palawisuth S, Manuskiatti W, Apinuntham C, Wanitphakdeedecha R, Cembrano KAG. Quantitative assessment of the long-term efficacy and safety of a 1064-nm picosecond laser with fractionated microlens array in the treatment of enlarged pores in Asians: a case-control study. Lasers Surg Med. 2022;54(3):348–54. https://doi.org/10.1002/lsm.23449.
41. Chang Y-S, Yang T-H, Li C-N. Histology changes of in vivo human skin after treatment with fractional 1064 nm Nd:YAG picosecond laser in different energy settings. Lasers Med Sci. 2022;37(3):2087–92. https://doi.org/10.1007/s10103-021-03396-w.
42. Tanghetti EA. The histology of skin treated with a picosecond alexandrite laser and a fractional lens array. Lasers Surg Med. 2016;48(7):646–52. https://doi.org/10.1002/lsm.22540.
43. Wat H, Yee-nam Shek S, Yeung CK, Chan HH. Efficacy and safety of picosecond 755-nm alexandrite laser with diffractive lens array for non-ablative rejuvenation in Chinese skin. Lasers Surg Med. 2019;51(1):8–13. https://doi.org/10.1002/lsm.23014.
44. Ma W, Si C, Kasyanju Carrero LM, Liu H-F, Yin X-F, Liu J, et al. Laser treatment for onychomycosis. Medicine (Baltimore). 2019;98(48):e17948. https://doi.org/10.1097/MD.0000000000017948.

Update on Lasers and Energy-Based Devices for the Treatment of Vascular Lesions

2

Geraldine Hui Min Ong, Suzanne Wei Na Cheng, and Chee Leok Goh

Lasers and Energy-Based Devices for Treating Vascular Lesions

With recent advancements in the development of laser and energy-based device (EBD), many vascular anomalies can now be treated effectively with minimal complications, therefore improving patient satisfaction. However, to improve treatment outcomes and minimize complications, correct diagnosis, choice of treatment devices, choice of treatment protocols, and determination of vascular physiology and blood vessel calibers are extremely important.

The management of vascular anomalies should be tailored to the individual patient phenotype, lesion characteristics (persistent/transient erythema, papules/pustules, telangiectasia, etc.), and goals of treatment. When mutually agreed upon by the patient and clinician, achieving clear to almost clear skin should be the primary target when treating vascular anomalies. Combination therapy with different devices, or even with medical therapies, may be necessary to achieve better outcomes, e.g., the use of oral or topical β-blockers and other therapies in the treatment of infantile hemangioma.

A variety of lasers and energy-based devices have been demonstrated to be useful in the treatment of vascular anomalies. They include:

- Pulsed dye laser (585/595 nm)
- KTP laser (532 nm)
- Long-pulsed alexandrite laser (755 nm)
- Long-pulsed diode laser (900 nm)
- Long-pulsed Nd:YAG lasers (532/1064 nm)
- Copper vapor laser (510/578 nm)
- Intense pulsed light (500–1000 nm)

Pulsed dye laser (PDL) is the most commonly used vascular laser, followed by the long-pulsed Nd:YAG lasers and intense pulsed light (IPL).

Mechanism

Like the laser treatment of other conditions (e.g., pigmentary lesions), the concept of selective photothermolysis is important to ensure controlled destruction of the targeted blood vessel without causing significant injury to its surrounding tissues. Three crucial principles enable this to be achieved:

1. **Wavelength:** an appropriate wavelength that can penetrate to the depth of the blood vessel

G. H. M. Ong · S. W. N. Cheng (✉) · C. L. Goh
National Skin Centre, Singapore, Singapore

S. W. N. Cheng, C. L. Goh (eds.), *Updates on Lasers in Dermatology*, Updates in Clinical Dermatology, https://doi.org/10.1007/978-3-031-71155-8_2

and also that can be absorbed preferentially by oxyhemoglobin
2. **Fluence (energy):** must be sufficient to achieve destruction of the target vessel within the appropriate time interval
3. **Pulse duration:** must be shorter than or approximately equal to the vessel's thermal relaxation time (TRT), which is proportional to the square of the size of the blood vessel (in millimeters). Blood vessels encompass a wide range of TRTs, including capillaries (tens of microseconds), large venules of adult port-wine stains (up to tens of milliseconds), telangiectasias, and leg veins (hundreds of milliseconds)

The target chromophore in vascular lesions is oxyhemoglobin, which has three primary absorption peaks within the visible light spectrum: 418, 542, and 577 nm. Oxyhemoglobin absorbs the laser light, which is then converted to heat and transferred to the blood vessel wall, causing coagulation and vessel closure. As the skin is structurally dynamic, factors including the blood vessel depth, thickness, and skin phototype need to be considered. To minimize complications, the treatment parameters chosen should avoid certain structures such as the normal epidermal melanocytes, hair follicles, or epidermis as a whole (Fig. 2.1) [1].

Considerations When Using Lasers and Light Devices for Vascular Lesions

While advances in lasers and energy-based devices have now enabled effective treatment of vascular anomalies, several factors must be taken into consideration to deliver the best outcomes possible. These include:

1. **Clinical assessment:** Confirm the correct diagnosis.
2. **Ascertain the type of vascular lesions to be treated including:**

   - Characteristics (e.g., port-wine stain, hemangioma, angioma, spider angioma, telangiectasia threads, diffuse erythema)
   - Diameter of the blood vessels
   - Depth of the blood vessels
   - Color of the lesions (oxyhemoglobin vs. methemoglobin)

3. **Choice of vascular laser/device:** e.g., PDL, IPL, long-pulsed Nd:YAG, KTP
4. **Skin phototype:** more conservative settings should be used in patients with darker skin phototypes due to the risk of post-inflammatory hyperpigmentation.

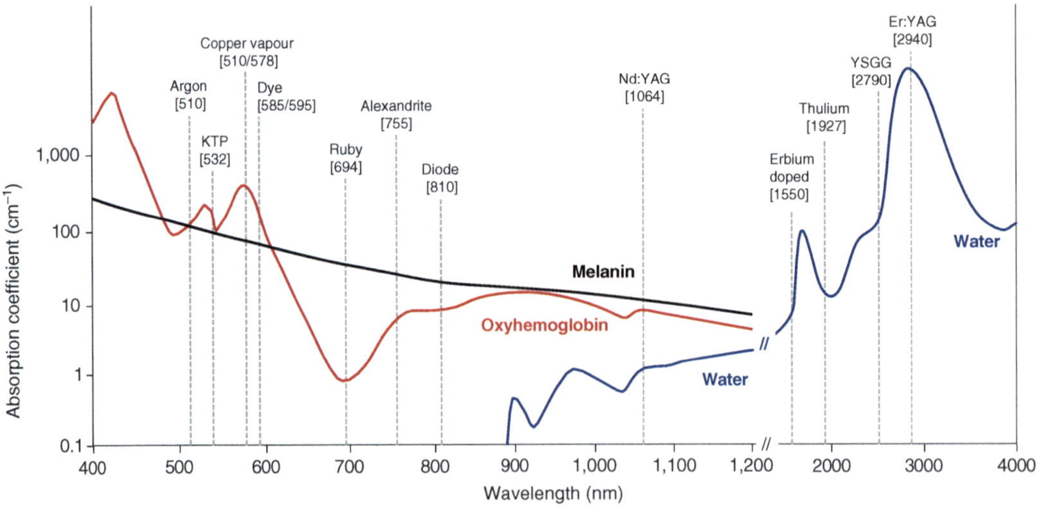

Fig. 2.1 Absorption spectra of the three main skin chromophores

5. **Treatment protocol used, taking into consideration:**

   - Fluence
   - Pulse width
   - Spot size
   - Filter selection (for IPL)
   - Skin cooling

6. **Post-laser skin care**

Types of Lasers and Light Devices for Treating Vascular Lesions

The treatment of port-wine stain and infantile hemangioma using vascular lasers will be described in detail at the end of this chapter.

Pulsed Dye Laser (585/595 nm)

Indication: All vascular anomalies

Including port-wine stains, infantile hemangiomas, angiomas, telangiectatic vessels and diffuse erythema, and venous lakes

First-generation pulsed dye lasers (PDLs) produced in the 1980s produced light at 577 nm, while modern-generation PDLs produce 585–600 nm light that has a greater depth of penetration. There is absorption by oxyhemoglobin and deoxyhemoglobin, as well as by melanin. The most frequently used PDL emits a wavelength of 585 or 595 nm, targeting oxyhemoglobin and leading to the destruction of blood vessels. The device allows the operator to adjust the fluence, pulse duration, and spot size to optimize treatment.

Several studies have confirmed the safety and efficacy of PDL in removing vascular anomalies [2]. It is often a preferred laser to treat all vascular anomalies. PDL has been utilized with an excellent safety profile in skin phototypes I–III. In a study of 75 subjects of skin phototypes IV and V, PDL demonstrated improvement in vascular anomalies with frequent transient hyperpigmentation (30%, typically lasting 6–8 weeks).

Very small and deep vessels are less likely to respond to PDL treatment. While PDL represents the standard initial laser treatment for port-wine stains, a reported 20–30% of vascular anomalies show resistance [3]. Resistant or deep port-wine stains are sometimes treated with alternative lasers in an effort to enhance clearance.

PDL emits wavelengths of 585 or 595 nm—close to the absorption peaks of oxyhemoglobin. It has a tunable pulse duration of 450 μs to 40 ms to treat vessels of various calibers. Its spot size varies from 3 to 12 mm and additionally has an elliptical spot (10 × 3 mm) to treat linear telangiectatic threads. The large spot size of >10 mm allows for deeper penetration and a gentler vascular coagulation. It also allows large areas to be treated quickly and is useful when treating large port-wine stains and superficial hemangiomas.

PDL is also a preferred device to treat the diffuse erythema of erythematotelangiectatic rosacea. Cryogen cooling allows larger spot size and higher fluence to be used with minimal tissue injury especially in patients with skin of color. PDL is reported to achieve 50% reduction in erythema, 55% reduction in flushing, and 75% reduction in telangiectasia following one to three treatments. For large telangiectatic threads, long pulse (10–40 ms depending on vessel caliber) and stacking may be needed to achieve the visible end point of vessel blanching or transient purpura. Complete clearance was seen in ten patients, and eight patients displayed more than 80% improvement after ultra-long-pulse PDL (ULPDL) treatment. ULPDL treatment delivered using a 3 mm × 10 mm elliptical spot was nonpurpuric and highly effective in the treatment of nasal telangiectasia resistant to KTP laser and PDL (pulse width < 10 ms) [4]. The preferred settings for ULPDL are 595 nm, 40 ms, double pulse, and 30:20 dynamic cooling device (DCD).

A double-blind, randomized, controlled split face study comparing the effectiveness of a 595 nm PDL and a 0.3 ms 1064 nm Nd:YAG laser in 16 patients with diffuse facial erythema showed slightly more improvement for the PDL treatment arm. PDL reduced facial redness by 6.4% more from baseline than Nd:YAG ($p = 0.0199$). Nd:YAG laser was associated with

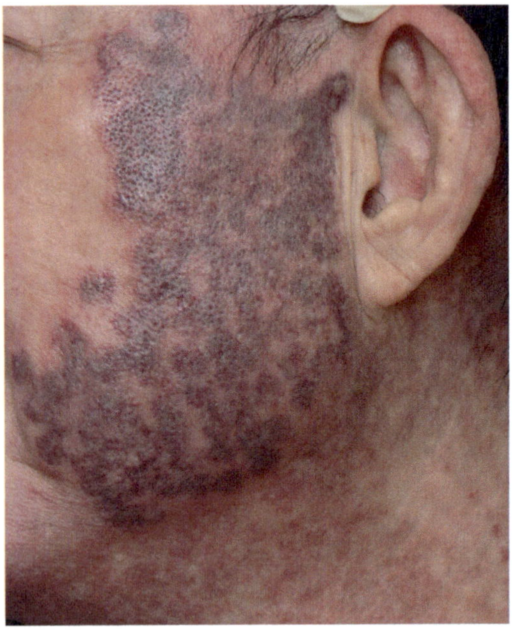

Fig. 2.2 Marked purpura is seen immediately post pulsed dye laser. A short pulse duration of 1.5 ms was used. The purpura resolved 2 weeks later without sequelae

less pain ($p = 0.0028$). Subjects rated redness as improvement by 52% with PDL versus 34% with Nd:YAG ($p = 0.031$) [5].

PDL can be used for venous lakes although optimal results are achieved with long-pulsed Nd:YAG laser [6]. In a case series of eight patients testing the effect of the 595 nm PDL with venous lakes on the lower lip, no adverse effects were noted, but there was one recurrence 4 months after treatment. 62.5% (5/8) of patients showed incomplete resolution of their lesions, and only 25% (2/8) of patients showed complete clearance. Therefore, while PDLs with longer wavelengths may penetrate deeper into the dermis while maintaining selectivity, they require higher fluence levels in order to remain effective. Furthermore, the authors administered pulse durations of 1.5 ms, corresponding to the duration necessary for the treatment of port-wine stain (PWS). However, venous lakes encompass a larger area than the vasculature of PWS, thereby potentially requiring longer pulse durations to optimize results. Therefore, length of pulse durations, in addition to oxyhemoglobin's peak absorption at wavelengths below 595 nm, may contribute to the suboptimal results observed in this study [7].

The most common complication of PDL is purpura, which occurs especially when a short pulse width (0.45 ms) is used (Fig. 2.2). Subpurpuric treatment using longer pulse width protocol requires more than two to six treatments to achieve similar effects (although this is preferred when treating darker skin types). When treating diffuse facial erythema, larger spot sizes of 10–12 mm performed with two to three passes help to prevent reticulation. Other complications include transient dyspigmentation and, rarely, vesiculation, crusting, and scarring.

Frequency-Doubled Neodymium-Doped Yttrium Aluminum Garnet (Nd:YAG) and Potassium Titanyl Phosphate Lasers (532 nm)

Indication: Superficial telangiectasias, cherry angiomas, venous malformations

Frequency-doubled neodymium-doped yttrium aluminum garnet (Nd:YAG) and potassium titanyl phosphate lasers produce 532 nm green light. Because of absorption by melanin, its use is primarily in skin phototypes I–III. With a limited penetration depth due to the shorter wavelength, these lasers have been primarily successful in treating superficial small-caliber vascular lesions. This laser is a frequency-doubled 1064 nm Nd:YAG laser. The KTP laser emits green light at 532 nm wavelength, which is well absorbed by hemoglobin but penetrates relatively superficially. A millisecond pulse width of 15–30 ms is utilized. The KTP laser is effective against small superficial telangiectatic vessels of up to 1 mm diameter due to its short wavelength. It has been reported that 40% of patients observed a reduction of >70% of telangiectasia after a single treatment [8]. KTP lasers may cause dyschromia and textural changes when used on darker skin because there is significant absorption by melanin at 532 nm. Thus, patients with darker skin types or tanned skin may have increased risk of side effects with a 532 nm laser beam, including epidermal burns, hypopigmentation, and hyperpigmentation.

Long-Pulsed Alexandrite Lasers and Diode Lasers

Indication: Leg telangiectasias, venous malformations, port-wine stains

Alexandrite lasers fall in the near-infrared category, having a 755 nm wavelength. With a 50–75% increased depth of penetration, near-infrared laser use for vascular anomalies is primarily for dark or resistant lesions [9]. A retrospective study of 20 patients with either hypertrophic or PDL-resistant capillary malformation treated with alexandrite laser alone or in combination with other lasers such as PDL showed that most had a moderate response, while some had mild or no response. Diode lasers (800–940 nm) may similarly be used to treat vascular malformations, although they are more often used for venous lakes or for endovenous ablation [10].

Long-Pulsed Neodymium-Yttrium Aluminum Garnet Laser (1064 nm LPNd:YAG)

Indication: Large and deep telangiectatic vessels, venous lakes, diffuse erythema

The LPNd:YAG laser is a solid-state laser with primary 1064 nm wavelength. It is the preferred laser for laser-assisted hair removal in skin of color. However, LPNd:YAG laser is also effective for the treatment of deep vascular lesions because of its long 1064 nm wavelength (Figs. 2.3 and 2.4). LPNd:YAG lasers have the highest depth of penetration of the vascular-selective lasers and the lowest epidermal melanin absorption. It can penetrate 6–10 mm into the skin. Because higher fluences are generally required, complication rates of pigmentary change and scarring are higher than with PDL in published studies (0–4.3%) [11]. Epidermal cooling is mandatory, typically by cryogen spray or contact cooling to provide epidermal protection.

LPNd:YAG lasers are typically used to treat vascular anomalies in patients with skin phototypes V–VI or for hypertrophic or resistant port-wine stains. In addition, they have shown efficacy in treating vascular blebs associated with port-wine stains [12]. In a retrospective study of 130 patients with vascular anomalies treated with LPNd:YAG laser, 2%, 15%, 64%, and 19% of patients experienced 25%, 25–49%, 50–75%, and >75% lesion clearance, respectively. Darker port-wine stains showed greater response than lighter port-wine stains [13]. In another study, LPNd:YAG laser (1064 nm) had demonstrated improvement in hypertrophy, with good-to-excellent improvements seen in the majority of the 32 patients studied. Adverse effects were more frequent, however, with hypopigmentation seen in 14 and scarring in 7 of the 32 subjects [14].

The 1064 nm LPNd:YAG laser wavelength is absorbed by hemoglobin and methemoglobin and can cause deep vessel destruction. It may be more

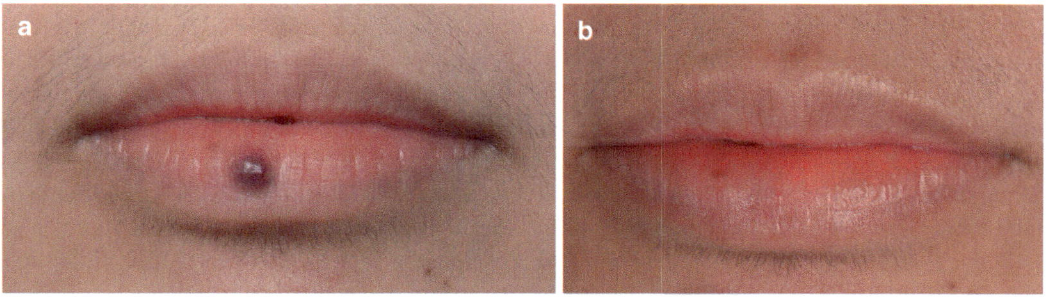

Fig. 2.3 Treatment of venous lake using long-pulsed Nd:YAG 1064nm laser. (**a**) Baseline (**b**) Complete clearance achieved 2 months later, after 1 treatment session

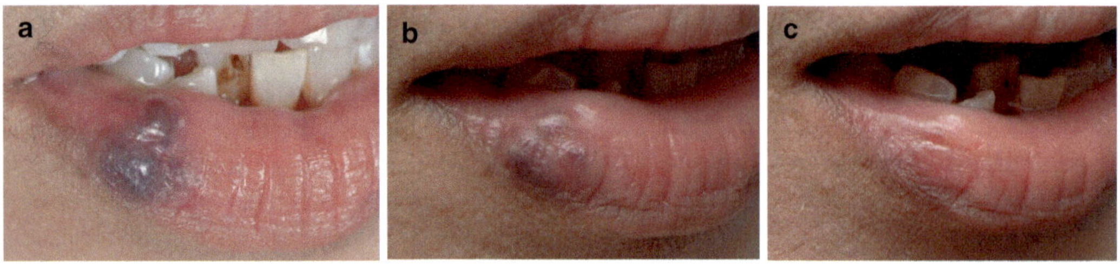

Fig. 2.4 Treatment of venous lake using long-pulsed Nd:YAG 1064nm laser. (**a**) Baseline (**b**) Partial clearance after 2 treatments (**c**) Complete clearance after 3 sessions

effective than PDL in destroying the deeper bluish vessels. Several reports have confirmed that LPNd:YAG laser is effective for the destruction of large nasal telangiectatic vessels. A study compared the efficacy of LPNd:YAG (1064 nm) and PDL in treating rosacea-associated nasal telangiectasia where each patient was treated with PDL on the left side of the nasal bridge, and LPNd:YAG laser on the right side, three times with 4-week intervals. The study concluded that good improvement was seen in six PDL and seven LPNd:YAG patients, and excellent improvement in five PDL and four LPNd:YAG patients. There was no significant difference ($p = 0.62$) between the groups. Overall improvement was similar; however, LPNd:YAG laser induced a greater response in thick, dilated vessels, while erythema with mild telangiectasia was more responsive to PDL [15].

LPNd:YAG laser can be used in the treatment of venous lakes. In a study of 16 patients, venous lakes less than 1 cm in size located on the lip and oral mucosa were treated using a 2 W of power, a 7 mm spot size, and 10-s pulse durations. The patients showed slight swelling, which lasted for 1–2 days with complete healing and reepithelialization 2–4 weeks posttreatment. They did not show any common side effects like dyspigmentation, scars, atrophy, or wrinkled texture [16]. In another study of 31 patients, the LPNd:YAG 1064 nm laser was tested on 31 patients with venous lakes on the lower lip and some extending intraorally. Three patients had previously been treated with excision, one with cryotherapy, and one with PDL—all of which did not respond to therapy. At 12-month follow-up, 83.8% (26/31) of patients showed complete resolution, while 12.9% (4/31) of patients showed signs of recurrence. If the lesion does not respond immediately to treatment, then the fluence level may be increased; however, caution must be taken if the initial fluence exceeds 80 J/cm^2 [17].

LPNd:YAG laser treatment carries a higher risk of potential collateral damage around vessels (such as burns) and pain during the procedure. This must be considered when using this laser to destroy large vessels especially when used on the skin of color. To avoid overheating the epidermis and causing textural changes, it is important to ensure that the skin surface of the field treated is adequately cooled with contact cooling, cryogen, or air cooling (before, during, and after the laser procedure). It is imperative to carefully check the vessel response after each laser shot. Stacking must be done with caution.

Copper Vapor Laser (510/578 nm CVL)

Indication: Superficial telangiectatic vessels of various sizes

The CVL is a dual-wavelength laser for treating pigmentary and vascular lesions. The wavelengths of light emitted by a CVL are 510 and 578 nm, targeting melanin and oxyhemoglobin, respectively. In contrast to other yellow light lasers, the CVL emits a train of pulses with a duration of 20–25 ns and 10,000–15,000 pulses/s. Because of the very short gap between each pulse of light, the biological effect of the CVL is similar to that of a continuous wave laser.

CVL has been reported to improve rhinophyma. A case report of a 52-year-old Caucasian male with typical clinical signs of rhinophyma revealed successful management with three sessions of CVL treatment. Such treatment resulted in restoration of the natural appearance of the nose, including removal of dysplastic superficial skin vessels, resolution of inflammation, decline in sebum production, and resolution of nasal hypertrophy [18].

Intense Pulsed Light (IPL 500–1200 nm)

Indication: Port-wine stains, superficial and small telangiectatic vessels, mild diffuse erythema

IPL is a non-laser flashlamp that produces noncoherent broadband light with wavelengths in the range of 500–1200 nm. It delivers a broad spectrum of wavelengths with filters used to remove unwanted wavelengths, adjusted to the patient's skin type and lesion depth. IPL has been shown in many studies to be efficacious in treating superficial vascular lesions in photoaging, rosacea and vascular anomalies, and dyschromia. It can also be used for light-assisted hair removal.

IPL has tunable pulse widths ranging from 0.5 to 150 ms. The variable pulse width allows the targeting of different sized vessels at different depths. The large spot size of the IPL facilitates the treatment of large areas of the face and is useful for treating the diffuse erythema and flushing of rosacea.

In one report, an average of two treatments resulted in facial clearing of 75–100% in the majority of patients (93%). Subsequent reports have confirmed the effectiveness of IPL in treating erythematotelangiectatic rosacea [19]. A recent study reported that short-pulsed (1.5 ms) IPL and PDL with two treatment sessions 4 weeks apart were similarly effective for decreasing facial erythema when non-purpuragenic low fluence was used. The IPL was faster and did not require consumables. An average of 60% improvement on the side treated with IPL was observed as opposed to 45% on the other side. In a study comparing non-purpuragenic PDL with IPL for facial erythema, telangiectasia, and symptoms of facial erythema rosacea, three monthly sessions were performed with initial PDL settings of 10 mm spot size, 7 J/cm^2, and 6 ms pulse duration, and initial IPL settings of 560 nm filter, a pulse train of 2.4 ms, and 6.0 ms in duration separated by a 15 ms delay, and a starting fluence of 25 J/cm^2; results showed that PDL and IPL produced a significant reduction in cutaneous erythema, telangiectasia, and patient-reported associated symptoms [19].

Complications including purpura, edema, and burns from IPL treatment are uncommon, and there is generally little downtime if correct patient selection is performed. Patients with darker skin types, e.g., types V and VII, are not suitable for IPL treatment as epidermal melanin in darker skin types tends to pick up the shorter IPL wavelengths and burn the skin. Similarly, patients with tanned skin should postpone IPL treatment until the skin color returns to normal.

To avoid burns, appropriate cutoff filters should be used for different skin types and depths of penetration. For example, for type II–III skin phototypes, a cutoff filter of 515 nm is safe, but for type IV skin phototype, a cutoff filter of more than 550 nm should be used. The variable pulse duration (0.5–100 ms) allows the targeting of vessels of different sizes at different depths. The large spot size of IPL sapphire tip reduces treatment time and allows bigger areas to be treated which is especially useful for treating diffuse facial erythema. It is important to note that treatment efficacy and settings of different brands of IPL devices vary and are not interchangeable.

Common Vascular Lesions Treated with Vascular Lasers

Port-wine stains and small hemangiomas are often encountered in the young requiring vascular laser treatment. Telangiectasias, superficial flushing and telangiectasias in rosacea, poikiloderma of Civatte, angiomas, spider veins, and venous lakes are more commonly encountered in adults seeking vascular laser treatment. Recently, vascular lasers have also been reported to clear bruising and purpura effectively.

Port-Wine Stains (PWSs)

The most common indication for the use of vascular lasers is to treat port-wine stains (PWSs).

PWSs are congenital vascular malformations characterized by ectasia of capillary and postcapillary venules in the skin and mucosa [20]. The incidence of PWS in newborns is approximately 0.3–0.5%, and they affect about 25 million people worldwide [21–23]. PWS can occur alone or as part of vascular syndromes such as Sturge-Weber syndrome, Klippel-Trenaunay syndrome, Proteus syndrome, and phakomatosis pigmentovascularis.

PWSs present at birth as pink to red well-demarcated irregular patches on the face, which can be unilateral, bilateral, or centrally located, and may affect the mucosa as well. Without treatment, the patches typically darken with age and may eventually become hypertrophic and nodular (Figs. 2.5 and 2.6). As the majority (70–80%) of PWSs occur on the face and neck which is cosmetically undesirable, it can have a significant psychological impact on patients. A retrospective study analyzed 425 patients with facial PWS and reported that 65% of all patients with PWS developed hypertrophic or nodular lesions in the fifth decade of life. In addition, the mean age of hypertrophy was noted to be 37 years old [24]. Another study showed that 60% of patients with PWS had soft tissue or bony hypertrophy, or nodule formation by the age of 9 years old [25].

Vascular lasers and energy-based devices are the standard of care for PWS, with the pulsed dye laser (PDL) being widely considered the first-line treatment. Other lasers such as the long-pulsed 755 nm alexandrite, long-pulsed 900 nm diode, and long-pulsed 1064 nm Nd:YAG laser, as well as intense pulsed light (IPL), can also be used. Regardless of the choice of laser, treatment is guided by the principle of selective photothermolysis which is to target the subsurface blood vessels without injury to the epidermis and other structures.

PDL (585 nm/595 nm) has the longest history of efficacy and safety for treating PWS, and many studies support this device as the gold standard. Even for infants, PDL is considered the standard of care and is safe. As PWSs are progressive vascular skin malformations that can result in progressive vascular thickening, soft tissue hypertrophy, and proliferative nodules that may bleed or cause discomfort, it is important to consider treating the patient as early as possible.

It is important to discuss the expected clinical outcomes of PDL with patients or their families as these can vary. Patients should have realistic expectations as complete PWS clearance is difficult to achieve. PDL can still achieve 50–90% clearance with majority being able to achieve more than 50% lightening [26]. Most patients require eight to ten treatments or more for optimal results, and touch-up treatments are often needed even after the initial successful lightening [27].

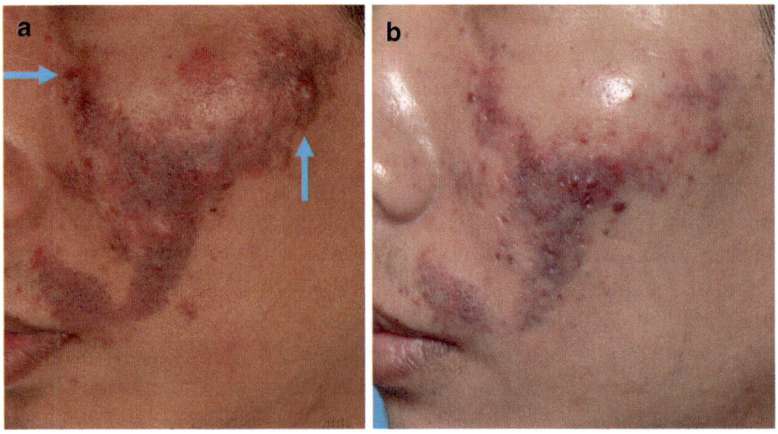

Fig. 2.5 Adult port wine stain with hypertrophy and nodules, treated with pulsed dye laser. (**a**) Baseline (**b**) Moderate improvement after 6 sessions of PDL. The lateral cheek responded better than the central face. The nodules (blue arrows) were excised

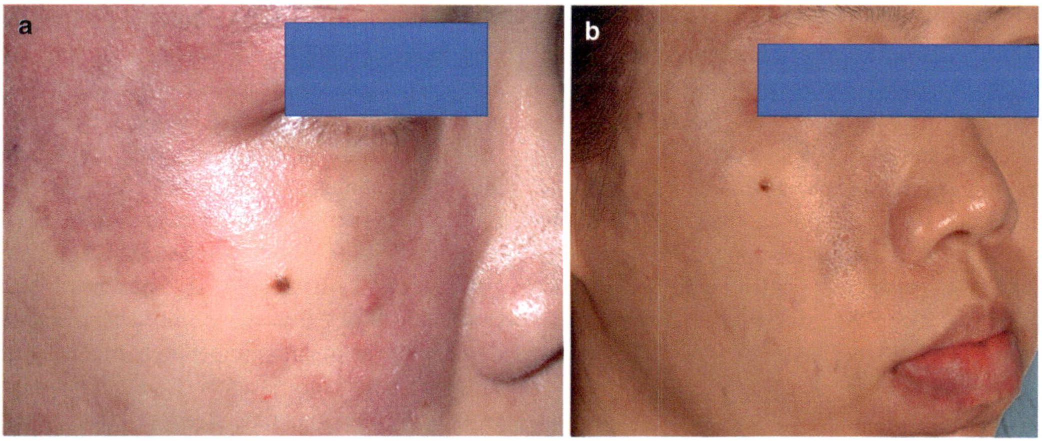

Fig. 2.6 Adult port wine stain treated with pulsed dye laser. (**a**) Baseline (**b**) Significant lightening after 11 sessions. Note soft tissue hypertrophy of the lower lip

Several factors influence the treatment outcomes. Patients with lighter skin types have better treatment responses [28]. PWSs on the face and neck respond better than those on the extremities [29]. PWSs on the lateral face respond better than those on the central face [30, 31]. Proximal extremity lesions respond better than distal extremity lesions. The eyelids and neck are at higher risk for blistering and scarring, and this should be considered when selecting laser parameters. PWS associated with Sturge-Weber syndrome may be more resistant to laser. Pink, red, and reticular lesions respond better than purple and geographically shaped lesions. PWSs which have hypertrophied or become nodular are harder to treat than those that are flat and smooth without textural changes. Despite considering the factors listed, response is difficult to predict [26].

The interval between laser treatments can be decided based upon factors like the patient's age, skin type, PWS location, pain tolerance, and presence of hypertrophy or nodularity. There is no optimal interval established, and this should be tailored to the individual. A few small studies in infants have analyzed the interval between PDL treatment sessions, which range from 2 weeks to 3 months, but the studies do not provide a clear recommendation on shorter versus longer interval times. They do however demonstrate the safety of PDL even when performed at short intervals [32, 33]. Older children, adolescents, and adults may also benefit from shorter treatment intervals although this needs to be balanced against the risk of increased side effects. A small pilot study in adults suggested that 2-week treatment intervals resulted in greater lightening compared to 6-week intervals [34], but other studies have failed to show this benefit [35].

In darker skin types, vascular lasers and EBDs are still the first-line treatment for PWS. Greater caution is warranted however, since these patients experience a higher rate of adverse effects like persistent dyspigmentation, atrophy, and scarring. To minimize adverse effects, moderate fluences, less pulse overlap, and increased cooling are recommended [27]. It is also recommended that these patients have longer treatment intervals.

There are limitations to the PDL. Despite PDL being the gold standard for the treatment of PWS, only a minority can achieve complete clearance, and recurrence is common. In addition, deeper vascular lesions like the hypertrophic PWSs do not respond well to PDL as the 595 nm wavelength may not penetrate deep enough. PDL cannot treat PWS vessels that are deeper than 2 mm in the human skin, and lasers of other wavelengths may need to be utilized for these deeper PWS. Compared with the PDL, a 755 nm alexandrite laser penetrates 50–75% deeper into the skin with less absorption of epidermal melanin [32]. Additionally, the penetration depth of a

1064 nm Nd:YAG laser is 4–7 mm into the dermis [36]. These lasers can be considered as alternatives for purple and hypertrophic PWS.

Alternative therapies have been investigated for the treatment of PWSs that do not respond to traditional laser and energy-based devices. These alternatives include (a) adjuvant medications such as topical imiquimod and topical rapamycin with PDL, (b) photodynamic therapy, (c) surgery to debulk thick PWS, and (d) corrective cover-up products like concealers.

Infantile Hemangiomas (IHs)

Infantile hemangiomas are common benign tumors of infancy. Its incidence ranges from 3% to 10% of the population with a higher prevalence in females and Caucasians [37–40]. They are most commonly located on the head, neck, and trunk, but can occur anywhere throughout the body, including the extremities, spine, and visceral organs [41–43]. Potential complications of IH include pain, infection, ulceration, and functional impairment of internal organs.

Infantile hemangiomas have a well-described clinical trajectory, first undergoing early and late proliferative stages, followed by a slow involution stage. They often appear in the first few weeks of life as areas of pallor, followed by telangiectatic or faint red patches. They then grow rapidly in the first 3–6 months of life. Superficial lesions are bright red, protuberant, or with a smooth surface and sharply demarcated. Deep lesions are bluish and dome shaped. Infantile hemangiomas continue to grow until 9–12 months of age. Involution typically begins by the age of 1. An estimated 50% of infantile hemangiomas will show complete involution by the time a child reaches 5 years; 70% will have involute by 7 years; and 95% will have regressed by 10–12 years of age [44].

Most IHs can be managed conservatively. For small, superficial IHs, topical timolol maleate or PDL may be considered. However, those located in areas of particular concern (e.g., periorbital, oropharyngeal, preauricular, or parotid regions) or those typified by a large size, ulceration, segmental distribution, or prominent deep component often require rapid treatment to prevent permanent sequelae. Oral propranolol is the treatment of choice for high-risk and complicated IHs. Other systemic treatments include corticosteroids, sirolimus, and other β-blockers [45].

Laser therapy provides an additional treatment modality for residual and recurrent hemangiomas as well as for patients with contraindications to propranolol. There is also some evidence to suggest that early treatment of superficial IH with vascular lasers may arrest growth and help treat ulcerated IH [45].

The 585 nm/595 nm PDL is the most widely used device for superficial IH often in residual refractory IH after propranolol treatment. The longer wavelength 1064 nm Nd:YAG is required for medically refractory lesions with a deeper or subcutaneous component [46–48]. In mixed IH, combination therapy with PDL and Nd:YAG can be considered [49].

Studies on PDL treatments for IH have shown response rates of 80–90% [50, 51]. A study compared three treatments for facial segmental IH: concurrent propranolol and PDL (n = 12), propranolol followed by PDL (n = 5), and propranolol alone (n = 8). The difference in effectiveness between combined therapy, either concurrently or sequentially, and propranolol alone was statistically significant. The number of days of propranolol treatment until near-complete clearance was significantly lower ($p < 0.001$) for those receiving concurrent or sequential therapy than those receiving propranolol alone [52].

The 1064 nm Nd:YAG laser is able to reach a depth of up to 10 mm due to its longer wavelength and is used to treat deeper hemangiomas, which the PDL is unable to reach (PDL can only reach a depth of up to 1.2 mm). Two large studies on the combination therapy with PDL and Nd:YAG lasers for the treatment of IH have been published. In the first study comprising 25 patients with IH in the head and neck region, 72% of lesions healed completely, 16% healed with mild hyperpigmentation/loss of pigmentation or "structural skin changes," and 12% responded adequately [53]. In the second retrospective study, all 22 patients benefited from

PDL and Nd:YAG LP laser treatment, irrespective of the stage of IH development [54].

Side effects of the 1064 nm Nd:YAG laser include swelling, blistering, and crust formation which occurs more frequently compared to the PDL. On the other hand, purpura, hypopigmentation, and hyperpigmentation are more common with the PDL. Cooling is essential to protect the epidermis against thermal damage.

Vascular lasers can be combined with systemic or topical β-blockers for increased efficacy, without any appreciable increase in side effects [55, 56].

Conclusion

Advancements in lasers and light technology have significantly enhanced the effectiveness of treating vascular anomalies, reducing complications and ultimately leading to better patient outcomes and satisfaction. Achieving optimal results begins with accurately diagnosing the condition, including identifying the lesion's color (oxyhemoglobin or methemoglobin). This diagnosis then guides clinicians in selecting the most suitable laser device, such as PDL, LPNd:YAG laser, or IPL. Laser parameters are carefully tailored based on factors like blood vessel diameter, depth, site, and skin phototype. Among the most prevalent conditions treated with vascular lasers are port-wine stains and hemangiomas. Particularly in the case of port-wine stains, initiating treatment during early childhood can greatly enhance effectiveness. Proper pre-procedure counseling and management of patient expectations are crucial for ensuring patient satisfaction.

References

1. Anderson RR, Parrish JA. Selective photothermolysis: precise microsurgery by selective absorption of pulsed radiation. Science. 1983;220(4596):524–7.
2. Tan ST, Bialostocki A, Armstrong JR. Pulsed dye laser therapy for rosacea. Br J Plast Surg. 2004;57(4):303–10.
3. Savas JA, Ledon JA, Franca K, Chacon A, Nouri K. Pulsed dye laser resistant port-wine stains: mechanisms of resistance and implications for treatment. Br J Dermatol. 2013;168(5):941–53.
4. Madan V, Ferguson J. Using the ultra-long pulse width pulsed dye laser and elliptical spot to treat resistant nasal telangiectasia. Lasers Med Sci. 2010;25(1):151–4.
5. Alam M, Voravutinon N, Warycha M, Whiting D, Nodzenski M, Yoo S, West DP, Veledar E, Poon E. Comparative effectiveness of nonpurpuragenic 595-nm pulsed dye laser and microsecond 1064-nm neodymium:yttrium-aluminum-garnet laser for treatment of diffuse facial erythema: a double-blind randomized controlled trial. J Am Acad Dermatol. 2013;69(3):438–43.
6. Mlacker S, Shah VV, Aldahan AS, McNamara CA, Kamath P, Nouri K. Laser and light-based treatments of venous lakes: a literature review. Lasers Med Sci. 2016;31(7):1511–9.
7. Cheung ST, Lanigan SW. Evaluation of the treatment of venous lakes with the 595-nm pulsed-dye laser: a case series. Clin Exp Dermatol. 2007;32(2):148–50.
8. Becher GL, Cameron H, Moseley H. Treatment of superficial vascular lesions with the KTP 532-nm laser: experience with 647 patients. Lasers Med Sci. 2014;29:267–71.
9. Izikson L, Anderson RR. Treatment endpoints for resistant port wine stains with a 755 nm laser. J Cosmet Laser Ther. 2009;11(1):52–5.
10. Wall TL, Grassi AM, Avram MM. Clearance of multiple venous lakes with an 800-nm diode laser: a novel approach. Dermatol Surg. 2007;33(1):100–3.
11. McGill DJ, MacLaren W, Mackay IR. A direct comparison of pulsed dye, alexandrite, KTP and Nd:YAG lasers and IPL in patients with previously treated capillary malformations. Lasers Surg Med. 2008;40(6):390–8.
12. Brauer JA, Geronemus RG. Single-treatment resolution of vascular blebs within port wine stains using a novel 1,064-nm neodymium doped yttrium aluminum garnet laser. Dermatol Surg. 2013;39(7):1113–5.
13. Zhong SX, Liu YY, Yao L, et al. Clinical analysis of port-wine stain in 130 Chinese patients treated by long-pulsed 1064-nm Nd: YAG laser. J Cosmet Laser Ther. 2014;16(6):279–83.
14. Van Drooge AM, Bosveld B, van der Veen JP, de Rie MA, Wolkerstorfer A. Long-pulsed 1064 nm Nd:YAG laser improves hypertrophic port-wine stains. J Eur Acad Dermatol Venereol. 2013;27(11):1381–6.
15. Kwon WJ, Park BW, Cho EB, Park EJ, Kim KH, Kim KJ. Comparison of efficacy between long-pulsed Nd:YAG laser and pulsed dye laser to treat rosacea-associated nasal telangiectasia. J Cosmet Laser Ther. 2018;20(5):260–4.
16. Migliari D, Vieira RR, Nakajima EK, Azevedo LH. Successful management of lip and oral venous varices by photocoagulation with Nd:YAG laser. J Contemp Dent Pract. 2015;16(9):723–6.

17. John HE, Phen HS, Mahaffey PJ. Treatment of venous lesions of the lips and perioral area with a long-pulsed Nd:YAG laser. Br J Oral Maxillofac Surg. 2015;54:376–8.
18. Ponomarev IV, Topchiy SB, Klyuchareva SV, Pushkareva AE. Rhinophyma treatment by copper vapor laser with the computerized scanner. J Lasers Med Sci. 2019;10(2):153–6.
19. Tirico MCCP, Jensen D, Green C, Ross EV. Short pulse intense pulsed light versus pulsed dye laser for the treatment of facial redness. J Cosmet Laser Ther. 2020;22(2):60–4.
20. Liu L, Li X, Zhao Q, Yang L, Jiang X. Pathogenesis of port-wine stains: directions for future therapies. Int J Mol Sci. 2022;23(20):12139.
21. Alper JC, Holmes LB. The incidence and significance of birthmarks in a cohort of 4641 newborns. Pediatr Dermatol. 1983;1:58–68.
22. Lister T, Wright P, Chappell P. Spectrophotometers for the clinical assessment of port-wine stain skin lesions: a review. Lasers Med Sci. 2010;25:449–57.
23. Lister T, Wright PA, Chappell PH. Simulating light transport through skin for color prediction of port wine stain lesions: a review. J Biomed Opt. 2012;17:110901.
24. Geronemus RG, Ashinoff R. The medical necessity of evaluation and treatment of port-wine stains. J Dermatol Surg Oncol. 1991;17:76–9.
25. Lee JW, Chung HY, Cerrati EW, Teresa MO, Waner M. The natural history of soft tissue hypertrophy, bony hypertrophy, and nodule formation in patients with untreated head and neck capillary malformations. Dermatol Surg. 2015;41:1241–5.
26. Brightman LA, Geronemus RG, Reddy KK. Laser treatment of port-wine stains. Clin Cosmet Investig Dermatol. 2015;8:27–33.
27. Sabeti S, Ball KL, Burkhart C, Eichenfield L, Fernandez Faith E, Frieden IJ, Geronemus R, Gupta D, Krakowski AC, Levy ML, Metry D, Nelson JS, Tollefson MM, Kelly KM. Consensus statement for the management and treatment of port-wine birthmarks in Sturge-Weber syndrome. JAMA Dermatol. 2021;157(1):98–104.
28. Fitzpatrick RE, Lowe NJ, Goldman MP, Borden H, Behr KL, Ruiz-Esparza J. Flashlamp-pumped pulsed dye laser treatment of port-wine status. J Dermatol Surg Oncol. 1994;20:743–8.
29. Updyke KM, Khachemoune A. Port-wine stains: a focused review on their management. J Drugs Dermatol. 2017;116:1145–51.
30. Bae YSC, Alabdulrazzaq H, Brauer JA, Geronemus RG. Treatment of recalcitrant port-wine stains (PWS) using a combined pulsed dye laser (PDL) and radiofrequency (RF) energy device. J Am Acad Dermatol. 2017;76:321–6.
31. Yu W, Ma G, Qiu Y, et al. Why do port-wine stains (PWS) on the lateral face respond better to pulsed dye laser (PDL) than those located on the central face? J Am Acad Dermatol. 2016;74:527–35.
32. Anolik R, Newlove T, Weiss ET, et al. Investigation into optimal treatment intervals of facial port-Wine stains using the pulsed dye laser. J Am Acad Dermatol. 2012;67:985–90.
33. Swan BC, Robertson SJ, Tuxen A, et al. Pulsed dye laser treatment of capillary malformations in infants at 2-weekly versus 3-monthly intervals, reducing the need for general anaesthesia. Australas J Dermatol. 2017;58:214–8.
34. Tomson N, Lim SPR, Abdullah A, Lanigan SW. The treatment of port-wine stains with the pulsed-dye laser at 2-week and 6-week intervals: a comparative study. Br J Dermatol. 2006;154:676–9.
35. Yu W, Zhu J, Changc SJ, et al. Shorter treatment intervals of East Asians with port-wine stain with pulsed dye laser are safe and effective—a prospective side-by-side comparison. Photomed Laser Surg. 2018;36:37–43.
36. Li T, Jia R, Fan X. Classification and treatment of orbital venous malformations: an updated review. Front Med. 2019;13:547–55.
37. Jacobs AH, Walton RG. The incidence of birthmarks in the neonate. Pediatrics. 1976;58:218–22.
38. Pratt AG. Birthmarks in infants. AMA Arch Derm Syphilol. 1953;67:302–5.
39. Jacobs AH. Strawberry hemangiomas; the natural history of the untreated lesion. Calif Med. 1957;86:8–10.
40. Drolet BA, Esterly NB, Frieden IJ. Hemangiomas in children. N Engl J Med. 1999;341:273–4.
41. Iacobas I, Burrows PE, Frieden IJ, et al. LUMBAR: association between cutaneous infantile hemangiomas of the lower body and regional congenital anomalies. J Pediatr. 2010;157:795–801.e7.
42. Christison-Lagay ER, Burrows PE, Alomari A, et al. Hepatic hemangiomas: subtype classification and development of a clinical practice algorithm and registry. J Pediatr Surg. 2007;42:62–8.
43. Stockman A, Boralevi F, Taïeb A, Léauté-Labrèze C. SACRAL syndrome: spinal dysraphism, anogenital, cutaneous, renal and urologic anomalies, associated with an angioma of lumbosacral localization. Dermatology. 2007;214:40–5.
44. Leung AKC, Lam JM, Leong KF, Hon KL. Infantile hemangioma: an updated review. Curr Pediatr Rev. 2021;17(1):55–69.
45. Wirth F, Lowitt M. Diagnosis and treatment of cutaneous vascular lesions. Am Fam Physician. 1998;57:765.
46. Chen W, Liu S, Yang C, Yang S. Clinical efficacy of the 595 nm pulsed dye laser in the treatment of childhood superficial hemangioma—analysis of 10-year application in Chinese patients. J Dermatol Treat. 2015;26(1):54–8.
47. Shen L, Zhou G, Zhao J, et al. Pulsed dye laser therapy for infantile hemangiomas: a systemic review and meta-analysis. QJM. 2015;108(6):473–80.
48. Zhong SX, Tao YC, Zhou JF, Liu YY, Yao L, Li SS. Infantile hemangioma: clinical characteristics and efficacy of treatment with the long-pulsed

1,064-nm neodymium-doped yttrium aluminum garnet laser in 794 Chinese patients. Pediatr Dermatol. 2015;32(4):495–500.
49. Hartmann F, Lockmann A, Gronemeyer LL, et al. Nd:YAG and pulsed dye laser therapy in infantile haemangiomas: a retrospective analysis of 271 treated haemangiomas in 149 children. J Eur Acad Dermatol Venereol. 2017;31(8):1372–9.
50. Patil U, Dhami L. Overview of lasers. Indian J Plast Surg. 2008;41:S101–13.
51. Chinnadurai S, Sathe NA, Surawicz T. Laser treatment of infantile hemangioma: a systematic review. Lasers Surg Med. 2016;48:221–33.
52. Reddy KK, Blei F, Brauer JA, et al. Retrospective study of the treatment of infantile hemangiomas using a combination of propranolol and pulsed dye laser. Dermatol Surg. 2013;39:923–33.
53. Saafan AM, Salah MM. Using pulsed dual-wavelength 595 and 1064 nm is more effective in the management of hemangiomas. J Drugs Dermatol. 2010;9:310–4.
54. Alcántara-González J, Boixeda P, Truchuelo-Díez MT, Pérez-García B, Alonso-Castro L, Jaén Olasolo P. Infantile hemangiomas treated by sequential application of pulsed dye laser and Nd:YAG laser radiation: a retrospective study. Actas Dermosifiliogr. 2013;104:504–11.
55. Chinnadurai S, Sathe NA, Surawicz T. Laser treatment of infantile hemangioma: a systematic review. Lasers Surg Med. 2016;48(3):221–33.
56. Feng H, Kauvar ANB. Successful treatment of a residual, thick, infantile hemangioma in a darker phototype pediatric patient using the 755-nm long-pulsed alexandrite laser. Dermatol Surg. 2017;43(12):1514–6.

Lasers for the Treatment of Pigmentary Disorders

3

Felix Paolo J. Lizarondo and Woraphong Manuskiatti

Introduction

Pigmentary disorders of the skin are a heterogenous and complex set of skin diseases that greatly impact the quality of life of affected patients. While a variety of treatment ranging from topical therapy to surgery can address most benign pigmented lesions, lasers have emerged as minimally invasive, viable tools in treating those conditions. Understanding the pathogenesis of various pigmented disorders and the basic principles of lasers is crucial in optimizing laser selection when treating hyperpigmentation disorders. This chapter reviews the essentials of selection of lasers for common pigmentary disorders and gives an update of the current evidence for the efficacy of lasers in common benign pigmented lesions.

Types of Lasers Used in Pigmentary Disorders

With a variety of lasers to choose from, deciding on which one to use can be a daunting task. A comprehensive understanding of the theory of selective photothermolysis is critical to understand and select among the currently available lasers that address pigmentary disorders. In order to eliminate a target with little collateral damage, the wavelength chosen has to be selectively absorbed by a specific target chromophore, and the pulse duration less than its thermal relaxation time (TRT) [1]. In pigmentary disorders, the most common chromophore is melanin, which has a wide absorption spectrum from 200 to 1200 nm wavelength [2]. On a cellular level, melanin is located within the melanosomes which is the target of pigment-specific lasers. The approximate size of melanosomes is 0.5–1 μm with corresponding TRTs of 250–1000 ns [1, 3, 4]. Thus, pigment-specific lasers have wavelengths in the absorption spectrum of melanin with pulse durations in nanoseconds and picoseconds. Other types of lasers that are used for pigmentary disorders include less specific pigment and ablative and nonablative lasers (Table 3.1).

Currently available pigment-specific lasers with pulse duration in the nanosecond range include the 532 nm Q-switched neodymium-doped:yttrium aluminum garnet laser or Nd:YAG (QSNYL 532), 694 nm Q-switched ruby laser (QSRL), 755 nm Q-switched alexandrite laser (QSAL), and 1064 nm Q-switched Nd:YAG laser (QSNYL 1064). The picosecond lasers include the 532 nm picosecond Nd:YAG laser (PSNYL 532), 755 nm picosecond alexandrite laser (PSAL), and 1064 nm picosecond Nd:YAG laser (PSNYL 1064). Novel picosecond lasers include 670 nm Nd:YAG and 730 and 785 nm titanium-

F. P. J. Lizarondo · W. Manuskiatti (✉)
Siriraj Skin Laser Center, Department of Dermatology, Faculty of Medicine Siriraj Hospital, Mahidol University, Bangkok, Thailand

S. W. N. Cheng, C. L. Goh (eds.), *Updates on Lasers in Dermatology*, Updates in Clinical Dermatology, https://doi.org/10.1007/978-3-031-71155-8_3

Table 3.1 Commonly used lasers and EBDs for the treatment of pigmentary disorders

Pigment-specific lasers	Less specific pigment lasers	Ablative lasers	Nonablative lasers
Q-switched 694 nm ruby laser (QSRL)	Long-pulsed 694 nm ruby laser (LPRL)	2940 nm Erbium:yttrium aluminum garnet (Er:YAG) laser	1550 nm erbium-doped laser
Q-switched 755 nm alexandrite laser (QSAL)	Long-pulsed 755 nm alexandrite laser (LPAL)	10,600 nm carbon dioxide (CO_2) laser	1927 nm thulium laser
Q-switched Nd:YAG laser (QSNYL) 532 and 1064 nm	Long-pulsed 532 and 1064 nm Nd:YAG laser		Intense pulsed light (IPL)
Picosecond alexandrite laser (PSAL)	Pulsed dye laser		
Picosecond Nd:YAG laser (PSNYL) 532 nm and 1064 nm	Diode laser		

sapphire. The pigment-specific lasers eliminate melanin via the photoacoustic or photomechanical effect. This occurs when the energy delivered by lasers creates shock waves that fragment the melanosomes. Q-switched lasers also have a photothermal effect, which is the primary mechanism of most lasers in the skin [3, 5]. With picosecond lasers primarily operating via a photoacoustic mechanism, there is better confinement of the energy delivered compared to Q-switched lasers. This chapter mainly focuses on pigment-specific lasers since they are currently the lasers of choice for pigment removal in most cases. Other pigment lasers target non-melanin pigment, e.g., tattoo ink of different colors which are sensitive to different wavelengths, e.g., 532 nm for red pigment and 755 nm for green pigment.

Less specific pigment lasers include the long-pulsed counterparts of 694 nm ruby (LPSRL), 755 nm alexandrite (LPAL), 1064 nm Nd:YAG (LPNYL 1064), and 810 nm diode. Even though they are well within the melanin absorption wavelength, they are considered less selective because the pulse widths of these lasers are in the millisecond range, much longer than the TRTs of melanosomes. When used to treat pigmented lesions, there is a higher risk of causing damage to the proximate tissue due to the longer pulse widths. This effect has been utilized in hair removal wherein melanin serves as a chromophore, and the pigmented hair follicle is designated as the target for laser treatment. In treating pigmented lesions, long-pulsed lasers are less effective and have higher complication rates compared to their Q-switched counterparts [6]. Another example of less specific pigment lasers is the 595 nm pulsed dye laser (PDL), which is primarily used to treat vascular lesions. They are typically used with compression to blanch the vessels so that the pigment in the lesions can be targeted like in a solar lentigines [7]. Although not a laser, another example of a light-based device that can be used to remove lesions such as lentigines and ephelides is the intense pulsed light (IPL) which produces a polychromatic light (515–1200 nm) [6].

Nonspecific removal of pigmented lesions can also be achieved with ablative lasers such as the 2940 nm erbium:yttrium aluminum garnet (Er:YAG), 2790 nm yttrium scandium gallium garnet (YSGG), and 10,600 nm carbon dioxide (CO_2) lasers. The chromophore for these lasers is water, which vaporizes tissue, leading to the ablation of the epidermis and papillary dermis. CO_2 laser has the greatest depth of penetration, while Er:YAG laser has the most superficial effect [8]. Such ablative procedures risk scarring and postinflammatory hyperpigmentation (PIH).

Nonablative fractional lasers, such as the 1550 nm erbium-doped and 1927 nm thulium laser, have also been used to treat pigmentary disorders. These lasers target the water in the dermis with sparing of the epidermis. Improvement of the pigmentation is thought to occur via the elimination of microscopic epidermal necrotic debris (MENDs) that contains the pigment [9]. These MENDs initially start in the subgranular layer and undergo transepidermal elimination within 7 days [9]. Some dermal content has also been demonstrated in the MENDs [10].

General Principles in Choosing Laser Parameters

Aside from determining which laser to use, one must also be adept in adjusting the settings of the chosen device. The approximate location of the melanin is a major determinant of what device and what laser parameters to use. The target chromophores may be in epidermis, dermis, or both areas, depending on the pathology of the pigmented lesion. Aside from the location of the chromophore, one must also be cognizant of the baseline skin color, which may cause complication and affect treatment outcome. This also has implications in individuals with tanned skin, as darker skin tones are more susceptible to adverse events. Delaying treatment until their tan has faded is often recommended. Consideration of these factors is important when optimizing laser parameters, including wavelength, pulse duration, spot size, and fluence, for safe and effective delivery of laser treatments for pigmented disorders.

Wavelength

Melanin has a higher/stronger absorption at shorter wavelengths of light, with decreasing absorption characteristics at longer wavelengths (see Chap. 2, Fig. 3.1). Beyond 1100 nm, its absorption is considered negligible [2]. Within the melanin absorption range, shorter wavelength light penetrates the skin more superficially than longer wavelength light. Shorter wavelength lasers are effective in treating epidermal lesions, while longer wavelength lasers target upper dermal lesions. A clinical example is using a 532 nm Nd:YAG laser to treat superficial lesions like solar lentigines and using a 1064 nm Nd:YAG laser to treat deeper lesions such as a nevus of Ota. Balancing between the absorption and penetration of the laser can be challenging in dermal lesions especially in darker skin phototypes. When employing 694 nm ruby and 755 nm alexandrite lasers to address dermal lesions in individuals with skin of color, transient hypopigmentation or hyperpigmentation may occur because the light can be absorbed by epidermal melanin during the treatment.

Pulse Duration

Melanosomes have a TRT of 250–1000 ns; hence, current pigment-specific lasers utilize short pulse durations in the nanosecond (e.g., Q-switched lasers) and picosecond range. In tattoo removal, the superiority of picosecond lasers over Q-switched lasers has been established [11]. Picosecond lasers generate a more pronounced photomechanical effect on tattoo ink particles, exhibiting superior energy confinement and thereby mitigating potential side effects. Recent research has centered on examining the safety and efficacy of picosecond lasers for pigmented lesions. There have also been comparisons between Q-switched and picosecond lasers. Further discussion of the findings from these pertinent studies will be presented in the clinical indications section.

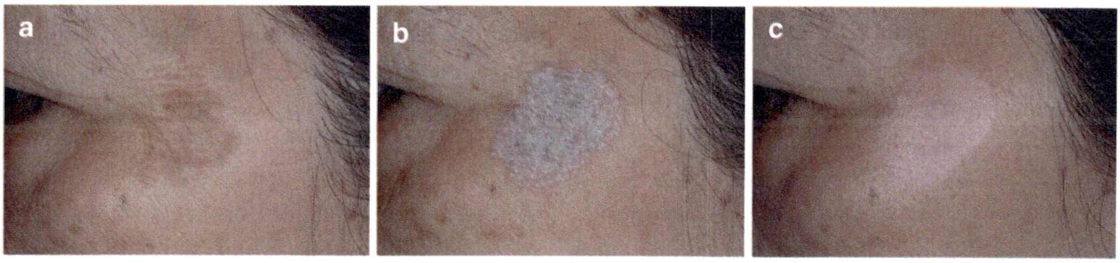

Fig. 3.1 Solar lentigo. (**a**) Before, (**b**) a clinical endpoint of immediate whitening of the lesions after laser irradiation, and (**c**) 2 weeks posttreatment with a 532 nm Q-switched Nd:YAG laser, transient hypopigmentation is observed, which typically resolves spontaneously within the subsequent 4–6 weeks

Spot Size

Adjusting the spot size goes beyond ensuring efficient coverage of all treatment areas. The scattering of the laser light, determined by the spot size, directly impacts the depth of penetration into the skin. Smaller spot sizes exhibit increased scatter, resulting in more superficial penetration. Conversely, larger spot sizes penetrate deeper due to reduced light scattering. Therefore, smaller spot sizes are preferable for treating superficial epidermal lesions like solar lentigines, while larger spot sizes are better suited for deeper dermal lesions such as nevus of Ota and acquired bilateral nevus of Ota-like macules (ABNOMs). An important consideration is that adjusting spot sizes to reach the desired depth of the pigmented lesion also affects fluence. When reducing the spot size by 50%, there is a corresponding fourfold increase in fluence [3]. Consequently, when using smaller spot sizes, it becomes necessary to decrease the fluence to maintain a comparable energy density achieved with a larger spot size.

Fluence

Fluence, also called energy density, is defined as the energy delivered by a laser over an area. Adjusting this parameter is critical in making sure that the desired clinical effect can be achieved. If the fluence is too low, improvement of the pigmented lesions might not be appreciated. However, if the fluence is too high, there is a higher risk of adverse events. In pigmented lesions, the clinical endpoint after laser treatment serves as a guide to determine the proper fluence. As an example, in epidermal lesions treated with Q-switched lasers, the endpoint is usually immediate whitening, which is thought to be from the steam formation brought about by the melanosome destruction [12]. When using picosecond lasers, a milder clinical endpoint can be considered sufficient since these lasers are able to target melanosomes with less surrounding tissue damage [12]. A test spot is usually treated to a desired clinical endpoint, and once achieved, similar settings can be applied for the rest of the lesions. It is crucial to avoid pulse stacking in test spots when determining endpoints to prevent adverse events. When treating the remaining lesions, it is essential to maintain a consistent clinical endpoint and carefully monitor for any adverse events, such as blistering and tissue splattering, that might have developed in previously treated areas. Furthermore, it may be suitable to adjust the fluence per area when treating lesions that extend across anatomical boundaries, such as a nevus of Ota involving both the temple and eyelids.

Clinical Indications

Prior to performing lasers on any pigmented lesion, it is essential to conduct thorough due diligence to confirm its benign nature. If there is any suspicion of a malignancy, laser treatment should not be undertaken. Once the benign nature of the lesion is ascertained, a comprehensive assessment of the skin must be done to estimate the potential for adverse events. Aside from determining the skin phototype and history of tanning as discussed in the previous section, the presence of melasma and prior untoward reactions to laser treatments should be noted since these factors contribute significantly to the risk of postinflammatory hyper- or hypopigmentation. In addition, patients should receive counseling regarding the appearance of wounds, encompassing crusting, erythema, and edema, which typically persists for approximately 1 week. Blistering can be brought about by using a high fluence and is best prevented by using the appropriate settings to reach an optimal clinical endpoint. Other rare side effects of laser treatment include textural alteration and hypertrophic or keloid formation. Another uncommon but important side effect is the blue gray pigmentation called chrysiasis, which can be seen in patients who previously underwent systemic gold therapy usually for rheumatoid arthritis or psoriatic arthritis and subsequently underwent Q-switched laser treatment [13]. Aside from doing preoperative counseling, patients also must be given postoperative instructions in advance as well. They should be advised to avoid excessive sun expo-

Table 3.2 Classification of common pigmentary disorders based on the location of pigment

Epidermal disorders	Dermal disorders	Mixed epidermal-dermal disorders
Lentigines (solar lentigo and lentigo simplex)	Nevus of Ota	Melasma
Ephelides	Acquired bilateral nevus of Ota-like macules (ABNOM) or Hori nevus	Postinflammatory hyperpigmentation
Café au lait macules (CALMs)		Periorbital hyperpigmentation
Seborrheic keratosis		Melanocytic nevus
		Nevus spilus
		Becker's nevus

sure and practice photoprotection measures such as regular application of a broad-spectrum sunscreen. Addressing these considerations before initiating any laser treatments will reassure the patient about the natural course of recovery. This, in turn, enables them to make necessary adjustments to their activities and schedule postoperatively.

Proceeding with this section, we will discuss the pathology of benign pigmented disorders, followed by a presentation of current evidence for different types of lasers, with focus on pigment-specific lasers. A practical approach to organizing clinical indications for pigmentary lasers is to note the location of the melanosomes in various disorders: epidermal, dermal, and mixed epidermal-dermal disorders. This classification will be used in this section (Table 3.2).

Epidermal Disorders

Lentigines (Solar Lentigo and Lentigo Simplex)

Solar lentigines present as well-demarcated light-dark brown to black, round, oval, or irregularly shaped macules. Other terms for these include lentigo senilis or senile freckles. These are acquired through chronic sun exposure; hence, they distribute on the sun-exposed areas such as the face, chest, forearm, arm, and shins. Since these lesions are indicators of long-term UV damage, monitoring these patients for skin cancers should also be done [14]. Another type of lentigines is the lentigo simplex, which usually appears in childhood and is not associated with UV exposure [15]. They can appear anywhere on the body, including the mucosa, and have no predilection for UV-exposed areas. When these simple lentigines present multiply, they can be associated with a variety of syndromes such as LEOPARD syndrome (or Noonan syndrome with multiple lentigines) and Carney complex [15]. Histologically, there is basal layer hyperpigmentation associated with rete ridges that have bud-like extensions and larger keratinocytes within the lesion [14].

Some of the earliest lasers used to treat lentigines included argon and CO_2 lasers [16]. Other devices that have been used are the long-pulsed lasers, such as 595 nm pulsed dye laser (PDL) and 755 nm alexandrite laser, and intense pulsed light [17]. Currently, these devices have largely been supplanted by Q-switched and picosecond lasers that deliver energy in the nanosecond and picosecond range, respectively. QSNYL 532, QSRL, and QSAL have been used for a long time and have demonstrated efficacy and safety in eliminating lentigines [6]. Of note, QSRL has a higher risk of hypopigmentation than QSAL and QSNYL 532 due to the higher absorption of melanin in the 694 nm wavelength [6]. The clinical endpoint when using QS lasers to treat lentigines is immediate whitening of the epidermis without purpura (Fig. 3.1). Crusting is expected and falls off within a week, leaving a transient erythema. Temporary pigmentary changes, such as hyperpigmentation, are more common in darker skin phototypes. Usually, one or two sessions are needed to remove lentigines.

Picosecond (PS) lasers are increasingly being used to address lentigines to theoretically increase the effectiveness and improve the safety profile of laser treatment in lentigines. While clinical endpoints vary in different studies, Negishi et al. have suggested that milder endpoints can be used since picosecond laser can target the chromophores with less collateral damage [12]. This is important to keep in mind since the endpoint used, whether mild or intense whitening, has a great influence on the rates of efficacy and side effects. Most of the early evidence that demonstrated the utility of PSAL and PSNYL 532 came from retrospective studies that included some solar lentigines in their study population [18–21]. Various prospective studies using PSNYL 532, with varying pulse durations of 375, 450, 750, and 800 ps, have demonstrated that 80–100% clearance of solar lentigines can be achieved in one to two treatment sessions [12, 22–25]. Guss et al. noted that thicker lesions had suboptimal responses [23]. In terms of postinflammatory hyperpigmentation, PSNYL 532 had lower rates ranging from 0.8% to 10.2% [12, 22–24]. This is in contrast to QS lasers that had higher rates of postinflammatory hyperpigmentation of 25–47% [22, 26]. Transient hypopigmentation was also noted in 3.6–4.65% of cases [12, 24].

A number of studies have directly compared QS and PS lasers on solar lentigines and have demonstrated faster clearance rates with PSNYL 532 [27, 28] (Fig. 3.2). However, Vachiramon et al. noted similar clearance rates between QSNYL 532 and PSNYL 532 [29]. No difference in adverse events was noted in a few studies, but higher patient satisfaction was noted with PSNYL 532 [27, 29]. In contrast, Kim et al. showed that the postinflammatory hyperpigmentation rate was only 5% in PS laser compared to 30% QS laser, similar to previously presented data [28]. These studies provide preliminary evidence that PS laser may be superior to QS lasers especially in improving the postinflammatory hyperpigmentation rate (Fig. 3.3). This is important in patients with darker skin phototypes wherein post-laser pigmentary changes are more prominent.

Novel picosecond lasers have also demonstrated promising findings for solar lentigines such as the PS 670 nm Nd:YAG, which led to a 100% clearance with a single treatment [30]. PS 730 nm titanium-sapphire was also demonstrated to clear lentigines in 73–86% of patients [31–33]. Transient hyperpigmentation was noted in 11–20% of patients [32, 33]. PS 785 nm titanium-sapphire has also been used to treat a case of solar lentigo [34].

Ephelides

Ephelides, also known as freckles, present as well-demarcated 1–3 mm light-dark brown round, oval, or irregularly shaped macules on the sun-exposed areas such as the face, upper trunk, and dorsal aspects of the upper extremities. Important differentiating features from lentigines are that ephelides do not become as dark, usually fade with cessation of sun exposure, exhibit seasonal darkening during summer, and are more common among younger patients. While these are more common in Caucasian patients with blond or red hair with skin phototype I or II, these can also be found in various ethnicities. Patients with ephelides have an increased risk of developing melanoma [15]. Histologically, the epidermis is normal, but the basal keratinocytes demonstrate increased melanin content since ephelides are thought to occur from the increased functional capacity of the melanocytes induced by

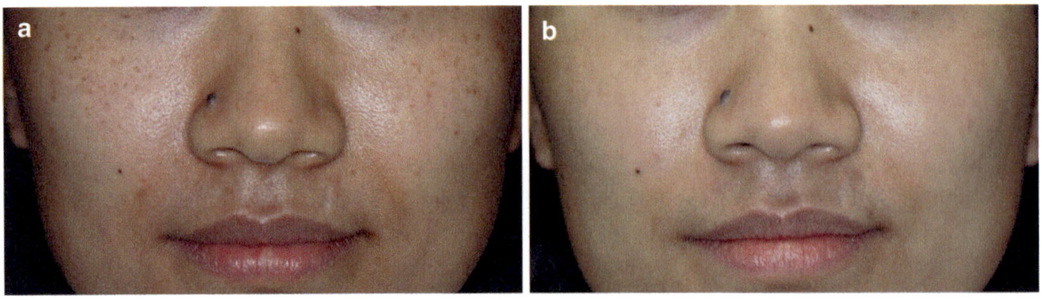

Fig. 3.2 Lentigines. (**a**) Before and (**b**) 6 weeks after single 532 nm picosecond laser treatment

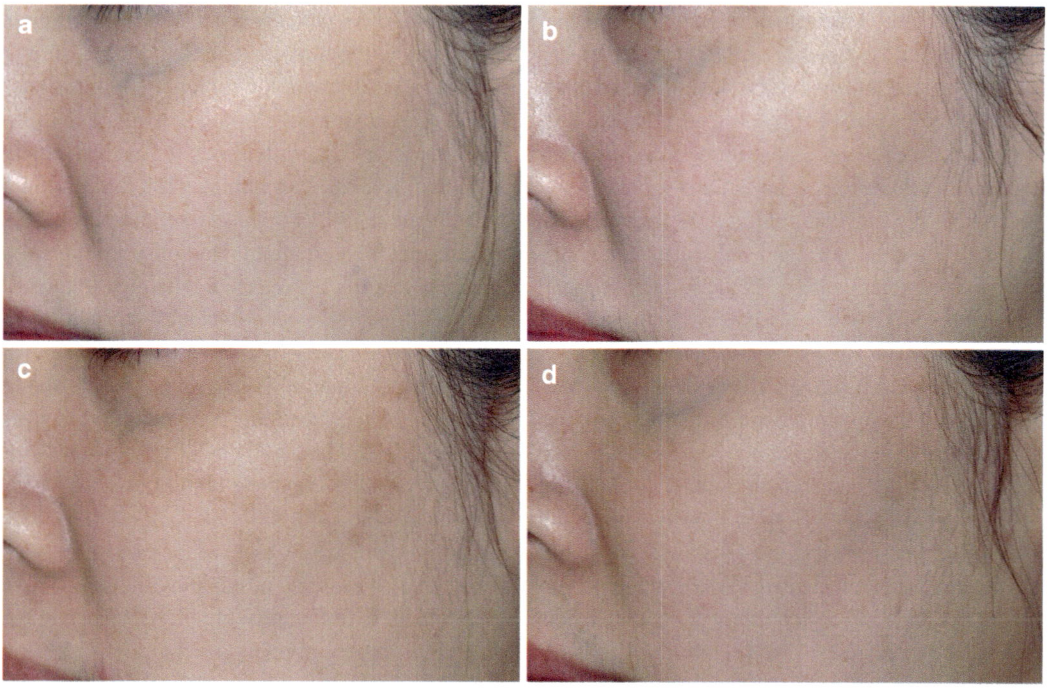

Fig. 3.3 Lentigines in an Asian patient with skin phototype III. (**a**) Before, (**b**) 6 weeks after treatment with a 532 nm picosecond laser, (**c**) the onset of postinflammatory hyperpigmentation (PIH) occurred 8 weeks after the treatment, and (**d**) the spontaneous resolution of PIH occurred at 7 months posttreatment

sun exposure [15]. Hence, consistent and correct sunscreen use is a cornerstone of the management of ephelides.

QSNYL 532, QSRL, and QSAL have all been utilized to address freckles [6, 16, 35]. Of note, 532 nm might be the better wavelength to use due to the higher pheomelanin content of ephelides [17]. Since freckles are more common among lighter skinned patients, any of the lasers can be used with minimal complications. If used on patients with higher skin phototypes or a different ethnicity, for example an Asian with phototype III or IV, there is a higher risk of postinflammatory hyperpigmentation. QSNYL 532 and QSAL have been used in Asians with transient pigmentary changes ranging from 10% to 25% [36, 37]. Using a long-pulsed alexandrite has been to shown to mitigate this risk to 6% [37].

Picosecond lasers have also been investigated in the treatment of freckles. A 450 ps PSNYL 532 was shown to improve 75% freckles in 1–3 sessions [22]. Novel picosecond lasers such as the PS 730 and 785 nm titanium-sapphire have also been demonstrated to be efficacious in a few cases [32, 38]. Various studies have compared PSAL and PSNYL 532 to their QS counterparts and showed that they have the same clearance and adverse event rates [39, 40]. However, PSNYL 532 demonstrated better clearance rates when measured using an imaging device and better pain tolerance as reported by patients with an overall low rate of hyperpigmentation and hypopigmentation at rates of 4.05% and 1.35%, respectively [40]. In contrast, one study showed that QSAL had better clearance and satisfaction rates than PSNYL 532 [41].

Café Au Lait Macules

Café au lait macules (CALMs) usually present during childhood as well-defined light-dark brown homogenous irregularly shaped macules and patches that range from 2 to 5 cm [15]. In 10–20% of the population, they are not associated with any syndromes although multiple lesions may serve as a marker of genodermatoses such as neurofibromatosis 1 and McCune-Albright syndrome [15]. Histologically, the epidermis is normal, but the basal keratinocytes have a slightly increased melanin content [15].

CALMs are especially difficult to treat because of varied response rates and propensity for recurrence posttreatment with QSNYL 532, QSRL, and QSAL [42–44]. Nonetheless, many studies are still being conducted to determine the efficacy of laser treatment for CALMs. Fractional QSRL has been utilized with most patients exhibiting at least 50% improvement after at least three sessions [45]. In a large study by Zhang et al. with 471 pediatric patients, QSAL had a 70.41% response rate with one to nine treatment sessions [46]. Better response and less recurrence have been noted with 510 nm pulsed dye and copper vapor laser [47, 48]. A case report demonstrated the possible utility of Er:YAG laser in an intractable case [49].

Although melanin has less absorption in QSNYL 1064 relative to QSNYL 532, various studies have investigated its role in CALMs. In a study comparing QSNYL 532 with QSNYL 1064, there was a trend to a better clearance with QSNYL 1064 [50]. Low-fluence QSNYL 1064 was demonstrated to induce >50% clearance in 74.4% of lesions without adverse events, despite being associated with a 17% recurrence rate [51]. This low-fluence QSNYL 1064 was shown to be comparable to QSAL [52]. Increasing the fluence in QSNYL 1064 has some promise that it can improve CALMs with a lower recurrence rate [53–55]. The number of treatments needed varied widely in the studies. In a study by Baek et al., 69% of CALM patients had achieved complete clearance without recurrence in the 12-month follow-up period with the treatment administered weekly for a total of 20–50 sessions [53]. Lin demonstrated that with three to five treatment sessions, patients can achieve fair to excellent improvement [54]. In a case series, Kim et al. noted that all four patients demonstrated marked to almost complete clearance when the treatment was administered every 2 weeks for a total of 12–24 sessions [55].

PSNYL 532 and PSAL have also been used to treat CALM in a few studies on benign pigmented lesions [18–22]. In a study by Artzi et al., 60% of patients had near-complete resolution of CALMs after treatment with PSNYL 532 with a 13% recurrence rate [56]. Cen et al. demonstrated that PSAL has the same efficacy with QSAL and QSNYL 532 in improving CALMs, but no postinflammatory pigmentary changes were seen in PSAL [57].

With all the various protocols and lasers presented in this section, CALMs remain challenging to treat since complete clearance is usually not achieved with all patients. In addition, treatments are still associated with a significant recurrence rate, although high-fluence QSNYL 1064 seems to be promising in this aspect. Patient selection may also be key in achieving treatment success as some factors that have been noted with a better response include a facial location of the CALM with a less than 16 cm^2 size and the CALM having irregular borders [51, 57, 58]. Multiple treatments (Fig. 3.4) are usually needed to achieve better results [46, 53, 55].

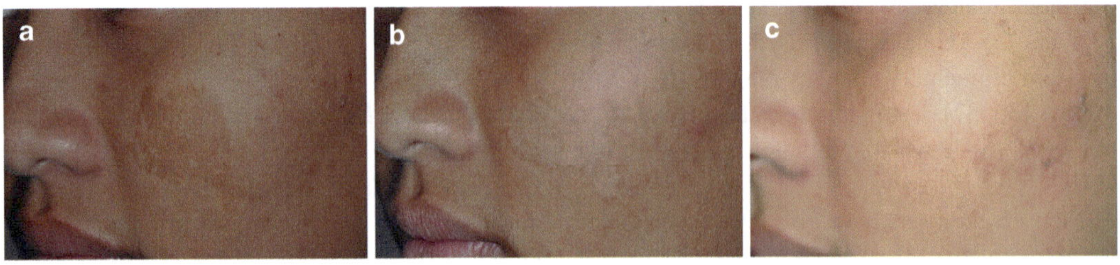

Fig. 3.4 A café au lait macule (CALM). (**a**) Before, (**b**) 4 months after the first 532 nm picosecond laser treatment, and (**c**) 1 year after three treatments

Seborrheic Keratosis

Seborrheic keratosis (SK) usually presents as well-demarcated round-oval-irregularly shaped light-dark brown to black verrucous papules and plaques with a stuck-on appearance. They can appear on any hair-bearing skin while sparing the mucous membranes, palms, and soles [14]. It usually presents in the fourth decade of life and is more common among Caucasians [14]. However, a variant called dermatosis papulosa nigra (DPN) is more common among patients with darker skin such as in Africans, Asians, and Hispanic ethnicity. UV exposure has been implicated as a factor in their development. Histologically, there are many different types, but hyperkeratosis, papillomatosis, and acanthosis are all present invariably [14].

SKs and DPNs are mainly removed for cosmetic concerns with shave excision, cryosurgery, electrodessication, and curettage. In recent years, ablative lasers have been commonly used to treat SKs and DPNs. The efficacy and safety of CO_2 laser in removing SKs and DP have been demonstrated [59–62]. The incidence of recurrence was seen in 28% in a few lesions of the patients [62]. While SKs and DPNs can generally be removed in one session with CO_2 laser, thicker lesions might need additional session (Fig. 3.5). Er:YAG laser can also be used to treat SKs [63, 64]. In a randomized intraindividual study by Zaresharifi et al., it was shown that the efficacy and patient satisfaction rates were comparable between electrodessication, CO_2, and Er:YAG laser [65].

Since some consider SKs to be along the spectrum of solar lentigines, pigment lasers (both pigment specific and less selective) have been utilized to treat SKs. Since SKs are thicker than solar lentigines, multiple treatments are usually needed to adequately clear them. PSAL has been used to treat SKs in a retrospective study [20]. LPAL has demonstrated to clear SKs with papular lesions requiring more treatment sessions [66, 67]. LPNYL 1064 has also been shown to improve DPNs [68, 69]. Other lasers that have been used to treat SKs and DPNs include the 532 nm diode laser, KTP, PDL, fractional 1927 thulium laser, and fractional 1550 nm erbium-doped laser [70–75].

Dermal Disorders

Nevus of Ota

Nevus of Ota, also known as oculodermal melanocytosis, presents during infancy or puberty as well-demarcated irregularly shaped bluish-gray confluent or mottled patches in the distribution of the trigeminal nerve. These are more common among patients with skin of color but can also present in Caucasians [15]. Most commonly affected areas include the forehead, temple, periorbital area, malar area, pre- and retroauricular area, nose, and conjunctiva [15]. If the lesions are distributed in the lateral cutaneous brachial and posterior supraclavicular nerves, such as in the

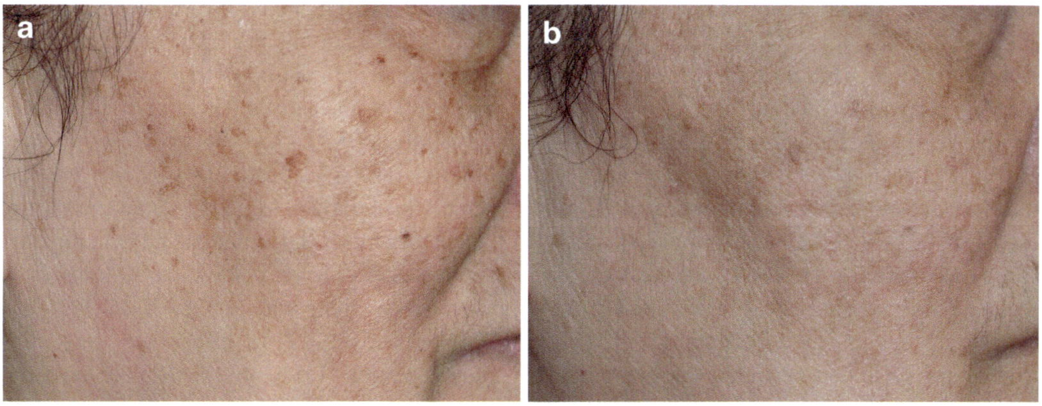

Fig. 3.5 Seborrheic keatosis (SK). (**a**) Before, and (**b**) 1 month after single CO_2 laser treatment in superpulse mode

scapular area, it is termed nevus of Ito. Histologically, there are melanocytes in the dermis, producing the characteristic color [15]. Since topical treatment is unable to address the melanocytes in the dermis, nevus of Ota is one of the skin conditions for which laser treatment is the primary choice of treatment.

QSRL, QSAL, and QSNYL 1064 have all been used to treat nevus of Ota [76–96]. Among the nanosecond lasers, QSNYL 1064 is considered the gold standard of treatment because it has a better safety profile since this wavelength is less absorbed by the epidermal melanin and able to penetrate and target the dermal melanin better compared to other QS lasers [17]. A recent meta-analysis has shown that QSNYL 1064 had the highest pooled success rate at 64% compared to QSAL and QSRL at 58% and 54%, respectively [97]. The same review noted that for the adverse events of pigment changes and scarring, QSNYL 1064 had the least pooled adverse event at 5% compared to QSAL and QSRL at 9% and 14%, respectively [97]. However, another meta-analysis has shown otherwise that QSAL had better efficacy and side effect profile compared to QSNYL 1064 [98]. The authors of the review did mention that the QSAL had longer treatment intervals and follow-up periods compared to QSNYL 1064 [98]. This is important to emphasize since nevus of Ota treatment intervals should be around 8–12 weeks to give enough time for the dermal macrophages to clear the pigment and for the skin to fully recover, minimizing adverse events [6]. It usually takes four to eight sessions to achieve significant improvement. The clinical endpoint for QS lasers when treating nevus of Ota is immediate whitening followed by delayed pinpoint purpura and edema.

Since Chesnut et al. initially described the use of PSAL in nevus of Ota, various case series and retrospective studies have demonstrated its efficacy [18–20, 99]. PSAL can improve nevus of Ota by at least 50% in 80% of the treated cases without permanent post-laser pigmentary changes in one to three sessions [100]. Other studies have also demonstrated a lower number of sessions needed to treat nevus of Ota with most studies noting one to four sessions with an average ranging from 2.2 to 2.5 sessions needed to induce at least 50% improvement [101–104]. Higher clearance of more than 75% can be achieved with PSAL in 40% of patients in two to three sessions [105]. Up to 88.89% of patients achieved moderate to marked improvement in one to four treatment sessions [104]. As much as 96.5% of pediatric patients achieved 95–100% clearance in around 4.3 treatment sessions with transient postinflammatory hyperpigmentation [106]. The high success rate seen in this study by Yang, CY et al. can be due to the fact that pediatric nevus of Ota patients respond better to laser treatment. Better clearance rates and less postinflammatory hyperpigmentation rates can be achieved if the treatment is started before the age of 5 [107].

While most studies have been conducted with focus mostly on PSAL, a few studies have been done on other picosecond lasers as well. PSNYL 1064 was demonstrated to treat nevus of Ota in one to three sessions [107, 108]. Improvement ranged from 50% to 94% with a 6.25% transient postinflammatory hyperpigmentation rate with bluish lesions responding better than brownish lesions [108]. In a case report of a brownish biopsy-proven nevus of Ota that was recalcitrant to QSAL and PSNYL 1064, PSNYL 532 proved to be successful in clearing the lesion [109]. This suggests that brownish and bluish lesions are better treated with PSNYL 532 and PSNYL 1064, respectively. Other picosecond lasers that have been reported to improve nevus of Ota are the PS 730 and 780 nm titanium-sapphire lasers [110].

Comparing QS and PS lasers' efficacy and safety in nevus of Ota has also been undertaken. In a randomized controlled trial with PS alexandrite and QS alexandrite, Ge et al. have demonstrated that PSAL had better clearance rate achieved with less treatment sessions and less pain compared to QSAL [111]. Transient postinflammatory hyperpigmentation and hypopigmentation rates were lower in PSAL at 26% and 21%, respectively, compared to QSAL at 34% and 47%, respectively [111]. In another prospective study comparing QSAL to PSAL, they have also shown similar findings that clearance was achieved faster with 4.2 treatment sessions in

PSAL compared to 5.4 treatment sessions in QSAL [112]. Additionally, there were no reported cases of pigmentary changes in PSAL compared to QSAL group that reported one case each of hyperpigmentation and hypopigmentation [112].

The endpoint used for PS lasers on nevus of Ota varied depending on the study that did report them; most studies on PSAL used mild surface whitening/blanching, while others used mild erythema without pinpoint purpura [20, 100–102]. One study that used PSNYL 1064 used mild purpura as an endpoint [108]. Similar to other indications, milder clinical endpoints in PS lasers are utilized compared to their QS counterparts. In the studies that compared QSAL to PSAL, one employed mild whitening for PSAL [111]. In another study, the same endpoint of immediate whitening was used for both QSAL and PSAL [112]. Since these PS lasers are relatively new compared to QS, this variety of endpoints are expected since the optimal endpoints for nevus of Ota treatment were investigated alongside their efficacy.

The breadth of experience on the safety and efficacy of QSRL, QSAL, and QSNYL 1064 has made the treatment of nevus of Ota possible, improving the quality of life of these patients. With the advent of PSAL and PSNYL 1064, emerging evidence of faster clearance rates and better safety profile has made these lasers a viable alternative (Fig. 3.6). Future randomized controlled studies can provide further evidence on PS lasers, especially head-to-head trials with their QS counterparts.

Hori Nevus

Hori nevus, also known as acquired bilateral nevus of Ota-like macules or ABNOMs, presents as well-demarcated round or irregularly shaped grayish blue to brown macules most commonly on the bilateral zygomatic area. Less commonly, it can also present on the upper eyelid, forehead, and nose [113]. It usually affects adult Asian females, although it can also be found in males. Histologically, there are scattered dendritic and stellate-shaped melanocytes in the papillary dermis [113, 114]. Its etiology is still uncertain but has been attributed to a possible latent dermal melanocytosis triggered by aging or epidermal atrophy [113]. A possible reason for its persistence is the presence of extracellular sheath protecting the melanocytes in the dermis [114]. It has also been noted that ABNOM lesions progressively become more grey with time [115, 116]. The reason for this has not been fully elucidated yet but most likely represents a progressive down migration of the melanocytes, which has likely implications in the choice of laser treatment.

Like in nevus of Ota, topical therapies are ineffective, and lasers are the primary mode of treatment. QSRL, QSAL, QSNYL 532, and 1064 have all been used to treat ABNOMs. The clinical endpoints used in the different studies are immediate whitening without purpura and minimal punctate bleeding. QSAL has been shown to clear ABNOM in 28–35% of cases, with majority of the patients achieving at least 50% clearance in various studies [35, 43, 117]. Postinflammatory hyperpigmentation rate ranged from 12.5% to as high as 80%, while postinflammatory hypopigmentation rate was 50% [35, 117]. QSRL has been shown to clear ABNOM in all treated patients with a 50% transient hyperpigmentation rate [118]. Combination treatment with CO_2 laser with QSRL has also been reported with good results with hyperpigmentation and hypopigmentation that completely resolved in the follow-up period [119]. Pretreatment for 4–6 weeks with tretinoin 0.1% aqueous gel and hydroquinone 5% with lactic acid 7% ointment led to all patients experiencing good to excellent clearance in two to three sessions with QSRL [120]. QSRL has also been shown to be effective when administered in a fractional mode [121].

QSNYL 1064 has been demonstrated to effectively clear ABNOMs in 50–100% of cases with temporary hyperpigmentation ranging from 6.8% to 50% [122–124]. The use of lower fluences while using QSNYL 1064 compared to the previous studies has demonstrated that 26–50% had good to excellent improvement when treated for at least one to two sessions but had a 73% hyperpigmentation rate that resolved within 2–6 months

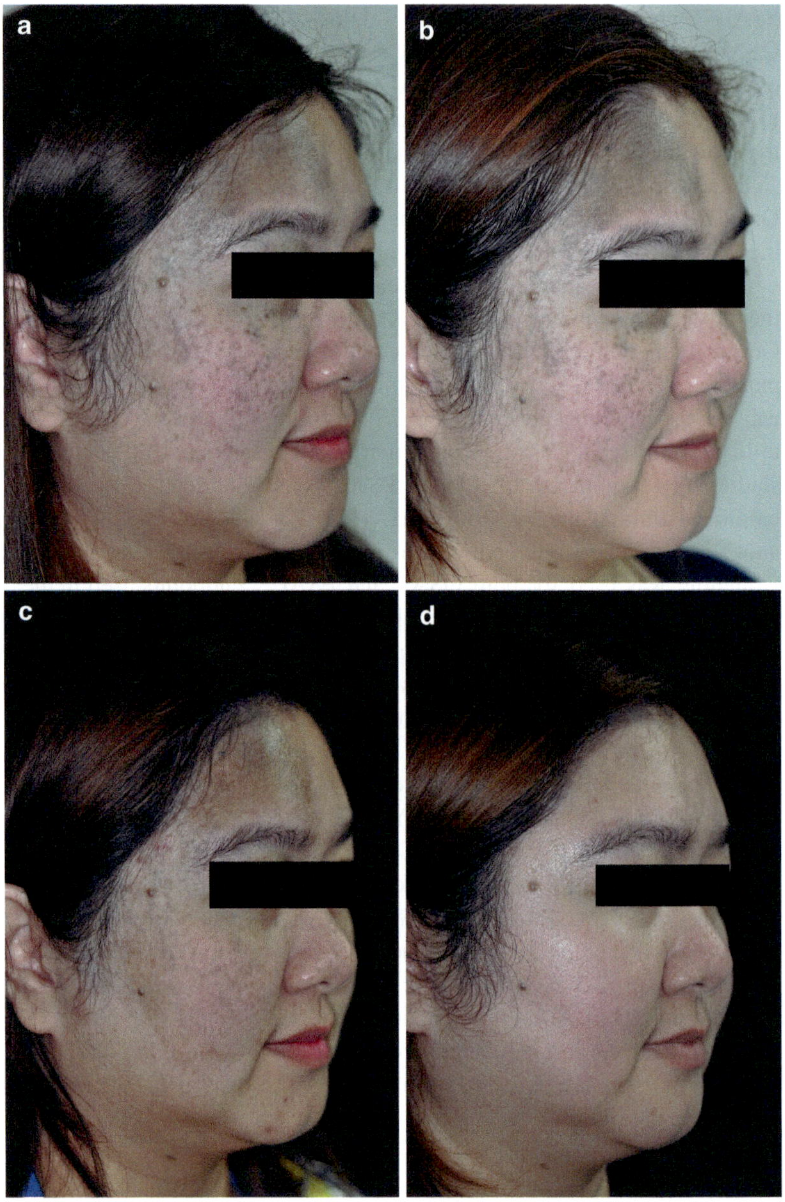

Fig. 3.6 Nevus of Ota. (**a**) Before), (**b**) 3 months after single 1064 nm picosecond laser treatment, (**c**) 3 months after the second laser treatment, and (**d**) 6 months after 6 ps laser treatments

[125]. Another study used a low-fluence QSNYL 1064 and demonstrated that 80% had at least 50% improvement but without any incidence of hyperpigmentation or hypopigmentation [126]. Combination of QSNYL 532 with QSNYL 1064 might be more useful in lesions that are brownish gray than bluish gray but was associated with more transient hyperpigmentation [127]. QSNYL 1064 was also combined with Er:YAG wherein all patients achieved at least 80% improvement [128]. Additionally, using cold air during treatment has been shown to worsen postinflammatory hyperpigmentation when used in treating ABNOM and should be avoided [129].

Among the QS lasers, in a retrospective study done on 685 patients by Zeng et al., the authors noted that QSNYL 1064 laser had the highest efficacy at 52.5% compared to 51.9% and 39.5% of the QSAL and QSRL, respectively [116]. The number of treatments required to completely

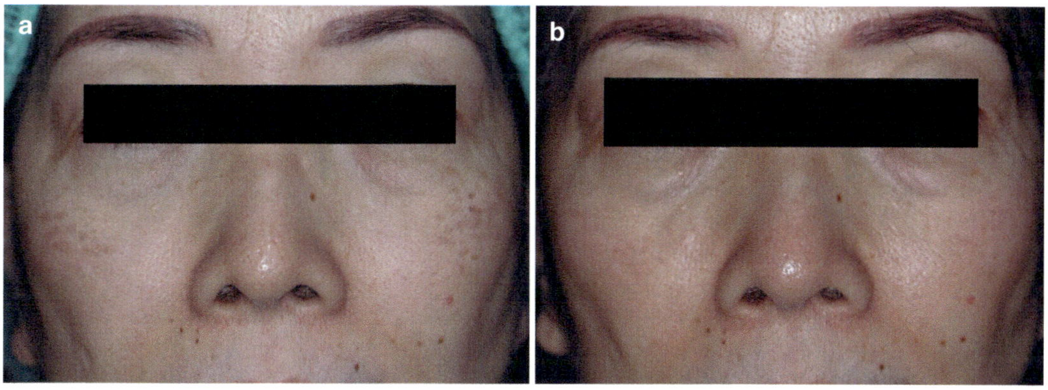

Fig. 3.7 Hori nevus. (**a**) Before, and (**b**) 6 months after six treatments with a 1064 nm picosecond laser

remove the lesions was the least for QSAL at 2.42 ± 1.48 compared to 2.65 ± 1.54 and 4.24 ± 2.19 for the QSRL and QSNYL 1064, respectively [116]. QSAL also had the lowest incidence of hyperpigmentation at 27.5% compared to 30.5% and 43.7% of QSNYL 1064 and QSRL, respectively [116]. Taking all of those factors into consideration, the authors recommend the QSAL to treat ABNOM [116].

PSAL and PSNYL 1064 have also been reported to improve Hori nevus [19, 130]. The clinical endpoint used in most studies was slight or mild immediate whitening without purpura [104]. In a retrospective study by Koh et al., the severity index of Hori nevus was improved from 2.6 ± 0.5 to 1.1 ± 0.4 with an average of 3.82 sessions that ranged from one to six sessions using PSAL without any incidence of permanent hyperpigmentation or hypopigmentation [102]. In a retrospective study that treated dermal lesions including 28 Hori nevi, 88.89% achieved moderate to marked improvement in one to four treatment sessions with one case of hypopigmentation and two cases of hyperpigmentation [104]. In another retrospective study on 265 patients with ABNOMs, Ding et al. noted that greater than 90% clearance can be achieved in 8.89%, 30.99%, 56.65%, and 60.00% of cases in one, two, three, and four treatment sessions, respectively [131]. Transient hyperpigmentation was observed in 22.67% in the same study which resolved in 6–12 months [131]. Combination of PSNYL 1064 with PSNYL 532 and 595 nm Nd:YAG was also reported to improve Hori nevus [132, 133].

Direct comparison of PS laser to their QS counterparts has also been studied. Three sessions of PSAL administered every 6 months had better clearance scores, less pain, and lower rates of postinflammatory hyperpigmentation compared to QSAL [134]. PSNYL 1064 also had better clearance compared to QSNYL 1064 with >50% clearance rate at 87.2% and 57.2%, respectively [27]. An extended follow-up period of 9 months after the last treatment using PSNYL 1064 noted that further clearance was achieved even without additional treatment [135]. This highlights the importance of allowing enough time to see the full effect of laser treatments, especially in dermal pigmented lesions such as ABNOMs and nevus of Ota (Fig. 3.7).

Mixed Epidermal-Dermal Disorders

Melasma

Melasma commonly presents in middle-aged women of Asian, Hispanic, or African descent as well-demarcated irregularly shaped light-dark brown patches on the malar area, forehead, nose, chin, or upper lip, and less commonly on the forearms or chest [136]. Although less frequent, it can also be found in men. It has a complex pathogenesis, with UV, genetics, and hormones contributing to the disease. Recent advances in the elucidation of its pathogenesis have viewed melasma as a photoaging disorder wherein fibroblasts and endothelial cells contribute to the melanocytic activation in many ways such as reduced Wnt inhibitory factor-1 (WIF-1) gene expression and endothelin receptor B activation, respectively [137–139]. Clinically, melasma can be classified into three types: epidermal, dermal, or epidermal-dermal. Wood's lamp enhancement of the lesion has been used to differentiate between the types: epidermal if with enhancement, dermal if without enhancement, and epidermal-dermal if both patterns are present. Histologically, there is melanin deposition in both the epidermis and dermis [140]. In addition, solar elastosis and increased vascularity have also been demonstrated [141, 142].

The mainstay of melasma therapy is a topical tyrosinase inhibitor usually formulated in combination with retinoids and steroids (such as hydroquinone/HQ 4%, tretinoin 0.05%, and fluocinolone acetonide 0.1% cream). This topical treatment is initiated with the consistent use of a sunscreen with UVA and UVB coverage. Addition of visible light coverage can also be considered [143]. Discontinuing hormone therapy as applicable should be done as well. Despite all these measures, the treatment of melasma remains challenging; hence, adjunct treatments are continuously being investigated. One of the frequently studied interventions is laser treatment. While most lasers do offer improvement, these are not considered a first-line treatment since they can cause postinflammatory hyperpigmentation or hypopigmentation, worsening, or even recurrence of melasma. Therefore, it is imperative that these risks are thoroughly explained to the patient prior to initiating any laser treatment.

Earlier use of QS lasers in melasma has been associated with recurrence and constant postinflammatory hyperpigmentation [17, 144–146]. This has prompted modification of the regimen to use lower fluences, which has been shown to affect stage IV melanosomes, a process called subcellular-selective photothermolysis [147]. Also known as laser toning, this low-fluence Q-switched treatment is one of the most extensively studied laser treatments for melasma. A systematic review of studies done on low-fluence QS 1064 nm Nd:YAG laser(LFQSNY) noted that when used as monotherapy, LFQSNY showed improvement in both objective and subjective measures when performed in 5–15 sessions with spot sizes ranging from 6 to 10 mm and fluences ranging from 0.5 to 3.8 J/cm^2 [148]. Low-fluence QS alexandrite (LFQSA) has been shown to be equivalent in efficacy [149]. The wide range of what is defined as low fluence in addition to the various treatment protocols is a challenge in interpreting current data. Recurrence usually measured around 3 months posttreatment reported rates of 0% (no recurrence) to as high as 81% [148]. An important side effect of LFQSNY is mottled hypopigmentation or punctate leukoderma (Fig. 3.8), of which risk factors include a relatively higher fluence, short treatment intervals, and increased total number of treatments [148]. Its reported incidence ranges from 0.5% to 13.6% [150–152]. Spontaneous improvement of mottled hypopigmentation can occur over 2–3 years in only less than 10% of affected patients [153]. Narrowband UVB treatment and excimer laser have been reported to improve this side effect from LFQSNY [154, 155]. Although current data shows that melasma can be improved with LFQS, a thorough risk-benefit assessment will likely limit the suitability of this treatment to patients with recalcitrant melasma.

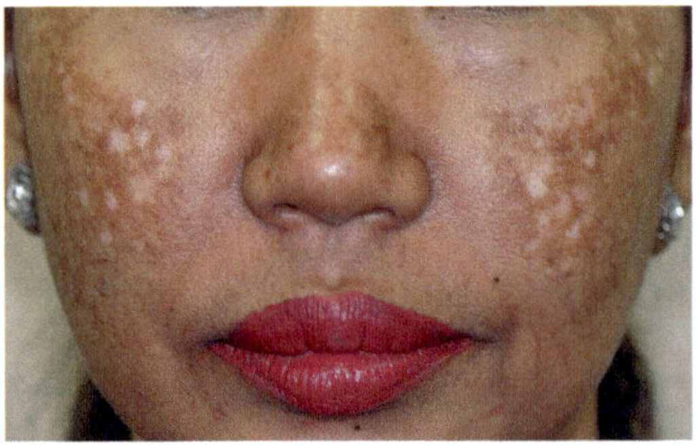

Fig. 3.8 Punctate leukoderma or mottled hypopigmentation observed following a series of eight treatment sessions with low-fluence QS 1064 nm Nd:YAG laser

PSNYL 1064 and PSAL have also been investigated for melasma. PSNYL 1064 has been reported to work in melasma with up to 75% of patients reporting at least >50% improvement in the 3-month follow-up period without incidence of mottled hypopigmentation, although recurrence is still an issue [21, 22]. PSNYL 1064 immediately followed by a PSNYL 595 in the same session induced at least >50% improvement 1 week after the last treatment in 77% of patients without post-laser pigmentary changes; however, this was not sustained at 18th-week follow-up [156]. PSNYL 1064 administered biweekly for six sessions showed moderate-excellent improvement at the 3-month follow-up [157]. The addition of PSAL to hydroquinone 2% cream did not have an additional benefit and was associated with a 15% incidence of postinflammatory hyperpigmentation in the PSAL, which was not seen in the group that only used hydroquinone [158]. PSNYL 1064 was shown to be superior to PSAL and hydroquinone 2% cream, which was seen as early as 2 months after follow-up and was sustained at the 6-month follow-up [159]. Recurrence rates were 5%, 10%, and 5% for PSNYL 1064, PSAL, and HQ, respectively; transient hyperpigmentation was seen in 5% in all groups, while hypopigmentation was only seen in 5% of HQ group [159].

Direct comparisons of PS with QS lasers have also been studied in a few trials. Four monthly treatments using PSAL had faster and better clearance than QSNYL 1064 at the 3-month follow-up without adverse events noted [160]. PSNYL 1064 was noted to have decreased melasma severity scores and better pain scores compared to QSNYL 1064 but was not statistically significant; no adverse events were reported, and similar recurrence rate of 12.5% was noted [161, 162]. In sum, PS lasers seem to improve melasma with improved rates of mottled hypopigmentation compared to QS lasers. However, recurrence is still an issue necessitating proper counseling on patients if this treatment is done.

Delivering the energy of the picosecond lasers using a fractional mode can possibly improve melasma via the formation of microscopic epidermal necrotic debris (MENDs), which eliminates the pigment transepidermally over a few days. Fractional PSNYL 1064 has demonstrated sustained significant improvement in the melasma score without any adverse pigmentary changes [163]. Fractional PSAL demonstrated that 80% of patients had good-moderate improvement in the 1-month follow-up, with only 5% incidence of transient hyperpigmentation [164]. Fractional PSAL administered 3-monthly intervals and 5-monthly intervals compared to a combination cream (fluocinolone acetonide 0.01%, HQ 4%, and tretinoin 0.05%) was shown to be comparable with improvement rates of 53%, 38%, and 50%, respectively, with 18% incidence of transient hyperpigmentation observed only with the PSAL administered five times [165]. Fractional PSAL (8 mm) had better clearance rates than flat optics (4 mm) at 75.7% compared to 52.7% improvement, respectively, with less recurrence rates at 5% and 16%, respectively [166]. Hypopigmentation was seen in 21% of cases in the flat optic group which lasted for more than 6 months [166]. On the other hand, another study using fractional PSAL and full beam/flat optics both at 8 mm demonstrated that both were equally effective and noted lower transient hyperpigmentation rates in the full beam mode without reports of hypopigmentation [167]. While fractional delivery of PS seems to be effective, more studies are needed to determine its utility.

With endothelial cells implicated also in the pathogenesis of melasma, vascular lasers have also been used to target the increased vascularity seen in melasma patients. The use of copper bromide plus/yellow laser (578 nm with 511 nm) decreased melasma area and severity index (MASI) scores with concomitant decrease in telangiectasia at the 6-month follow-up period with decreased immunohistochemical markers Melan-A, CD34, endothelin-1, and VEGF [168]. In contrast, another study has shown that copper bromide laser was not effective and noted that while initial improvement was seen after three treatments, this was not sustained after three more treatments were administered [169]. Another study noted that the addition of copper bromide laser to topical treatment with hydroquinone (HQ) 5%, dexamethasone acetate 0.1%, and retinoic acid 0.1% cream had less improvement of the MASI scores compared to just topical therapy [170]. PDL 595 nm in combination with HQ

4%, fluocinolone acetonide 0.01%, and tretinoin 0.05% was shown to work mostly in melasma patients with skin type II or III, with one patient demonstrating sustained improvement of up to 3 years [171, 172]. Combining PDL 595 nm with a fractional low-powered diode led to a >50% improvement of melasma in 54% of patients in a follow-up period ranging from 26 up to 249 days [173]. Adding PDL into QSNYL can be beneficial if patients demonstrated increased vascularity on dermoscopy [174]. Another device that can be utilized is IPL, although not a laser, which is also proposed to target the vascular component of melasma similar to PDL [17, 175–177]. IPL has also been shown to improve melasma in combination with topical therapies including combination cream (hydroquinone 4%, tretinoin 0.05%, and triamcinolone acetonide 0.1% cream), topical tranexamic acid, and collagen repair dressing [178–180].

With solar elastosis being a feature of melasma and fibroblasts being implicated in its pathogenesis, lasers that promote dermal remodeling have been found to be effective in improving melasma. Nonablative fractional lasers such as 1550 nm have been demonstrated to improve melasma and were found to be comparable to 15% trichloroacetic acid peel and a combination cream (HQ 5%, tretinoin 0.05%, and triamcinolone acetonide 0.1% cream) [181–183]. 1410 nm laser was also found to be effective especially when using a lower coverage of 5% [184]. Early studies on 1927 nm thulium laser showed efficacy with minimal side effects with sustained response up to 12 months [185, 186]. A particular advantage noted with 1927 nm thulium was the early response seen with 48.5% of patients having at least 50% improvement as early as 2 weeks after three treatments that were spaced apart every 2–4 weeks. However, 21% of patients still experienced recurrence at the 6-month follow-up period [187]. In contrast, another study using fractional 1927 nm thulium laser demonstrated that MASI was improved as early as 1 month, and sustained improvement was seen at the 6-month follow-up without recurrence [188]. A weekly regimen of fractional 1927 nm thulium laser with topical tranexamic acid showed similar findings with sustained improvement up to 3 months without adverse events [189].

Ablative lasers have also been used in melasma. CO_2 in combination with QSAL has been used with some success [190, 191]. Low-power fractional CO_2 has demonstrated efficacy with the addition of intradermal tranexamic acid having a marginal benefit [192]. In another study, fractional CO_2 has also been demonstrated to improve melasma in combination with various adjunct therapies such as oral tranexamic acid and laser toning with CO_2, QSNYL 1064, and PSNYL 1064 [193]. Aside from CO_2, Er:YAG was also shown to improve melasma, with epidermal melasma having the best response [194–196].

Postinflammatory Hyperpigmentation (PIH)

Postinflammatory hyperpigmentation is a common acquired pigmentary disorder that arises after the resolution of inflammatory skin disorders such as eczema and arthropod bites. In some instances, the preceding inflammation can be transient or subclinical [136]. It can also come from any injury to the skin, including procedures such as laser treatments. While it can occur to anyone, it is more commonly seen in darker skin types. It can be divided into two main types: epidermal PIH which presents with light-dark brown macules or patches and dermal PIH that presents with bluish-gray macules or patches [136]. It can also present with both features having a mixed epidermal and dermal PIH. The darkening associated with PIH comes from inflammation-induced melanocytic activation in the epidermis, and if the basal layer of the epidermis is damaged, pigmentary incontinence can occur. Histologically, there is increased melanin in the epidermis in epidermal PIH while there are dermal melanophages in dermal PIH [136].

When considering laser treatment for PIH, the underlying skin condition must be controlled to prevent new hyperpigmentation from appearing. In addition, judicious sunscreen use should be advised to patients if the PIH is located in sun-exposed areas since UV exposure can worsen it. The prognosis of PIH largely depends on the location of the pigment since epidermal PIH can resolve without any intervention in a few months or years while dermal PIH tends to have a protracted course and sometimes can be permanent [197]. Nonetheless, since PIH affects the quality of life of patients, treatment is usually undertaken. Epidermal PIH can be treated with topical whitening agents or chemical peels, while dermal PIH can be treated with lasers [198]. In cases of mixed epidermal and dermal PIH, combination of treatments is appropriate to maximize therapy. When treating PIH with lasers, it is important to counsel patients that the response of PIH to laser is variable with a risk of nonresponse or even worsening.

The early use of QSRL had some variable success in lightening PIH [144, 145, 199]. Like in melasma, this prompted the modification to utilize low fluence in treating PIH. A few case series reported the sustained improvement of PIH with low-fluence QSNYL 1064 (LFQSNYL) [200, 201]. Various studies using LFQSNYL 1064 on post-acne hyperpigmentation noted that 86.7–100% of patients had at least 50% improvement [202, 203]. The addition of either QSNYL 1064 or PDL to topical therapy had better response rates than either treatment alone [204]. The addition of tranexamic acid to LFQSNYL 1064 was also reported to be beneficial in PIH from contact dermatitis [203]. QSNYL 1064 has also shown efficacy in a few case series done on axillary hyperpigmentation [205–207]. A method called medium-fluence QSNYL 1064 was used in persistent PIH, which demonstrated at least 50% improvement in 73% of treated patients [208]. PSAL has also been reported to improve PIH [18, 20, 209, 210]. Less selective pigment lasers and devices that have been used to treat PIH also include 578 and 511 nm copper bromide laser/light-emitting diode, variable pulsed light (VPL), and IPL [211–214].

Fractional lasers have been reported to improve PIH presumably by the transepidermal elimination of pigment via the creation of MENDs. 1550 nm Erbium-doped lasers have been reported to improve PIH [215, 216]. However, one study did not see significant improvement in PIH patients treated with 1550 nm erbium-doped laser [217]. Fractional 1927 nm thulium lasers have also been demonstrated to improve different types of PIH such as cupping, dermatitis, acne, and post-laser [218, 219]. In a retrospective study done on PIH mostly from chemical peels done on skin types IV–VI, fractional 1927 nm diode laser improved the lesions by 43.24% [220]. Fractional CO_2 was also reported to improve PIH that resulted from acne and from waxing [221, 222].

Periorbital Hyperpigmentation

Periorbital hyperpigmentation (POH) presents as ill- or well-defined light-dark brown-bluish patches in the bilateral infraorbital area but can also be found in the upper eyelids as well. Other terms for this include dark circles, raccoon eyes, periorbital melanosis, and idiopathic cutaneous hyperchromia of the orbital region [223]. Its pathogenesis remains unclear but is thought to result from a variety of factors including melanin deposition, postinflammatory hyperpigmentation, superficial venous congestion, lax skin that produces shadowing, and swelling in the infraorbital area [224]. Ranu et al. proposed a classification system for POH: constitutional, vascular, PIH, shadow effects, and other. Constitutional POH presents with brownish skin approximating the orbital rim and commonly includes the upper and lower eyelids. This is more common in Indians and Malays. Vascular POH presents with erythema-bluish discoloration and is more common in Chinese. POH from PIH can present with lichenification with a history of eczema, while POH from shadowing effects disappears with lighting. Other possible causes include dry skin, nutritional deficiencies, and chronic illnesses [225]. Histologically, POH has increased melanin in the epidermis and melanophages in the dermis with increased melanin of vellus hair follicles as well [223].

Targeting POH with pigment-specific lasers has been investigated. The efficacy of QSRL in lightening POH by at least 40–50% has been demonstrated in 50–88.9% of patients in various studies [224, 226]. However, transient hyperpigmentation and hypopigmentation rates were 29.4% and 5.9% of cases, respectively [224]. Fractional QSRL also improved POH by at least 50% in 93.33% of patients without postinflammatory pigmentary changes [227]. Full face resurfacing with CO_2 laser followed by QSAL improved POH by at least 75% in all patients which started to fade at 6–8 weeks after treatment [228]. LFQSNYL 1064 was demonstrated to lighten POH by at least 50% in 86.67% of patients without adverse events [229]. Fractional QSNYL 1064 also improved POH [230, 231]. In contrast, PS lasers delivered in a fractional mode such as PSNYL 532, PSNYL 1064, and PSAL did not have much effect in improving POH [232]. Full beam PSNYL 1064 has been demonstrated to improve POH although at relatively similar rates as their Q-switched counterparts [21].

For the venous component of POH, LPNYL 1064 was demonstrated to induce 100% clearance in all patients without postinflammatory pigmentary changes. A frequent side effect that was noted in 92.3% of patients was eyelid edema that lasted for 1–3 days [233]. While no visual changes were reported by the patients, Biesman cautioned that ocular injuries may occur with the use of LPNYL 1064 such as macular holes and uveitis, which were not adequately investigated in the previously mentioned study since it requires comprehensive ophthalmologic examination [234].

Nonselective removal of epidermal and dermal pigment in POH can also be done by ablative lasers and nonablative lasers via the formation of MENDs. A possible additional benefit in using these lasers is the stimulation of collagen production and improving the texture, partially addressing the skin laxity seen in some cases of POH. Fractionated 1550 erbium-doped laser was reported to improve POH in a case report [235]. CO_2 laser resurfacing was noted to lighten at least 50% in all patients with skin types I–III with transient hyperpigmentation incidence of 33% that lasted for 8 weeks [236]. It was also noted to be safe in patients with skin types III–VI, exhibiting greater improvement than patients with lighter skin types even if there was a 100% transient hyperpigmentation that resolved by the 12th-month follow-up period [237]. Fractional CO_2 also lightened POH significantly more than the combination of microneedling combined with trichloroacetic acid 10% peel [238]. 2970 nm Er:YAG was also demonstrated to improve POH by 72.5% in all patients without adverse events [239]. The addition of platelet-rich plasma to fractional Er:YAG was noted to be beneficial than Er:YAG alone [240].

Since more than one type of POH can exist in one patient, combining lasers with other interventions is a comprehensive way of improving POH. In a study by Goldman et al., they identified components of POH that were present in patients: eyelid fat pads, tear trough deformity, pigmentation, small blood vessels, and skin texture (lines and wrinkles). Lower eyelid blepharoplasty with fat pad resection was done for patients with severe deformities. Fat graft or hyaluronic acid fillers were performed for tear trough deformities. The pigmentation, blood vessels, and skin texture were addressed with QSNYL 532 or 1064, LPNYL 1064, and IPL or fractional CO_2, respectively. With the combination of these treatments, 83.7% of patients reported a good-excellent outcome [241]. In a study by Kounidas et al., they analyzed the etiology of patients that had tear trough/volume loss, vascular component, pigmentation, and wrinkles, and they treated them with hyaluronic acid fillers, LPNYL 1064, QSNYL 1064, and fractional CO_2, respectively [242]. For patients that had mixed types, multiple treatments were given, and analysis into three groups that were given fillers, lasers (LPNYL 1064, QSNYL 1064, or fractional CO_2), and both fillers and lasers was done. There was no statistically significant difference between the treatment groups, suggesting that making an accurate assessment of the etiology of POH followed by combination of treatment modalities can ensure patient satisfaction and POH improvement.

Melanocytic Nevus

Melanocytic nevi, which are proliferation of benign melanocytes, can be classified into two main types: congenital and acquired. Congenital melanocytic nevus (CMN) is commonly present at birth although a variant termed tardive congenital nevus develops later within 2 years of birth [15]. These well-demarcated round, oval, or irregularly shaped light-dark brown-black macules, papules, patch, or plaques can also have an associated hypertrichosis. Lesions in adults that are <1.5 cm, 1.5–20 cm, >20–40 cm, and >40 cm are termed small, medium, large, and giant CMNs. In newborns, lesions that are >6 cm and >9 cm on the trunk and scalp, respectively, are considered large and giant CMNs already. It is important to note the size of these lesions since large and giant CMNs are associated with a significantly higher risk of melanoma [15]. Neurocutaneous syndrome also occurs with multiple medium CMNs and those with large and giant CMNs especially when located posteriorly [15]. The other type of melanocytic nevus is the common acquired melanocytic nevi, which are usually present in early childhood, and its number peaks during the third decade of life and gradually decreases thereafter with older age [15]. These factors are mainly influenced by genetics and UV exposure [15]. Histologically, acquired melanocytic nevus can have the nests of melanocytes in the epidermis, dermis, or both in junctional, compound, and dermal nevi, respectively. In contrast to the common nevi that have melanocytes mainly in the papillary and upper reticular dermis, CMN histologically would have nests that are in the deep reticular dermis, along the adnexal structure, and can extend into the underlying subcutaneous fat and fascia [15].

Since CMNs have an increased risk of malignant transformation, surgical excision is usually offered. If the lesions are large, excision can be done serially or staged and closed with flaps or grafts or with the use of tissue expanders. Otherwise, lifelong monitoring should be done to monitor for any signs and symptoms suspicious for malignancy. Immediate histological examination should be done for any areas that are suspicious for malignant transformation. Common acquired nevi are usually removed for cosmetic concerns or for practical purposes if it is located in an area that is frequently traumatized. Histologic examination is also warranted if they develop any signs and symptoms suspicious for malignancy, as in CMNs. It is for these reasons that laser is not a first-line treatment for melanocytic nevi, whether congenital or acquired. Since the nests of melanocytes can be located deep in the dermis, complete removal of lesions is difficult to achieve; hence, recurrence can occur. Complications such as scarring and dyspigmentation are possible when trying to remove the deeper parts of the melanocytic nevi. Laser treatment can also lead to pseudomelanoma, a phenomenon initially described after incomplete excision of nevi [243–245]. While the risk of melanoma after laser treatment is still not fully established, there have been reported cases of melanoma arising in melanocytic nevi previously treated with lasers [246–248]. In cases wherein surgical excision is not feasible, these risks must be thoroughly explained prior to initiating any laser treatment.

QS lasers have been used to treat melanocytic nevi since these can target melanocytes while their long-pulsed counterparts can target the larger nests of melanocytes. Most studies have reported the efficacy of QSRL and normal mode RL (NMRL) [249–254]. Some have also combined QSRL and NMRL especially for the superficial intradermal type of CMN [255, 256]. CMNs with deeper component may not be responsive [257]. It is also important to do long-term follow-up even if the lesions clinically improve since recurrence can occur long after treatment [258]. Combining QSRL with other lasers such as QSNYL 1064, PDL, and CO_2 has also been reported to improve CMN [259–261]. QSAL, normal mode alexandrite laser (NMRL), and QSNYL 1064 have also been demonstrated to treat CMNs [262–266]. LPAL combined with LPNYL 1064 has been utilized in one case [267]. LPNYL 532 has been demonstrated to be effective in removing small acquired melanocytic nevi [268]. PSAL has also been used in a few cases [18, 20].

Melanocytic nevi can also be removed by ablative lasers. Er:YAG laser has been used to improve CMNs with minimal scarring [269–272]. While up to 80% of patients can maintain minimal repigmentation in a follow-up period of up to

3 years, deeper melanocytes of the CMN still remain unaffected [270]. Short-pulse Er:YAG laser was demonstrated histopathologically to clear 96% of treated acquired melanocytic nevi [273]. CO_2 laser was also used to treat CMNs but with a higher risk of hypertrophic scarring in as much as 50% of patients in one study [272, 274, 275]. Fractional CO_2 has been noted to have 85% clearance of AMNs after one session with a 4% recurrence rate after following up for 1 year [276].

Combination of CO_2 laser with pigment-selective lasers has also been investigated based on the theory that removing epidermal melanocytes can increase the efficacy of pigment-selective lasers in reaching the deeper components on the CMN. CO_2 laser combined with pigment-selective lasers such as QSRL demonstrated higher response rates than using QSRL alone [277]. QSNYL 532 and QSAL in combination with CO_2 laser showed some benefit [278–280]. In particular, combination with QSNYL 532 had an 87% satisfaction rate with 12.5% of patients exhibiting recurrence [281]. In contrast, combining QSNYL 532 or QSAL with CO_2 laser did not provide additional benefit [282]. The type and location can also predict the outcome of laser treatment with macular CMN on the trunk and mamillary CMN on the head and neck being more responsive to treatment [282]. Combination of CO_2 laser with QSNYL 1064 has also demonstrated efficacy in CMNs located on the nasal ala [283]. Er:YAG laser in combination with LPAL has also demonstrated efficacy in removing AMNs and CMNs although recurrence rate was 3% for CMNs within 6 months [284].

Nevus Spilus

Nevus spilus (NS), also known as speckled lentiginous nevus or zosteriform lentiginous nevus, presents as well-demarcated irregularly shaped light-dark brown patch with darker macules and papules randomly distributed within the patch. There is some controversy still whether these lesions are congenital or acquired but represent a field defect wherein any type of nevus can develop [15]. NS has been associated with melanoma with 0.13–0.2% risk with lesions that are congenital or appear during infancy, macules, and size greater than 4 cm as risk factors for malignant degeneration [285]. Histologically, the patch has melanocytic hyperplasia with elongated epidermal rete ridges, while the darker smaller macules and papules have features of junctional nevi, compound, dermal, blue, Spitz, or atypical nevi [15].

Monitoring for any suspicious malignant degeneration should be done regularly, and if any signs of melanoma are present, histological examination is warranted. While no treatment is usually necessary, surgery has been proposed to eliminate the risk of melanoma [286]. Aside from surgical management, various lasers have been tried to treat NS with varied success. QSRL, QSAL, QSNYL 532, and 1064 nm have all been demonstrated to improve NS in as much as 83% of patients [43, 287–290]. Leeuwen et al. noted that lentiginous spots cleared while the papules usually recurred [287]. In a study by Kar and Gupta using QSNYL 532 and 1064, 60% of patients had at least 50% improvement, but 13% noted worsening of the lesion [291]. Tang et al. demonstrated that the addition of fractional CO_2 to QSNYL 532 and 1064 led to all ten patients having an improvement of at least 50% although one patient developed hypertrophic scar [292]. PSAL has been used in case reports to treat NS [19, 20]. Both PDL and IPL have also been reported to improve NS [293, 294].

Becker's Nevus

Becker's nevus (BN), also known as Becker's melanosis, nevoid melanosis, or Becker's pigmentary hamartoma, presents usually in the second or third decade of life with well-demarcated irregularly shaped light to dark brown patches. The lesion can exhibit thickening and can be associated with hypertrichosis which ranges from being subtle to very thick coarse hairs [15]. The presence of hypertrichosis varies from 17% to 23.15% of cases [295, 296]. Becker's nevi are most commonly located on the upper outer quadrant of the anterior or posterior chest but can be found elsewhere in the body [15]. It can be associated with hypoplastic abnormalities, such as hypoplastic breast, in a Becker's nevus syndrome which is more common in females [15]. Histologically, it can be associated with acanthosis, papillomatosis, and hyperkeratosis with increased melanin content in the keratinocytes with dermal melanophages. The number of melanocytes is usually normal or slightly increased. It can also demonstrate a concomitant smooth muscle hamartoma [15].

Laser treatment of BN can be done by targeting the pigmentation, which is primarily epidermal with some dermal component, and by removing the associated hypertrichosis. The usual endpoint is whitening in treating the epidermal component while perifollicular erythema and hair singeing when performing hair removal. Pigment-specific lasers such as QSRL have been used to decrease the pigment with a clearance rate of up to 63% [290, 297, 298]. QSNYL 532 has also been used with 43% clearance rate and 25% fair response rate in various studies [290, 299]. QSAL was shown to improve >50% of the lesions in 34.2% of patients with 40.7% recurrence rate but with postinflammatory hyperpigmentation and hypopigmentation rates of 14.6% and 7.3%, respectively [300]. PSAL has also been reported to improve BN in a few case series [18, 20]. Compared to other lasers, PSAL was shown to have higher clearance rates than QSRL, QSNYL 532, QSAL, PSAL fractional, and PSNYL 1064 fractional, in descending order [301]. In the same study, the hyperpigmentation and hypopigmentation rates were 10.2% and 8.2%, respectively, for all the included treatments [301].

Pigment lasers that are less selective for melanosomes such as LP ruby laser (LPRL) and alexandrite laser (LPAL) are utilized to decrease the hair density and improve pigmentation [302, 303]. While all patients had at least a fair response and no recurrence was observed with LPAL, hypopigmentation was noted in some patients [303]. LPNYL 1064 combined with LPAL was reported to clear a case of BN but was associated with hypopigmentation [304]. Low-fluence 808–810 nm diode lasers have also been used to reduce hypertrichosis in BN [305]. 800 nm diode also demonstrated temporary efficacy for hypertrichosis since regrowth occurred in all patients within 6 months [306]. IPL, with 550 and 590 nm filters, has also been used with some success in reduction of both the pigment and hypertrichosis [307, 308]. BN without hypertrichosis has been noted to respond better than hypertrichotic BN [309]. While there was >75% improvement in both the pigmentation and hair reduction in a few cases, this was not sustained when followed up for 6 months [310]. IPL combined with 1550 nm has been reported to fare better than QSNYL 1064 in one case [311]. 577 nm Yellow laser has also been noted to improve pigmentation in a case report [312].

Nonablative lasers such as the 1550 Er:doped fiber laser have also been demonstrated to improve BN [313]. Its combination with an LPNYL 1064 to remove the hair has resulted in >75% clearance [314]. Adding LPNYL 1064 or LPAL to fractional 1550 nm led to at least 50–75% improvement in the majority of treated patients [315]. Fractional 1927 nm thulium laser has also been reported to induce very good to excellent clearance in all treated patients although partial recurrence and transient hypopigmentation were seen as well [316].

Ablative lasers have also been utilized in the treatment of BN. One session of Er:YAG was shown to induce complete clearance in 54% of patients, while the rest exhibited >50% clearance that was sustained after a 2-year follow-up period compared to 9% seen in QSNYL 1064 [317, 318]. Transient hypopigmentation was observed and resolved by 3 months [318]. A 10,600 nm fractional ablative laser demonstrated that 56% of patients had >50% improvement with 22% demonstrating worsening of the BN [319]. Multiple Er:YAG laser treatments led to moderate-good improvement in all patients in one study, but all of them experienced hypopigmentation [320].

Conclusion

When using lasers for pigmentary disorders, a key step in maximizing treatment is determining the location of the chromophore, which is the melanin located within the melanosomes. These structures can be located within the epidermis, dermis, or both. Keeping this in mind will allow one to choose and adjust the appropriate wavelength, pulse duration, spot size, and fluence to safely remove the pigment. Epidermal disorders respond to shorter wavelengths and smaller spot sizes since these parameters allow for a more superficial delivery of the energy. On the other hand, dermal disorders respond to longer wavelengths and larger spot sizes since these parameters allow for deeper delivery of the energy. Fluence settings are determined by the clinical endpoint, which varies per pigmentary disorder and the laser used. Specifically for pigmentary disorders, the advent of the Q-switched and picosecond lasers with pulse durations in subnanosecond range has led to a better confinement of the energy, offering a safe, effective, and minimally invasive way of pigment removal.

Among the epidermal disorders, solar lentigines and ephelides are highly responsive to the pigment-specific lasers (QSRL, QSAL, QSNYL 532, PSAL, and PSNYL 532) (Table 3.3). Seborrheic keratoses and dermatosis papulosa

Table 3.3 Summary of response of pigmentary disorders to various laser treatments

	Response to laser treatments
Epidermal disorders	
Lentigines	Highly responsive to PSAL, PSNYL 532, QSRL, QSAL, and QSNYL 532
Ephelides	Highly responsive to PSAL, PSNYL 532, QSRL, QSAL, and QSNYL 532
Café au lait macule	Variably responsive to PSAL, PSNYL 532, QSRL, QSAL, and QSNYL 532 and 1064
Seborrheic keratosis	Highly responsive to Er:YAG laser and CO_2 laser
Dermal disorders	
Nevus of Ota	Highly responsive to PSAL, PSNYL 1064, QSRL, QSAL, and QSNYL 1064
Hori nevus or acquired bilateral nevus of Ota-like macules (ABNOMs)	Highly responsive to PSAL, PSNYL 1064, QSRL, QSAL, and QSNYL 1064
Mixed epidermal-dermal disorders	
Melasma	Variably responsive to PSAL (full beam and fractional), PSNYL 1064 (full beam and fractional), low-fluence QSNYL 1064, and low-fluence QSAL
	Variably responsive to vascular lasers that target the vascular component of melasma such as copper/bromide laser and PDL
	Variably responsive to fractional ablative and nonablative lasers such as CO_2 laser, 1550 nm erbium-doped laser, and 1927 nm thulium laser
Postinflammatory hyperpigmentation	Variably responsive to PSAL, PSNYL 1064, and low-fluence QSNYL 1064
	Variably responsive to fractional ablative and nonablative lasers such as CO_2 laser, 1550 nm erbium-doped laser, and 1927 nm thulium laser
Periorbital hyperpigmentation	Variably responsive to QSRL, QSAL, QSNYL 1064, and PSNYL 1064
	Variably responsive to LPNYL 1064 laser that targets the venous component
	Variably responsive to fractional ablative and nonablative lasers such as CO_2 laser and 1550 nm erbium-doped laser
	Multimodality approach (e.g., hyaluronic acid fillers with laser treatment) might be beneficial in some patients
Melanocytic nevus	Variably responsive to QSRL, QSAL, and QSNYL 532 and 1064 since deeper components can remain after treatment. LP may be able to better target larger nests of melanocytes
	Variably responsive to ablative lasers since deeper components can remain after treatment
Nevus spilus	Variably responsive to QSRL, QSAL, and QSNYL 532 and 1064

(continued)

Table 3.3 (continued)

	Response to laser treatments
Becker's nevus	Variably responsive to QSRL, QSAL, QSNYL 532, PSAL (full beam and fractional), and fractional PSNYL 1064 Variably responsive to fractional ablative and nonablative lasers such as CO_2 laser, 2940 nm Er:YAG laser, 1550 nm erbium-doped laser, and 1927 nm thulium laser Hypertrichosis component highly responsive to LPRL, LPAL, and LPNYL 1064

nigra can be removed using ablative lasers. Cafe au lait macules have a variable response to the pigment-specific lasers (QSRL, QSAL, QSNYL 532 and 1064, PSAL, and PSNYL 532) and the other lasers that have been investigated. Among the dermal disorders, nevus of Ota and Hori nevus are both highly responsive to pigment-specific lasers (QSRL, QSAL, QSNYL 1064, PSAL, and PSNYL 1064), which are the gold standard of treatment. Mixed epidermal-dermal disorders, as a group, have a variable response to the pigment-specific and other types of lasers used. Included in this group are melasma, postinflammatory hyperpigmentation, periorbital hyperpigmentation, melanocytic nevi, nevus spilus, and Becker's nevus. In these mixed disorders, a thorough risk-benefit assessment can help in selecting patients that can benefit from laser treatment.

While a lot of research has been done for the laser treatment of pigmentary disorders, a major limitation is that most of the studies presented in this section are retrospective studies, case series, and uncontrolled prospective studies. Another limitation is that the treatment, assessment, and follow-up protocols used by the investigators varied widely per study. These limitations highlight the need for more large-scale, randomized comparative and controlled studies with long-term follow-up. These future studies will enable clinicians to deliver evidence-based laser treatments that ultimately improve the quality of life of affected patients.

References

1. Anderson RR, Parrish JA. Selective photothermolysis: precise microsurgery by selective absorption of pulsed radiation. Science. 1983;220:524–7.
2. Anderson RR, Parrish JA. The optics of human skin. J Invest Dermatol. 1981;77:13–9. https://doi.org/10.1111/1523-1747.ep12479191.
3. Allemann IB, Kaufman J. Laser principles. In: Allemann IB, Goldberg DJ, Itin P, Jemec G, editors. Basics in dermatological laser applications, Current problems in dermatology, vol. 42. 1st ed. Basel: Karger; 2011. p. 7–23.
4. Sakamoto FH, Avram MM, Anderson RR. Lasers and other energy technologies—principles & skin interactions. In: Bolognia JL, Schaffer J V, Cerroni L. Dermatology. 4. Elsevier; 2018. p. 2251–2259. doi:https://doi.org/10.1016/B978-0-7234-3571-6.00136-6.
5. Rohrer AT, Arndt KA, Hogan SR. Laser and light therapy for cutaneous hyperpigmentation. UpToDate.
6. Allemann IB, Goldberg DJ. Benign pigmented lesions. In: Allemann IB, Goldberg DJ, Itin P, Jemec G, editors. Basics in dermatological laser applications, Current problems in dermatology, vol. 42. 1st ed. Basel: Karger; 2011. p. 81–96.
7. Kono T, Chan HH, Groff WF, Sakurai H, Takeuchi M, Yamaki T, et al. Long-pulse pulsed dye laser delivered with compression for treatment of facial lentigines. Dermatol Surg. 2007;33:945–50.
8. Stewart N, Lim AC, Lowe PM, Goodman G. Lasers and laser-like devices: part one. Australas J Dermatol. 2013;54:173–83.
9. Laubach HJ, Tannous Z, Anderson RR, Manstein D. Skin responses to fractional photothermolysis. Lasers Surg Med. 2006;38:142–9.
10. Hantash BM, Bedi VP, Sudireddy V, Struck SK, Herron GS, Chan KF. Laser-induced transepidermal elimination of dermal content by fractional photothermolysis. J Biomed Opt. 2006;11:041115.
11. Ross EV, Naseef G, Lin C, Kelly M, Michaud N, Flotte TJ, et al. Comparison of responses of tattoos to picosecond and nanosecond Q-switched neodymium:YAG lasers. Arch Dermatol. 1998;134:167–71.
12. Negishi K, Akita H, Matsunaga Y. Prospective study of removing solar lentigines in Asians using a novel dual-wavelength and dual-pulse width picosecond laser. Lasers Surg Med. 2018;50:851–8.
13. Cohen PR, Ross EV. Q-switched alexandrite laser-induced chrysiasis. J Clin Aesthet Dermatol. 2015;8:48–53.

14. Requena L, Requena C, Clay C. Benign epidermal tumors and proliferations. In: Bolognia JL, Schaffer J V, Cerroni L, editors. Dermatology. 4. Elsevier; 2018. p. 1894–1916.
15. Balin SJ, Barnhill RL. Benign melanocytic neoplasms. In: Bolognia JL, Schaffer JV, Cerroni L, editors. Dermatology. 4th ed. Elsevier; 2018. p. 1954–88.
16. Polder KD, Landau JM, Vergilis-Kalner IJ, Goldberg LH, Friedman PM, Bruce S. Laser eradication of pigmented lesions: a review. Dermatol Surg. 2011;37:572–95.
17. Passeron T, Genedy R, Salah L, Fusade T, Kositratna G, Laubach HJ, et al. Laser treatment of hyperpigmented lesions: position statement of the European Society of Laser in Dermatology. J Eur Acad Dermatol Venereol. 2019;33:987–1005.
18. Levin MK, Ng E, Bae YSC, Brauer JA, Geronemus RG. Treatment of pigmentary disorders in patients with skin of color with a novel 755 nm picosecond, Q-switched ruby, and Q-switched Nd:YAG nanosecond lasers: a retrospective photographic review. Lasers Surg Med. 2016;48:181–7.
19. Chan JCY, Shek SYN, Kono T, Yeung CK, Chan HHL. A retrospective analysis on the management of pigmented lesions using a picosecond 755-nm alexandrite laser in Asians. Lasers Surg Med. 2016;48:23–9.
20. Alegre-Sanchez A, Jiménez-Gómez N, Moreno-Arrones ÓM, Fonda-Pascual P, Pérez-García B, Jaén-Olasolo P, et al. Treatment of flat and elevated pigmented disorders with a 755-nm alexandrite picosecond laser: clinical and histological evaluation. Lasers Med Sci. 2018;33:1827–31.
21. Mehrabi JN, Friedman O, Al-Niaimi F, Artzi O. Retrospective photographic review of nontattoo indications treated by picosecond laser. J Cosmet Dermatol. 2020;19:612–21.
22. Kung KY, Shek SYN, Yeung CK, Chan HHL. Evaluation of the safety and efficacy of the dual wavelength picosecond laser for the treatment of benign pigmented lesions in Asians. Lasers Surg Med. 2019;51:14–22.
23. Guss L, Goldman MP, Wu DC. Picosecond 532 nm neodymium-doped yttrium aluminium garnet laser for the treatment of solar lentigines in darker skin types: safety and efficacy. Dermatol Surg. 2017;43:456–9.
24. Chan MWM, Shek SYN, Yeung CK, Chan HHL. A prospective study in the treatment of lentigines in Asian skin using 532 nm picosecond Nd:YAG laser. Lasers Surg Med. 2019;51:767–73.
25. Friedmann DP, Timmerman A, Cahana Z. Prospective study of 532-nm picosecond laser for the treatment of pigmented lesions of the face and dorsal hands. Dermatol Surg. 2022;48:1215–9.
26. Wang CC, Sue YM, Yang CH, Chen CK. A comparison of Q-switched alexandrite laser and intense pulsed light for the treatment of freckles and lentigines in Asian persons: a randomized, physician-blinded, split-face comparative trial. J Am Acad Dermatol. 2006;54:804–10.
27. Ungaksornpairote C, Manuskiatti W, Junsuwan N, Wanitphakdeedecha R. A prospective, split-face, randomized study comparing picosecond to Q-switched Nd:YAG laser for treatment of epidermal and dermal pigmented lesions in Asians. Dermatol Surg. 2020;46:1671–5.
28. Kim JY, Yang J, Huh G, Choi YJ, Kim WS. A split-face, single-blinded, randomized controlled comparison of 532 nm picosecond neodymium-doped yttrium aluminum garnet laser versus 532 nm q-switched neodymium-doped yttrium aluminum garnet laser in the treatment of solar lentigines. Ann Dermatol. 2020;32:8–13.
29. Vachiramon V, Iamsumang W, Triyangkulsri K. Q-switched double frequency Nd:YAG 532-nm nanosecond laser vs. double frequency Nd:YAG 532-nm picosecond laser for the treatment of solar lentigines in Asians. Lasers Med Sci. 2018;33:1941–7.
30. Evangelista K, Manuskiatti W, Wanitphakdeedecha R, Techapichetvanich T. Clinical evaluation of safety and efficacy of a 670-nm picosecond laser for treatment of benign pigmented lesions in Asians. Dermatol Surg. 2021;47:e153–8.
31. Lee SJ, Han HS, Hong JK, Park KY, Seo SJ. Successful treatment of pigmentary disorders in Asians with a novel 730-nm picosecond laser. Lasers Surg Med. 2020;52:923–7.
32. Lipp MB, Angra K, Wu DC. Safety and efficacy of a novel 730 nm picosecond titanium sapphire laser for the treatment of benign pigmented lesions. Lasers Surg Med. 2021;53:429–34.
33. Kauvar ANB, Sun R, Bhawan J, Singh G, Ugonabo N, Feng H, et al. Treatment of facial and non-facial lentigines with a 730 nm picosecond titanium: sapphire laser is safe and effective. Lasers Surg Med. 2022;54:89–97.
34. Hong JK, Koh YG, Li K, Seo SJ, Seo SB, Park KY. Treatment of facial pigmented disorders with a 785-nm picosecond Ti:sapphire laser in Asians: a report of three cases. Dermatol Ther. 2022;35:e15919.
35. Wang CC, Chen CK. Effect of spot size and fluence on Q-switched alexandrite laser treatment for pigmentation in Asians: a randomized, double-blinded, split-face comparative trial. J Dermatolog Treat. 2012;23:333–8.
36. Rashid T, Hussain I, Haider M, Haroon TS. Laser therapy of freckles and lentigines with quasi-continuous, frequency-doubled, Nd:YAG (532 nm) laser in Fitzpatrick skin type IV: a 24-month follow-up. J Cosmet Laser Ther. 2002;4:81–5.
37. Ho SGY, Yeung CK, Chan NPY, Shek SY, Chan HHL. A comparison of Q-switched and long-pulsed alexandrite laser for the treatment of freckles and lentigines in oriental patients. Lasers Surg Med. 2011;43:108–13.

38. Chung HJ, McGee JS, Lee SJ. Successful treatment of ephelides in Asian skin using the picosecond 785-nm laser. J Cosmet Dermatol. 2020;19:1990–2.
39. Yang Y, Peng L, Ge Y, Lin T. Comparison of the efficacy and safety of a picosecond alexandrite laser and a Q-switched alexandrite laser for the treatment of freckles in Chinese patients. J Am Acad Dermatol. 2018;79:1155–6. https://doi.org/10.1016/j.jaad.2018.07.047.
40. Yang Y, Xia Z, Guo L, Wu Q, Zhang M, Zeng R, et al. Comparison of the efficacy and safety of a picosecond frequency-doubled 532-nm Nd:YAG laser and a Q-switched frequency-doubled 532-nm Nd:YAG laser for the treatment of ephelides: a randomized, split-lesion, double-center, controlled trial. J Cosmet Dermatol. 2023;22:712–4.
41. Ma S-Y, Gong Y-Q, Zhang W-J, Liang B-H, Li Y-M, Xie Z-M, et al. Split-face comparison of the efficacy of picosecond 532 nm Nd:YAG laser and Q-switched 755 nm Alexandrite laser for treatment of freckles. J Cosmet Laser Ther. 2022;24:22–7.
42. Grossman MC, Rox Anderson R, Farinelli W, Flotte TJ, Grevelink JM. Treatment of cafe au lait macules with lasers. Arch Dermatol. 1995;131:1416–20.
43. Kagami S, Asahina A, Watanabe R, Mimura Y, Shirai A, Hattori N, et al. Treatment of 153 Japanese patients with Q-switched alexandrite laser. Lasers Med Sci. 2007;22:159–63.
44. Shimbashi T, Kamide R, Hashimoto T. Long-term follow-up in treatment of solar lentigo and cafe-au-lait macules with Q-switched ruby laser. Aesthet Plast Surg. 1997;21:445–8.
45. Gu T, Yuan J, Zhang Y, Li YH, Wu Y, Gao XH, et al. A retrospective study of FQSRL and IPL in the treatment of Café-au-lait macule. J Dermatolog Treat. 2021;32:544–7. https://doi.org/10.1080/09546634.2019.1687813.
46. Zhang B, Chu Y, Xu Z, Sun Y, Li L, Han X, et al. Treatment of café-au-Lait spots using Q-switched alexandrite laser: analysis of clinical characteristics of 471 children in mainland China. Lasers Surg Med. 2019;51:694–700.
47. Alster TS. Complete elimination of large cafe-au-lait birthmarks by the 510-nm pulsed dye laser. Plast Reconstr Surg. 1995;96:1660–4.
48. Somyos K, Boonchu K, Somsak K, Panaddat L. Copper vapour laser treatment of cafe-au-lait macules. Br J Dermatol. 1996;135:964–8.
49. Alora MB, Arndt KA. Treatment of a café-au-lait macule with the erbium:YAG laser. J Am Acad Dermatol. 2001;45:566–8.
50. Zhuang Y, Huang M, Shen J, Wang L, Yang L, Jiang A, et al. Comparison of the efficacy and safety between a low-fluence 1064-nm Q-switched neodymium-doped yttrium aluminum garnet laser and a conventional Q-switched 532-nm laser for the treatment of cafe-au-lait macules in 40 Chinese children: a prospective, random. Lasers Med Sci. 2022;37:279–86.
51. Kim HR, Ha JM, Park MS, Lee Y, Seo YJ, Kim CD, et al. A low-fluence 1064-nm Q-switched neodymium-doped yttrium aluminium garnet laser for the treatment of café-au-lait macules. J Am Acad Dermatol. 2015;73:477–83. https://doi.org/10.1016/j.jaad.2015.06.002.
52. Cen Q, Zhu J, Zhou L, Yu W, Wu X, Liu Y, et al. Comparison of the safety and efficacy of low fluence Q-switched 1064-nm and conventional Q-switched 755-nm lasers in the treatment of café-au-lait macules: a prospective self-controlled trial. Lasers Surg Med. 2022;54:1051–9.
53. Baek JO, Park IJ, Lee KR, Ryu HR, Kim J, Lee S, et al. High-fluence 1064-nm Q-switched Nd:YAG laser: safe and effective treatment of café-au-lait macules in Asian patients. J Cosmet Dermatol. 2018;17:380–4.
54. Lin Y, Liu HX, Shi WH, Wang HX, Geng JH, Guo X, et al. Preliminary experience of the Q-switched 1064-nm neodymium:yttrium aluminum garnet laser in the treatment of café-au-lait macules. J Eur Acad Dermatol Venereol. 2019;33:e185–6.
55. Kim J, Hur H, Kim YR, Cho SB. Treatment of café-au-lait macules with a high-fluenced 1064-nm Q-switched neodymium:yttrium aluminum garnet laser. J Cosmet Laser Ther. 2018;20:17–20.
56. Artzi O, Mehrabi JN, Koren A, Niv R, Lapidoth M, Levi A. Picosecond 532-nm neodymium-doped yttrium aluminium garnet laser—a novel and promising modality for the treatment of café-au-lait macules. Lasers Med Sci. 2018;33:693–7.
57. Cen Q, Gu Y, Luo L, Shang Y, Rao Y, Zhu J, et al. Comparative effectiveness of 755-nm picosecond laser, 755- and 532-nm nanosecond lasers for treatment of Café-au-Lait Macules (CALMs): a randomized, split-lesion clinical trial. Lasers Surg Med. 2021;53:435–42.
58. Belkin DA, Neckman JP, Jeon H, Friedman P, Geronemus RG. Response to laser treatment of café au lait macules based on morphologic features. JAMA Dermatol. 2017;153:1158–61.
59. Fitzpatrick RE, Goldman MP, Ruiz-Esparza J. Clinical advantage of the CO_2 laser superpulsed mode. J Dermatol Surg Oncol. 1994;20:449–56. https://doi.org/10.1111/j.1524-4725.1994.tb03215.x.
60. Bruscino N, Conti R, Campolmi P, Bonan P, Cannarozzo G, Lazzeri L, et al. Dermatosis Papulosa Nigra and 10,600-nm CO2 laser, a good choice. J Cosmet Laser Ther. 2014;16:114–6.
61. Furukawa F, Mizawa M, Shimizu T. Treatment of dermatosis papulosa nigra using a carbon dioxide laser. J Cosmet Dermatol. 2020;19:2572–5.
62. Ali FR, Bakkour W, Ferguson JE, Madan V. Carbon dioxide laser ablation of dermatosis papulosa nigra: high satisfaction and few complications in patients with pigmented skin. Lasers Med Sci. 2016;31:593–5. https://doi.org/10.1007/s10103-016-1906-y.

63. Drnovšek-Olup B, Vedlin B. Use of Er:YAG laser for benign skin disorders. Lasers Surg Med. 1997;21:13–9.
64. Khatri KA. Ablation of cutaneous lesions using an erbium:YAG laser. J Cosmet Laser Ther. 2003;5:150–3.
65. Zaresharifi S, Robati RM, Dadkhahfar S, Forouzanfar MM, Zaresharifi N. Efficacy and safety of cryotherapy, electrodesiccation, CO_2 laser, and Er:YAG laser in the treatment of seborrheic keratosis. Dermatol Ther. 2021;34:1–7.
66. Mehrabi D, Brodell RT. Use of the alexandrite laser for treatment of seborrheic keratoses. Dermatol Surg. 2002;28:437–9.
67. Kim YK, Kim DY, Lee SJ, Chung WS, Cho SB. Therapeutic efficacy of long-pulsed 755-nm alexandrite laser for seborrheic keratoses. J Eur Acad Dermatol Venereol. 2014;28:1007–11.
68. Schweiger ES, Kwasniak L, Aires DJ. Treatment of dermatosis papulosa nigra with a 1064 nm Nd:YAG laser: report of two cases. J Cosmet Laser Ther. 2008;10:120–2.
69. Badawi A, Ali FA, Tome M, Samy N. Treatment of dermatosis papulosa nigra with a 1064 nm Nd:YAG laser in dark skin with a 1-year follow-up. J Egypt Womens Dermatol Soc. 2015;12:156–61.
70. Culbertson GR. 532-nm diode laser treatment of seborrheic keratoses with color enhancement. Dermatol Surg. 2008;34:525–8.
71. Kundu RV, Joshi SS, Suh KY, Boone SL, Huggins RH, Alam M, et al. Comparison of electrodesiccation and potassium-titanyl-phosphate laser for treatment of dermatosis papulosa nigra. Dermatol Surg. 2009;35:1079–83.
72. Karadag AS, Ozkanli S, Mansuroglu C, Ozlu E, Zemheri E. Effectiveness of the pulse dye laser treatment in a Caucasian women with dermatosis papulosa nigra. Indian J Dermatol. 2015;60:321.
73. Garcia MS, Azari R, Eisen DB. Treatment of dermatosis papulosa Nigra in 10 patients: a comparison trial of electrodesiccation, pulsed dye laser, and curettage. Dermatol Surg. 2010;36:1968–72.
74. Polder KD, Mithani A, Harrison A, Bruce S. Treatment of macular seborrheic keratoses using a novel 1927-nm fractional thulium fiber laser. Dermatol Surg. 2012;38:1025–31.
75. Katz TM, Goldberg LH, Friedman PM. Dermatosis papulosa nigra treatment with fractional photothermolysis. Dermatol Surg. 2009;35:1840–3.
76. Geronemus RG. Q-switched ruby laser therapy of nevus of Ota. Arch Dermatol. 1992;128:1618–22.
77. Lowe NJ, Wieder JM, Sawcer D, Burrows P, Chalet M. Nevus of Ota: treatment with high energy fluences of the Q-switched ruby laser. J Am Acad Dermatol. 1993;29:997–1001. https://doi.org/10.1016/0190-9622(93)70280-7.
78. Lu Z, Fang L, Jiao S, Huang W, Chen J, Wang X. Treatment of 522 patients with nevus of Ota with Q-switched Alexandrite laser. Chin Med J (Engl). 2003;116:226–30.
79. Sami L, Changzheng H, Yan L. Factors affecting response, number of laser sessions and complications in nevus of Ota treated by Q-switched alexandrite laser: a retrospective study. G Ital Dermatol Venereol. 2016;151:160–8.
80. Chan HH, Leung RSC, Ying SY, Lai CF, Kono T, Chua JKH, et al. A retrospective analysis of complications in the treatment of nevus of Ota with the Q-switched alexandrite and Q-switched Nd:YAG lasers. Dermatol Surg. 2000;26:1000–6.
81. Aurangabadkar S. QYAG5 Q-switched Nd:YAG laser treatment of nevus of Ota: an Indian study of 50 patients. J Cutan Aesthet Surg. 2008;1:80.
82. Kar HK, Gupta L. 1064 nm Q switched Nd: YAG laser treatment of nevus of Ota: an Indian open label prospective study of 50 patients. Indian J Dermatol Venereol Leprol. 2011;77:565–70.
83. Chang CJ, Kou CS. Comparing the effectiveness of Q-switched Ruby laser treatment with that of Q-switched Nd:YAG laser for oculodermal melanosis (Nevus of Ota). J Plast Reconstr Aesthet Surg. 2011;64:339–45. https://doi.org/10.1016/j.bjps.2010.05.036.
84. Sethuraman G, Sharma V, Sreenivas V. Melanin index in assessing the treatment efficacy of 1064 nm Q switched Nd-Yag laser in nevus of Ota. J Cutan Aesthet Surg. 2013;6:189.
85. Choi CW, Kim HJ, Lee HJ, Kim YH, Kim WS. Treatment of nevus of Ota using low fluence Q-switched Nd: YAG laser. Int J Dermatol. 2014;53:861–5.
86. Liu Y, Zeng W, Geng S. A retrospective study on the characteristics of treating nevus of Ota by 1064-nm q-switched neodymium-doped yttrium aluminum garnet laser. Indian J Dermatol. 2016;61:347.
87. Yan L, Di L, Weihua W, Feng L, Ruilian L, Jun Z, et al. A study on the clinical characteristics of treating nevus of Ota by Q-switched Nd:YAG laser. Lasers Med Sci. 2018;33:89–93.
88. Watanabe S, Takahashi H. Treatment of nevus of Ota with the Q-switched ruby laser. N Engl J Med. 1994;331:1745–50. https://doi.org/10.1056/NEJM199412293312604.
89. Liu Y, Zeng W, Li D, Wang W, Liu F. A retrospective analysis of the clinical efficacies and recurrence of Q-switched Nd:YAG laser treatment of nevus of Ota in 224 Chinese patients. J Cosmet Laser Ther. 2018;20:410–4.
90. Taylor CR, Flotte TJ, Gange RW, Anderson RR. Treatment of nevus of Ota by Q-switched ruby laser. J Am Acad Dermatol. 1994;30:743–51. https://doi.org/10.1016/S0190-9622(08)81505-8.
91. Yang HY, Lee CW, Ro YS, Yu HJ, Kim YT, Kim JH, et al. Q-switched ruby laser in the treatment of nevus of Ota. J Korean Med Sci. 1996;11:165. https://doi.org/10.3346/jkms.1996.11.2.165.
92. Shimbashi T, Hyakusoku H, Okinaga M. Treatment of nevus of Ota by Q-switched ruby laser. Aesthet Plast Surg. 1997;21:118–21.

93. Ueda S, Isoda M, Imayama S. Response of naevus of Ota to Q-switched ruby laser treatment according to lesion colour. Br J Dermatol. 2000;142:77–83.
94. Kono T, Chan HHL, Eroçöçen AR, Kikuchi Y, Uezono S, Iwasaka S, et al. Use of Q-switched ruby laser in the treatment of nevus of Ota in different age groups. Lasers Surg Med. 2003;32:391–5.
95. Alster TS, Williams CM. Treatment of nevus of Ota by the Q-switched alexandrite laser. Dermatol Surg. 1995;21:592–6.
96. Kang W, Lee E, Choi GS. Treatment of Ota's nevus by Q-switched alexandrite laser: therapeutic outcome in relation to clinical and histopathological findings. Eur J Dermatol. 1999;9:639–43.
97. Williams NM, Gurnani P, Long J, Reynolds J, Pan Y, Suzuki T, et al. Comparing the efficacy and safety of Q-switched and picosecond lasers in the treatment of nevus of Ota: a systematic review and meta-analysis. Lasers Med Sci. 2021;36:723–33.
98. Yu P, Yu N, Diao W, Yang X, Feng Y, Qi Z. Comparison of clinical efficacy and complications between Q-switched alexandrite laser and Q-switched Nd:YAG laser on nevus of Ota: a systematic review and meta-analysis. Lasers Med Sci. 2016;31:581–91.
99. Chesnut C, Diehl J, Lask G. Treatment of nevus of Ota with a picosecond 755-nm alexandrite laser nevus. Dermatol Surg. 2015;41:508–10.
100. Ohshiro T, Ohshiro T, Sasaki K, Kishi K. Picosecond pulse duration laser treatment for dermal melanocytosis in Asians: a retrospective review. Laser Ther. 2016;25:99–104.
101. Sakio R, Ohshiro T, Sasaki K, Ohshiro T. Usefulness of picosecond pulse alexandrite laser treatment for nevus of Ota. Laser Ther. 2018;27:251–5.
102. Koh YP, Tan AWM, Chua SH. Treatment of laser-responsive dermal pigmentary conditions in type III-IV Asian skin with a 755-nm picosecond pulse duration laser: a retrospective review of its efficacy and safety. Dermatol Surg. 2020;46:e82–7.
103. Luo B, Kang L, Lu J. Successful and quick treatment of nevus of Ota with 755nm picosecond laser in Chinese. J Cosmet Laser Ther. 2020;22:93–5. https://doi.org/10.1080/14764172.2020.1740274.
104. Hu S, Yang C-S, Chang S-L, Huang Y-L, Lin Y-F, Lee M-C. Efficacy and safety of the picosecond 755-nm alexandrite laser for treatment of dermal pigmentation in Asians—a retrospective study. Lasers Med Sci. 2020;35:1377–83.
105. Peng L, Yang Y, Ge Y, Lin T. Picosecond alexandrite laser for nevus of Ota treatment in Chinese. J Eur Acad Dermatol Venereol. 2018;32:e276–7.
106. Yang CY, Shih IH, Huang YL, Hu S. Efficacy and safety of picosecond 755-nm alexandrite laser for treatment of nevus of Ota in Taiwanese children: a retrospective study. Lasers Surg Med. 2022;54:355–65.
107. Achavanuntakul P, Manuskiatti W, Wanitphakdeedecha R, Jantarakolica T. Early treatment initiation improves outcomes in nevus of Ota: a 10-year retrospective study. Am J Clin Dermatol. 2021;23:105–14.
108. Yang H, Guo L, Jia G, Gong X, Wu Q, Zeng R, et al. Treatment of nevus of Ota with 1064 nm picosecond Nd:YAG laser: a retrospective study. Dermatol Ther. 2021;34:1–5.
109. Jerdan K, Hsu JT, Schnurstein E. Successful treatment of Ota nevus with the 532-nm solid-state picosecond laser. Cutis. 2017;99:E29–31.
110. Loh TY, Wu DC. Novel application of the 730 and 785 nm picosecond titanium sapphire lasers for the treatment of nevus of Ota. Lasers Surg Med. 2021;53:1141–5.
111. Ge Y, Yang Y, Guo L, Zhang M, Wu Q, Zeng R, et al. Comparison of a picosecond alexandrite laser versus a Q-switched alexandrite laser for the treatment of nevus of Ota: a randomized, split-lesion, controlled trial. J Am Acad Dermatol. 2020;83:397–403. https://doi.org/10.1016/j.jaad.2019.03.016.
112. Imagawa K, Kono T, Hanai U, Groff WF, Komaba C, Tsunoda Y, et al. Prospective comparison study of a 550 picosecond 755 nm laser vs. a 50 ns 755 nm laser in the treatment of nevus of Ota. Lasers Med Sci. 2023;38:55.
113. Hori Y, Kawashima M, Oohara K, Kukita A. Acquired bilateral nevus of Ota-like macules. J Am Acad Dermatol. 1984;10:961–4.
114. Park JM, Tsao H, Tsao S. Acquired bilateral nevus of Ota-like macules (Hori nevus): etiologic and therapeutic considerations. J Am Acad Dermatol. 2009;61:88–93. https://doi.org/10.1016/j.jaad.2008.10.054.
115. Wang B, Xie HF, Tan J, Xie HJ, Xu LY, Ding R, et al. Induction of melasma by 1064-nm Q-switched neodymium:yttrium-aluminum-garnet laser therapy for acquired bilateral nevus of Ota-like macules (Hori nevus): a study on related factors in the Chinese population. J Dermatol. 2016;43:655–61.
116. Zeng R, Liu YZ, Lin T, Guo LF, Ge YP, Zhang ML, et al. Effects of Q-switched laser treatments on acquired bilateral nevus of Ota-like macules: a retrospective comparative study. Int J Dermatol Venereol. 2019;2:70–6.
117. Lam AYM, Wong DSY, Lam LK, Ho WS, Chan HHL. A retrospective study on the efficacy and complications of Q-switched alexandrite laser in the treatment of acquired bilateral nevus of Ota-like macules. Dermatol Surg. 2001;27:937–42.
118. Kunachak S, Leelaudomlipi P, Sirikulchayanonta V. Q-switched ruby laser therapy of acquired bilateral nevus of Ota-like macules. Dermatol Surg. 1999;25:938–41.
119. Manuskiatti W, Sivayathorn A, Leelaudomlipi P, Fitzpatrick RE. Treatment of acquired bilateral nevus of Ota-like macules (Hori's nevus) using a combination of scanned carbon dioxide laser followed by Q-switched ruby laser. J Am Acad Dermatol. 2003;48:584–91.
120. Momosawa A, Yoshimura K, Uchida G, Sato K, Aiba E, Matsumoto D, et al. Combined therapy

using Q-switched ruby laser and bleaching treatment with tretinoin and hydroquinone for acquired dermal melanocytosis. Dermatol Surg. 2003;29:1001–7.
121. Lee SJ, Nam SM, Cha HG, Park ES, Kim YB. The efficacy of a Q-switched 694-nm ruby fractional laser for treating acquired bilateral nevus of Ota-like macules. Arch Aesthetic Plast Surg. 2018;24:20.
122. Kunachak S, Leelaudomlipi P. Q-switched Nd:YAG laser treatment for acquired bilateral nevus of Ota-like maculae: a long-term follow-up. Lasers Surg Med. 2000;26:376–9.
123. Suh DH, Han KH, Chung JH. Clinical use of the Q-switched Nd:YAG laser for the treatment of acquired bilateral nevus of Ota-like macules (ABNOMs) in Koreans. J Dermatolog Treat. 2001;12:163–6.
124. Lee WJ, Han SS, Chang SE, Lee MW, Choi JH, Moon KC, et al. Q-switched ND:YAG laser therapy of acquired bilateral nevus of Ota-like macules. Ann Dermatol. 2009;21:255–60.
125. Polnikorn N, Tanrattanakorn S, Goldberg DJ. Treatment of Hori's nevus with the Q-switched Nd:YAG laser. Dermatol Surg. 2000;26:477–80.
126. Cho SB, Park SJ, Kim MJ, Bu TS. Treatment of acquired bilateral nevus of Ota-like macules (Hori's nevus) using 1064-nm Q-switched Nd:YAG laser with low fluence. Int J Dermatol. 2009;48:1308–12.
127. Ee HL, Goh CL, Khoo LSW, Chan ESY, Ang P. Treatment of acquired bilateral nevus of Ota-like macules (Hori's nevus) with a combination of the 532 nm Q-switched Nd:YAG laser followed by the 1,064 nm Q-switched Nd:YAG is more effective: prospective study. Dermatol Surg. 2006;32:34–40.
128. Tian BWCA. Novel treatment of Hori's nevus: a combination of fractional nonablative 2,940-nm Er:YAG and low-fluence 1,064-nm Q-switched Nd:YAG laser. J Cutan Aesthet Surg. 2015;8:227–9.
129. Manuskiatti W, Eimpunth S, Wanitphakdeedecha R. Effect of cold air cooling on the incidence of postinflammatory hyperpigmentation after Q-switched Nd:YAG laser treatment of acquired bilateral nevus of Ota-like macules. Arch Dermatol. 2007;143:1139–43.
130. Kim SY, Park J, Kim H, Cho SB. Long-term follow-up of 1,064-nm picosecond-domain neodymium:yttrium-aluminum-garnet laser treatment for acquired bilateral nevus of Ota-like macules. Med Lasers. 2017;6:93–8.
131. Ding H, Yang Y, Guo L, Lin T. Use of a picosecond alexandrite laser for treating acquired bilateral nevus of Ota-like macules in Chinese patients. Lasers Surg Med. 2020;52:935–9.
132. Wong THS. Picosecond laser treatment for acquired bilateral nevus of Ota-like macules. JAMA Dermatol. 2018;154:1226–8.
133. Suk D, Cho KSB. Improvement in acquired bilateral nevus of Ota-like macules with picosecond-domain wavelength-converted 595-nm neodymium:yttrium aluminium garnet laser treatment. Med Lasers. 2016;5:111–4.
134. Yu W, Zhu J, Yu W, Lyu D, Lin X, Zhang Z. A split-face, single-blinded, randomized controlled comparison of alexandrite 755-nm picosecond laser versus alexandrite 755-nm nanosecond laser in the treatment of acquired bilateral nevus of Ota–like macules. J Am Acad Dermatol. 2018;79:479–86. https://doi.org/10.1016/j.jaad.2017.12.053.
135. Phothong W, Manuskiatti W, Wongdama S, Gulfan MC. Long-term follow-up for 1,064-nm nanosecond and picosecond laser treatment of acquired bilateral nevus of Ota-like macules. Dermatol Surg. 2022;48:1008–9.
136. Chang MW. Disorders of hyperpigmentation. In: Bolognia JL, Schaffer JV, Cerroni L, editors. Dermatology. 4th ed. Elsevier; 2018. p. 1115–43.
137. Kim JY, Lee TR, Lee AY. Reduced WIF-1 expression stimulates skin hyperpigmentation in patients with melasma. J Invest Dermatol. 2013;133:191–200. https://doi.org/10.1038/jid.2012.270.
138. Regazzetti C, De Donatis GM, Ghorbel HH, Cardot-Leccia N, Ambrosetti D, Bahadoran P, et al. Endothelial cells promote pigmentation through endothelin receptor B activation. J Invest Dermatol. 2015;135:3096–104.
139. Passeron T, Picardo M. Melasma, a photoaging disorder. Pigment Cell Melanoma Res. 2018;31:461–5. https://doi.org/10.1111/pcmr.12684.
140. Grimes PE, Yamada N, Bhawan J. Light microscopic, immunohistochemical, and ultrastructural alterations in patients with melasma. Am J Dermatopathol. 2005;27:96–101.
141. Kim EH, Kim YC, Lee ES, Kang HY. The vascular characteristics of melasma. J Dermatol Sci. 2007;46:111–6.
142. Kang WH, Yoon KH, Lee ES, Kim J, Lee KB, Yim H, et al. Melasma: histopathological characteristics in 56 Korean patients. Br J Dermatol. 2002;146:228–37.
143. Boukari F, Jourdan E, Fontas E, Montaudié H, Castela E, Lacour JP, et al. Prevention of melasma relapses with sunscreen combining protection against UV and short wavelengths of visible light: a prospective randomized comparative trial. J Am Acad Dermatol. 2015;72:189–190.e1.
144. Taylor CR, Anderson RR. Ineffective treatment of refractory melasma and postinflammatory hyperpigmentation by Q-switched ruby laser. J Dermatol Surg Oncol. 1994;20:592–7.
145. Kopera D, Hohenleutner U. Ruby laser treatment of melasma and postinflammatory hyperpigmentation. Dermatol Surg. 1995;21:994.
146. Trivedi MK, Yang FC, Cho BK. A review of laser and light therapy in melasma. Int J Womens Dermatol. 2017;3:11–20. https://doi.org/10.1016/j.ijwd.2017.01.004.
147. Mun JY, Jeong SY, Kim JH, Han SS, Kim IH. A low fluence Q-switched Nd:YAG laser modifies the 3D structure of melanocyte and ultrastructure of melanosome by subcellular-selective photothermolysis. J Electron Microsc (Tokyo). 2011;60:11–8.

148. Lee YS, Lee YJ, Lee JM, Han TY, Lee JH, Choi JE. The low-fluence Q-switched Nd:YAG laser treatment for melasma: a systematic review. Medicina (B Aires). 2022;58:936.
149. Fabi SG, Friedmann DP, Niwa Massaki AB, Goldman MP. A randomized, split-face clinical trial of low-fluence Q-switched neodymium-doped yttrium aluminum garnet (1,064 nm) laser versus low-fluence Q-switched alexandrite laser (755 nm) for the treatment of facial melasma. Lasers Surg Med. 2014;46:531–7.
150. Kim MJ, Cho SB, Kim JS. Melasma treatment in Korean women using a 1064-nm Q-switched Nd:YAG laser with low pulse energy. Clin Exp Dermatol. 2009;34:847–50.
151. Wattanakrai P, Mornchan R, Eimpunth S. Low-fluence q-switched neodymium-doped yttrium aluminum garnet (1,064 nm) laser for the treatment of facial melasma in Asians. Dermatol Surg. 2010;36:76–87.
152. Choi CP, Yim SM, Seo SH, Ahn HH, Kye YC, Choi JE. Retrospective analysis of melasma treatment using a dual mode of low-fluence Q-switched and long-pulse Nd:YAG laser vs. low-fluence Q-switched Nd:YAG laser monotherapy. J Cosmet Laser Ther. 2015;17:2–8.
153. Kim JE, Chang SE, Yeo UC, Haw S, Kim IH. Histopathological study of the treatment of melasma lesions using a low-fluence Q-switched 1064-nm neodymium:yttrium-aluminium-garnet laser. Clin Exp Dermatol. 2013;38:167–71.
154. Chan NPY, Ho SGY, Shek SYN, Yeung CK, Chan HH. A case series of facial depigmentation associated with low fluence Q-switched 1,064nm Nd:YAG laser for skin rejuvenation and melasma. Lasers Surg Med. 2010;42:712–9.
155. Namkoong S, Kim JS, Kim JY, Gye J, Chung J, Choi HI, et al. Systematized inflammatory linear verrucous epidermal nevus. Korean J Dermatol. 2012;50:464–7.
156. Choi YJ, Nam JH, Kim JY, Min JH, Park KY, Ko EJ, et al. Efficacy and safety of a novel picosecond laser using combination of 1 064 and 595 nm on patients with melasma: a prospective, randomized, multicenter, split-face, 2% hydroquinone cream-controlled clinical trial. Lasers Surg Med. 2017;49:899–907.
157. Kim YJ, Suh HY, Choi ME, Jung CJ, Chang SE. Clinical improvement of photoaging-associated facial hyperpigmentation in Korean skin with a picosecond 1064-nm neodymium-doped yttrium aluminum garnet laser. Lasers Med Sci. 2020;35:1599–606.
158. Manuskiatti W, Yan C, Gulfan MCB, Techapichetvanich T, Wanitphakdeedecha R. Combination of a 755-nm picosecond laser and hydroquinone 2% cream versus hydroquinone 2% cream alone for the treatment of melasma: a randomized, split-face, and controlled trial. Lasers Surg Med. 2022;54:1245–50.
159. Liang S, Shang S, Zhang W, Tan A, Zhou B, Mei X, et al. Comparison of the efficacy and safety of picosecond Nd:YAG laser (1,064 nm), picosecond alexandrite laser (755 nm) and 2% hydroquinone cream in the treatment of melasma: a randomized, controlled, assessor-blinded trial. Front Med. 2023;10:1–10.
160. Lee MC, Lin YF, Hu S, Huang YL, Chang SL, Cheng CY, et al. A split-face study: comparison of picosecond alexandrite laser and Q-switched Nd:YAG laser in the treatment of melasma in Asians. Lasers Med Sci. 2018;33:1733–8.
161. Hong JK, Shin SH, Park SJ, Seo SJ, Park KY. A prospective, split-face study comparing 1,064-nm picosecond Nd:YAG laser toning with 1,064-nm Q-switched Nd:YAG laser toning in the treatment of melasma. J Dermatolog Treat. 2022;33:2547–53. https://doi.org/10.1080/09546634.2022.2033674.
162. Feng J, Huang L. Comparison of picosecond and nanosecond Nd:YAG 1064-nm lasers in the treatment of melasma: a Split-face randomized clinical trial. Plast Reconstr Surg. 2023;151:772–7. https://doi.org/10.1097/PRS.0000000000009994.
163. Chalermchai T, Rummaneethorn P. Effects of a fractional picosecond 1,064 nm laser for the treatment of dermal and mixed type melasma. J Cosmet Laser Ther. 2018;20:134–9. https://doi.org/10.1080/14764172.2017.1376098.
164. Chen YT, Lin ET, Chang CC, Lin BS, Chiang HM, Huang YH, et al. Efficacy and safety evaluation of picosecond alexandrite laser with a diffractive lens array for treatment of melasma in Asian patients by VISIA imaging system. Photobiomodul Photomed Laser Surg. 2019;37:559–66.
165. Wang YJ, Lin ET, Chen YT, Chiu PC, Lin BS, Chiang HM, et al. Prospective randomized controlled trial comparing treatment efficacy and tolerance of picosecond alexandrite laser with a diffractive lens array and triple combination cream in female Asian patients with melasma. J Eur Acad Dermatol Venereol. 2020;34:624–32.
166. Polnikorn N, Tanghetti E. Treatment of refractory melasma in Asians with the picosecond alexandrite laser. Dermatol Surg. 2020;46:1651–6.
167. Manuskiatti W, Yan C, Tantrapornpong P, Cembrano KAG, Techapichetvanich T, Wanitphakdeedecha R. A prospective, split-face, randomized study comparing a 755-nm picosecond laser with and without diffractive lens array in the treatment of melasma in Asians. Lasers Surg Med. 2021;53:95–103.
168. Lee HI, Lim YY, Kim BJ, Kim MN, Min HJ, Hwang JH, et al. Clinicopathologic efficacy of copper bromide plus/yellow laser (578 nm with 511 nm) for treatment of melasma in Asian patients. Dermatol Surg. 2010;36:885–93.
169. Eimpunth S, Wanitphakdeedecha R, Triwongwaranat D, Varothai S, Manuskiatti W. Therapeutic outcome of melasma treatment by dual-wavelength (511 and 578 nm) laser in patients with skin phototypes III–V. Clin Exp Dermatol. 2014;39:292–7.

170. Ghorbel HH, Boukari F, Fontas E, Montaudié H, Bahadoran P, Lacour JP, et al. Copper bromide laser vs. triple-combination cream for the treatment of melasma: a randomized clinical trial. JAMA Dermatol. 2015;151:791–2.
171. Passeron T, Fontas E, Kang HY, Bahadoran P, Lacour JP, Ortonne JP. Melasma treatment with pulsed-dye laser and triple combination cream: a prospective, randomized, single-blind, split-face study. Arch Dermatol. 2011;147:1106–8.
172. Passeron T. Long-lasting effect of vascular targeted therapy of melasma. J Am Dermatol. 2013;69:e141–2. https://doi.org/10.1016/j.jaad.2013.02.022.
173. Geddes ERC, Stout AB, Friedman PM. Retrospective analysis of the treatment of melasma lesions exhibiting increased vascularity with the 595-nm pulsed dye laser combined with the 1927-nm fractional low-powered diode laser. Lasers Surg Med. 2017;49:20–6.
174. Kong SH, Suh HS, Choi YS. Treatment of melasma with pulsed-dye laser and 1,064-nm Q-switched Nd:YAG laser: a split-face study. Ann Dermatol. 2018;30:1–7.
175. Hassan AM, Elfar NN, Rizk OM, Eissa NY. Pulsed dye laser versus intense pulsed light in melasma: a split-face comparative study. J Dermatolog Treat. 2018;29:725–32. https://doi.org/10.1080/09546634.2018.1441487.
176. Wang CC, Hui CY, Sue YM, Wong WR, Hong HS. Intense pulsed light for the treatment of refractory melasma in Asian persons. Dermatol Surg. 2004;30:1196–200.
177. Li YH, Chen JZS, Wei HC, Wu Y, Liu M, Xu YY, et al. Efficacy and safety of intense pulsed light in treatment of melasma in Chinese patients. Dermatol Surg. 2008;34:693–701.
178. Goldman MP, Gold MH, Palm MD, Colón LE, Preston N, Johnson LA, et al. Sequential treatment with triple combination cream and intense pulsed light is more efficacious than sequential treatment with an inactive (control) cream and intense pulsed light in patients with moderate to severe melasma. Dermatol Surg. 2011;37:224–33.
179. Chung JY, Lee JH, Lee JH. Topical tranexamic acid as an adjuvant treatment in melasma: side-by-side comparison clinical study. J Dermatolog Treat. 2016;27:373–7.
180. Chen J, Liu J, Wu J. Treatment of melasma by a combination of intense pulsed light with advanced optimal pulse technology and human-like collagen repair dressing: a case series study. Medicine (Baltimore). 2022;101:E29492.
181. Rokhsar CK, Fitzpatrick RE. The treatment of melasma with fractional photothermolysis: a pilot study. Dermatol Surg. 2005;31:1645–50.
182. Kroon MW, Wind BS, Beek JF, Wietze Van Der Veen JP, Nieuweboer-Krobotová L, Bos JD, et al. Nonablative 1550-nm fractional laser therapy versus triple topical therapy for the treatment of melasma: a randomized controlled pilot study. J Am Acad Dermatol. 2011;64:516–23.
183. Hong SP, Han SS, Choi SJ, Kim MS, Won CH, Lee MW, et al. Split-face comparative study of 1550 nm fractional photothermolysis and trichloroacetic acid 15% chemical peeling for facial melasma in Asian skin. J Cosmet Laser Ther. 2012;14:81–6.
184. Wanitphakdeedecha R, Keoprasom N, Eimpunth S, Manuskiatti W. The efficacy in melasma treatment using a 1410 nm fractional photothermolysis laser. J Eur Acad Dermatol Venereol. 2014;28:293–7.
185. Polder KD, Bruce S. Treatment of melasma using a novel 1,927-nm fractional thulium fiber laser: a pilot study. Dermatol Surg. 2012;38:199–206.
186. Niwa Massaki ABM, Eimpunth S, Fabi SG, Guiha I, Groff W, Fitzpatrick R. Treatment of melasma with the 1,927-nm fractional thulium fiber laser: a retrospective analysis of 20 cases with long-term follow-up. Lasers Surg Med. 2013;45:95–101.
187. Rho N-K. Treatment of melasma using a novel 1,927 nm fractional thulium laser: a retrospective analysis of 68 Korean patients. Med Lasers. 2017;6:10–6.
188. Kurmuş G, Tatlıparmak A, Aksoy B, Koç E, Aşiran Serdar Z, Ergin C. Efficacy and safety of 1927 nm fractional thulium fiber laser for the treatment of melasma: a retrospective study of 100 patients. J Cosmet Laser Ther. 2019;21:408–11. https://doi.org/10.1080/14764172.2019.1683581.
189. Wanitphakdeedecha R, Sy-Alvarado F, Patthamalai P, Techapichetvanich T, Eimpunth S, Manuskiatti W. The efficacy in treatment of facial melasma with thulium 1927-nm fractional laser-assisted topical tranexamic acid delivery: a split-face, double-blind, randomized controlled pilot study. Lasers Med Sci. 2020;35:2015–21.
190. Nouri K, Bowes L, Chartier T, Romagosa R, Spencer J. Combination treatment of melasma with pulsed CO_2 laser followed by Q-switched alexandrite laser: a pilot study. Dermatol Surg. 1999;25:494–7.
191. Angsuwarangsee S, Polnikorn N. Combined ultrapulse CO_2 laser and Q-switched alexandrite laser compared with Q-switched alexandrite laser alone for refractory melasma: Split-face design. Dermatol Surg. 2003;29:59–64.
192. Tawfic SO, Abdel Halim DM, Albarbary A, Abdelhady M. Assessment of combined fractional CO_2 and tranexamic acid in melasma treatment. Lasers Surg Med. 2019;51:27–33.
193. Kim C, Gao JC, Moy J, Lee HS. Fractional CO_2 laser and adjunctive therapies in skin of color melasma patients. JAAD Int. 2022;8:118–23. https://doi.org/10.1016/j.jdin.2022.02.010.
194. Manaloto RMP, Alster T. Erbium:YAG laser resurfacing for refractory melasma. Dermatol Surg. 1999;25:121–3.
195. Attwa E, Khater M, Assaf M, Haleem MA. Melasma treatment using an erbium: YAG laser: a clinical, immunohistochemical, and ultrastructural study. Int J Dermatol. 2015;54:235–44.

196. Garg S, Vashisht KR, Makadia S. A prospective randomized comparative study on 60 Indian patients of melasma, comparing pixel Q-switched NdYAG (1064 nm), super skin rejuvenation (540 nm) and ablative pixel erbium YAG (2940 nm) lasers, with a review of the literature. J Cosmet Laser Ther. 2019;21:297–307. https://doi.org/10.1080/14764172.2019.1605447.
197. Silpa-archa N, Kohli I, Chaowattanapanit S, Lim HW, Hamzavi I. Postinflammatory hyperpigmentation: a comprehensive overview: epidemiology, pathogenesis, clinical presentation, and noninvasive assessment technique. J Am Acad Dermatol. 2017;77:591–605. https://doi.org/10.1016/j.jaad.2017.01.035.
198. Chaowattanapanit S, Silpa-archa N, Kohli I, Lim HW, Hamzavi I. Postinflammatory hyperpigmentation: a comprehensive overview: treatment options and prevention. J Am Acad Dermatol. 2017;77:607–21. https://doi.org/10.1016/j.jaad.2017.01.036.
199. Mitra A, Yeung R, Sheehan-Dare R, Wilson CL. Lentiginous hyperpigmentation confined to resolved psoriatic plaques and treated with a Q-switched ruby laser. Clin Exp Dermatol. 2006;31:298–9.
200. Cho S, Park S, Kim J, Kim M, Bu T. Treatment of post-inflammatory hyperpigmentation using 1064-nm Q-switched Nd:YAG laser with low fluence: report of three cases. J Eur Acad Dermatol Venereol. 2009;23:1206–7. https://doi.org/10.1111/j.1468-3083.2009.03123.x.
201. Kim S, Cho KH. Treatment of procedure-related postinflammatory hyperpigmentation using 1064-nm Q-switched Nd:YAG laser with low fluence in Asian patients: report of five cases. J Cosmet Dermatol. 2010;9:302–6.
202. Kim S, Cho KH. Treatment of facial postinflammatory hyperpigmentation with facial acne in Asian patients using a Q-switched neodymium-doped yttrium aluminum garnet laser. Dermatol Surg. 2010;36:1374–80.
203. Lee YB, Park SM, Kim JW, Yu DS. Combination treatment of low-fluence Q-switched Nd:YAG laser and oral tranexamic acid for post-inflammatory hyperpigmentation due to allergic contact dermatitis to henna hair dye. J Cosmet Laser Ther. 2016;18:95–7.
204. Ho SGY, Yeung CK, Chan NPY, Shek SY, Kono T, Chan HHL. A retrospective analysis of the management of acne post-inflammatory hyperpigmentation using topical treatment, laser treatment, or combination topical and laser treatments in oriental patients. Lasers Surg Med. 2011;43:1–7.
205. Ghannam S, Al Otabi FK, Frank K, Cotofana S. Efficacy of low-fluence Nd:YAG 1064 nm laser for the treatment of post-inflammatory hyperpigmentation in the axillary area. J Drugs Dermatol. 2017;16:1118–23.
206. Robredo IGC. Q-switched 1064nm Nd:YAG laser in treating axillary hyperpigmentation in Filipino women with skin types IV-V. J Drugs Dermatol. 2020;19:66–9.
207. Amornpetkul W, Kanokrungsee S, Kamanamool N, Udompataikul M, Rojhirunsakool S. Comparison between the use of intense pulsed light and Q-switched neodymium-doped yttrium aluminum garnet laser for the treatment of axillary hyperpigmentation. J Cosmet Dermatol. 2021;20:2785–93. https://doi.org/10.1111/jocd.13981.
208. Feng J, Huang L. Treatment of permanent post-inflammatory hyperpigmentation with medium-fluence medium-spot-size setting in Q-switched Nd:YAG 1064 nm laser: a novel treatment parameters setting strategy. J Cosmet Dermatol. 2022;21:1300–2.
209. Ren R, Bao S, Qian W, Zhao H. 755-nm alexandrite picosecond laser with a diffractive lens array or zoom handpiece for post-inflammatory hyperpigmentation: two case reports with a three-year follow-up. Clin Cosmet Investig Dermatol. 2021;14:1459–64.
210. Ren R, Zhao H. A case report on the use of 755-nm alexandrite picosecond laser in the treatment of post-inflammatory hyperpigmentation in the nose. J Cosmet Dermatol. 2022;21:2046–8.
211. Ho WS, Chan HH, Ying SY, Chan PC, Burd A, King WWK. Prospective study on the treatment of postburn hyperpigmentation by intense pulsed light. Lasers Surg Med. 2003;32:42–5.
212. Park KY, Choi SY, Mun SK, Kim BJ, Kim MN. Combined treatment with 578-/511-nm copper bromide laser and light-emitting diodes for post-laser pigmentation: a report of two cases. Dermatol Ther. 2014;27:121–5.
213. Augustyniak A, Erkiert-Polguj A, Rotsztejn H. Variable pulsed light treatment of melasma and post-inflammatory hyperpigmentation-a pilot study. J Cosmet Laser Ther. 2015;17:15–9.
214. Park JH, Kim JI, Kim WS. Treatment of persistent facial postinflammatory hyperpigmentation with novel pulse-in-pulse mode intense pulsed light. Dermatol Surg. 2016;42:218–24.
215. Katz TM, Goldberg LH, Firoz BF, Friedman PM. Fractional photothermolysis for the treatment of postinflammatory hyperpigmentation. Dermatol Surg. 2009;35:1844–8.
216. Rokhsar CK, Ciocon DH. Fractional photothermolysis for the treatment of postinflammatory hyperpigmentation after carbon dioxide laser resurfacing. Dermatol Surg. 2009;35:535–7.
217. Kroon MW, Wind BS, Meesters AA, Wolkerstorfer A, Wietze Van Der Veen JP, Bos JD, et al. Non-ablative 1550 nm fractional laser therapy not effective for erythema dyschromicum perstans and postinflammatory hyperpigmentation: a pilot study. J Dermatolog Treat. 2012;23:339–44.
218. Lee SJ, Chung WS, Lee JD, Kim HS. A patient with cupping-related post-inflammatory hyperpigmentation successfully treated with a 1,927 nm thulium fiber fractional laser. J Cosmet Laser Ther. 2014;16:66–8.

219. Alharbi MA. 1927 nm thulium laser successfully treats postinflammatory hyperpigmentation in skin of color. Dermatol Res Pract. 2021;2021:1–5.
220. Bae YSC, Rettig S, Weiss E, Bernstein L, Geronemus R. Treatment of post-inflammatory hyperpigmentation in patients with darker skin types using a low energy 1,927 nm non-ablative fractional laser: a retrospective photographic review analysis. Lasers Surg Med. 2020;52:7–12.
221. Oram Y, Akkaya AD. Refractory postinflammatory hyperpigmentation treated fractional CO_2 laser. J Clin Aesthet Dermatol. 2014;7:42–4.
222. Tawfic SO, Abdel Hay R, Salim H, Elmasry MF. Tranexamic acid versus fractional carbon dioxide laser in post-acne hyperpigmentation. Dermatol Ther. 2021;34(6):e15103.
223. Nayak C, Giri A, Zambare U. A study of clinicopathological correlation of periorbital hyperpigmentation. Indian Dermatol Online J. 2018;9:245.
224. Lowe NJ, Wieder JM, Shorr N, Boxrud C, Saucer D, Chalet M. Infraorbital pigmented skin. Dermatol Surg. 1995;21:767–70.
225. Ranu H, Thng S, Goh BK, Burger A, Goh CL. Periorbital hyperpigmentation in Asians: an epidemiologic study and a proposed classification. Dermatol Surg. 2011;37:1297–303.
226. Watanabe S, Nakai K, Ohnishi T. Condition known as "dark rings under the eyes" in the Japanese population is a kind of dermal melanocytosis which can be successfully treated by Q-switched ruby laser. Dermatol Surg. 2006;32:785–9.
227. Xu TH, Li YH, Chen JZS, Gao XH, Chen HD. Treatment of infraorbital dark circles using 694-nm fractional Q-switched ruby laser. Lasers Med Sci. 2016;31:1783–7. https://doi.org/10.1007/s10103-016-2050-4.
228. Manuskiatti W, Fitzpatrick RE, Goldnan MP. Treatment of facial skin using combinations of CO_2, Q-switched alexandrite, flashlamp-pumped pulsed dye, and Er:YAG lasers in the same treatment session. Dermatol Surg. 2000;26:114–20.
229. Xu T-H, Yang Z-H, Li Y-H, Chen JZ, Guo S, Wu Y, et al. Treatment of infraorbital dark circles using a low-fluence Q-switched 1,064-nm laser. Dermatol Surg. 2011;37:797–803.
230. Nilforoushzadeh MA, Heidari-Kharaji M, Alavi S, Zolghadr S, Mahmoudbeyk M, Nikkhah N. Comparison of carboxy therapy and fractional Q-switched ND:YAG laser on periorbital dark circles treatment: a clinical trial. Lasers Med Sci. 2021;36:1927–34.
231. Alavi S, Goodarzi A, Nilforoushzadeh MA, Mansouri P, Jafari MA, Hejazi S, et al. Evaluation of efficacy and safety of low-fluence Q-switched 1064-nm laser in infra-orbital hyperpigmentation based on biometric parameters. J Lasers Med Sci. 2022;13:19–22.
232. Vanaman Wilson MJ, Jones IT, Bolton J, Larsen L, Wu DC, Goldman MP. Prospective studies of the efficacy and safety of the picosecond 755, 1,064, and 532 nm lasers for the treatment of infraorbital dark circles. Lasers Surg Med. 2018;50:45–50.
233. Ma G, Lin XX, Hu XJ, Jin YB, Chen H. Treatment of venous infraorbital dark circles using a long-pulsed 1,064-nm neodymium-doped yttrium aluminum garnet laser. Dermatol Surg. 2012;38:1277–82.
234. Biesman B. Commentary: treatment of venous infraorbital dark circles using a long-pulsed 1,064-nm neodymium-doped yttrium aluminum garnet laser. Dermatol Surg. 2012;38:1283.
235. Moody MN, Landau JM, Goldberg LH, Friedman PM. Fractionated 1550-nm erbium-doped fiber laser for the treatment of periorbital hyperpigmentation. Dermatol Surg. 2012;38:139–42.
236. West TB, Alster TS. Improvement of infraorbital hyperpigmentation following carbon dioxide laser resurfacing. Dermatol Surg. 1998;24:615–6.
237. Alster TS, Hirsch RJ. Single-pass CO_2 laser skin resurfacing of light and dark skin: extended experience with 52 patients. J Cosmet Laser Ther. 2003;5:39–42.
238. Zamanian A, Azizi M, Ghasemi M, Behrangi E, Naeji S. Comparing the effectiveness of fractional CO_2 laser and the combination therapy with microneedling and topical 10% trichloroacetic acid to remove infra-orbital dark circles in Tehran women. J Cosmet Laser Ther. 2019;21:61–4.
239. Park KY, Oh IY, Moon NJ, Seo SJ. Treatment of infraorbital dark circles in atopic dermatitis with a 2790-nm erbium: yttrium scandium gallium garnet laser: a pilot study. J Cosmet Laser Ther. 2013;15:102–6.
240. Nilforoushzadeh MA, Heidari-Kharaji M, Alavi S, Mahmoudbeyk M, Torkamaniha E, Peyrovan A, et al. Assessing the effectiveness of the combination therapy with fractional Er-YAG laser and platelet-rich plasma in treatment of periorbital dark circles patients: a clinical trial. J Cosmet Dermatol. 2021;20:3526–36.
241. Goldman A, Goldust M, Wollina U. Periorbital hyperpigmentation—dark circles under the eyes; treatment suggestions and combining procedures. Cosmetics. 2021;8:1–12.
242. Kounidas G, Kastora S, Rajpara S. Decoding infraorbital dark circles with lasers and fillers. J Dermatolog Treat. 2022;33:1563–7. https://doi.org/10.1080/09546634.2020.1855297.
243. Kornberg R. Pseudomelanoma: recurrent melanocytic nevus following partial surgical removal. Arch Dermatol. 1975;111:1588–90. https://doi.org/10.1001/archderm.111.12.1588.
244. Dummer R, Kempf W, Burg G. Pseudo-melanoma after laser therapy. Dermatology. 1998;197:71–3.
245. Hwang K, Lee WJ, Lee S II. Pseudomelanoma after laser therapy. Ann Plast Surg. 2002;48:562–4.
246. Woodrow SL, Burrows NP. Malignant melanoma occurring at the periphery of a giant congenital naevus previously treated with laser therapy. Br J Dermatol. 2003;149:886–8.

247. Zipser MC, Mangana J, Oberholzer PA, French LE, Dummer R. Melanoma after laser therapy of pigmented lesions—circumstances and outcome. Eur J Dermatol. 2010;20:334–8.
248. Delker S, Livingstone E, Schimming T, Schadendorf D, Griewank KG. Melanoma diagnosed in lesions previously treated by laser therapy. J Dermatol. 2017;44:23–8. https://doi.org/10.1111/1346-8138.13484.
249. Goldberg DJ, Stampien T, Response T, Erythematosus L. Q-switched ruby laser treatment of congenital nevi. Arch Dermatol. 1995;131:621–3.
250. Heidi A, Arielle N, Geronemus G, Waldorf HA, Kauvar AN, Geronemus RG. Treatment of small and medium congenital nevi with the Q-switched ruby laser. Arch Dermatol. 1996;132:301–4.
251. Ueda S. Normal-mode ruby laser for treating congenital nevi. Arch Dermatol. 1997;133:355. https://doi.org/10.1001/archderm.1997.03890390095013.
252. Vibhagool C, Byers HR, Grevelink JM. Treatment of small nevomelanocytic nevi with a Q-switched ruby laser. J Am Acad Dermatol. 1997;36:738–41.
253. Imayama S, Ueda S. Long- and short-term histological observations of congenital nevi treated with the normal-mode ruby laser. Arch Dermatol. 1999;135:1211–8.
254. Duke D, Byers HR, Sober AJ, Anderson RR, Grevelink JM. Treatment of benign and atypical nevi with the normal-mode ruby laser and the Q-switched ruby laser: clinical improvement but failure to completely eliminate nevomelanocytes. Arch Dermatol. 1999;135:290–6.
255. Kono T, Erçöçen AR, Chan HHL, Kikuchi Y, Nozaki M. Effectiveness of the normal-mode ruby laser and the combined (normal-mode plus Q-switched) ruby laser in the treatment of congenital melanocytic nevi: a comparative study. Ann Plast Surg. 2002;49:476–85.
256. Kono T, Erçöçen AR, Nozaki M. Treatment of congenital melanocytic nevi using the combined (normal-mode plus Q-switched) ruby laser in Asians: clinical response in relation to histological type. Ann Plast Surg. 2005;54:494–501.
257. Helsing P, Mørk G, Sveen B. Ruby laser treatment of congenital melanocytic naevi—a pessimistic view. Acta Derm Venereol. 2006;86:235–7.
258. Minakawa S, Takeda H, Korekawa A, Kaneko T, Urushidate S, Sawamura D. Q-switched ruby laser therapy and long-term follow-up evaluation of small to medium-sized congenital melanocytic naevi. Clin Exp Dermatol. 2012;37:438–40.
259. Grevelink JM. Clinical and histological responses of congenital melanocytic nevi after single treatment with Q-switched lasers. Arch Dermatol. 1997;133:349. https://doi.org/10.1001/archderm.1997.03890390089012.
260. Funayama E, Sasaki S, Furukawa H, Hayashi T, Yamao T, Takahashi K, et al. Effectiveness of combined pulsed dye and Q-switched ruby laser treatment for large to giant congenital melanocytic naevi. Br J Dermatol. 2012;167:1085–91.
261. Funayama E, Yamamoto Y, Oyama A, Murao N, Hayashi T, Maeda T, et al. Combination laser therapy as a non-surgical method for treating congenital melanocytic nevi from cosmetically sensitive locations on the body. Lasers Med Sci. 2019;34:1925–8.
262. Rosenbach A, WIlliams CM, Alster TS. Comparison of the Q-switched alexandrite (755 nm) and Q-switched Nd:YAG (1064 nm) lasers in the treatment of benign melanocytic nevi. Dermatol Surg. 1997;23:239–44.
263. Reda AM, Taha IR, Riad HA. Clinical and histological effect of a single treatment of normal mode alexandrite (755 nm) laser on small melanocytic nevi. J Cosmet Laser Ther. 1999;1:209–15.
264. Sohn S, Kim S, Kang WH, Chan HHL. Recurrent pigmented macules after Q-switched alexandrite laser treatment of congenital melanocytic nevus. Dermatol Surg. 2004;30:898–907.
265. Kim S, Kang WH. Treatment of congenital nevi with the Q-switched alexandrite laser. Eur J Dermatol. 2005;15:92–6.
266. Kim YJ, Whang KU, Choi WB, Kim HJ, Hwang JY, Lee JH, et al. Efficacy and safety of 1,064 nm Q-switched Nd:YAG laser treatment for removing melanocytic nevi. Ann Dermatol. 2012;24:162–7.
267. Cho SB, Ahn KJ, Oh D, Kim H, Yoo KH. Sequential delivery of long-pulsed 755-nm alexandrite laser and long-pulsed 1,064-nm neodymium:yttrium-aluminum-garnet laser treatment for pigmented disorders. Skin Res Technol. 2019;25:683–92.
268. Alshami MA. Long-pulsed 532-nm Nd:YAG laser treatment for small acquired melanocytic nevi in a single session: an 8-year study on 350 Yemeni patients. J Cosmet Laser Ther. 2014;16:14–20.
269. Lapière K, Ostertag J, Krekels G, Van De Kar T. A neonate with a giant congenital naevus: New treatment option with the erbium:YAG laser. Br J Plast Surg. 2002;55:440–2.
270. Ostertag JU, Quaedvlieg PJF, Kerckhoffs FEMJ, Vermeulen AHM, Bertleff MJOE, Venema AW, et al. Congenital naevi treated with erbium:YAG laser (Derma K) resurfacing in neonates: clinical results and review of the literature. Br J Dermatol. 2006;154:889–95.
271. Rajpar SF, Abdullah A, Lanigan SW. Er:YAG laser resurfacing for inoperable medium-sized facial congenital melanocytic naevi in children. Clin Exp Dermatol. 2007;32:159–61.
272. Gu Y, Chang SJ, Ma G, Wang Y, Zhu J, Chen H, et al. Treatment of congenital melanocytic nevi in the eyelid and periorbital region with ablative lasers. Ann Plast Surg. 2019;83:S65–9.
273. Baba M, Bal N. Efficacy and safety of short-pulse erbium:YAG laser in the treatment of acquired melanocytic nevi. Dermatol Surg. 2006;32:256–60.
274. Reynolds N, Kenealy J, Mercer N. Carbon dioxide laser dermabrasion for giant congenital melanocytic nevi. Plast Reconstr Surg. 2003;111:2209–14.

275. Horner BM, El-Muttardi NS, Mayou BJ. Treatment of congenital melanocytic naevi with CO_2 laser. Ann Plast Surg. 2005;55:276–80.
276. Köse O. Carbon dioxide ablative laser treatment of acquired junctional melanocytic nevi. J Cosmet Dermatol. 2021;20:491–6.
277. Park SH, Koo SH, Choi EO. Combined laser therapy for difficult dermal pigmentation: resurfacing and selective photothermolysis. Ann Plast Surg. 2001;47:31–6.
278. Dave R, Mahaffey PJ. Combined early treatment of congenital melanocytic naevus with carbon dioxide and NdYag lasers. Br J Plast Surg. 2004;57:720–4.
279. Chong SJ, Jeong E, Park HJ, Lee JY, Cho BK. Treatment of congenital nevomelanocytic nevi with the CO_2 and Q-switched alexandrite lasers. Dermatol Surg. 2005;31:518–21.
280. Mandal A, Al-Nakib K, Quaba AA. Treatment of small congenital nevocellular naevi using a combination of ultrapulse carbon dioxide laser and Q-switched frequency-doubled Nd-YAG laser. Aesthet Plast Surg. 2006;30:606–10.
281. Al-Hadithy N, Al-Nakib K, Quaba A. Outcomes of 52 patients with congenital melanocytic naevi treated with ultrapulse carbon dioxide and frequency doubled Q-switched Nd-Yag laser. J Plast Reconstr Aesthet Surg. 2012;65:1019–28. https://doi.org/10.1016/j.bjps.2012.03.003.
282. August PJ, Ferguson JE, Madan V. A study of the efficacy of carbon dioxide and pigment-specific lasers in the treatment of medium-sized congenital melanocytic naevi. Br J Dermatol. 2011;164:1037–42.
283. Zeng Y, Ji C, Zhan K, Weng W. Treatment of nasal ala nodular congenital melanocytic naevus with carbon dioxide laser and Q-switched Nd:YAG laser. Lasers Med Sci. 2016;31:1627–32. https://doi.org/10.1007/s10103-016-2028-2.
284. Lee SE, Choi JY, Hong KT, Lee KR. Treatment of acquired and small congenital melanocytic nevi with combined Er:YAG laser and long-pulsed alexandrite laser in asian skin. Dermatol Surg. 2015;41:473–80.
285. Brito MH, Dionísio CS, Fernandes CM, Ferreira JC, Rosa MJ, Garcia MM. Synchronous melanomas arising within nevus spilus. An Bras Dermatol. 2017;92:107–9.
286. Casanova D, Bardot J, Aubert JP, Andrac L, Magalon G. Management of nevus spilus. Pediatr Dermatol. 1996;13:233–8.
287. Leeuwen R, Bastiaens MT, Grevelink JM. Management of nevus spilus with laser. Pediatr Dermatol. 1997;14:155–6. https://doi.org/10.1111/j.1525-1470.1997.tb00227.x.
288. Grevelink JM, González S, Bonoan R, Vibhagool C, Gonzalez E. Treatment of nevus spilus with the Q-switched ruby laser. Dermatol Surg. 1997;23:365–9.
289. Moreno-Arias GA, Bulla F, Vilata-Corell JJ, Camps-Fresneda A. Treatment of widespread segmental nevus spilus by Q-switched alexandrite laser (755 nm, 100 nsec). Dermatol Surg. 2001;27:841–4.
290. Tse Y, Levine VJ, McClain SA, Ashinoff R. The removal of cutaneous pigmented lesions with the Q-switched ruby laser and the Q-switched neodymium:yttrium-Aluminum-garnet laser. J Dermatol Surg Oncol. 1994;20:795–800. https://doi.org/10.1111/j.1524-4725.1994.tb03707.x.
291. Kar H, Gupta L. Treatment of nevus spilus with Q switched Nd:YAG laser. Indian J Dermatol Venereol Leprol. 2013;79:243.
292. Tang M, Cheng Y, Yang C, Liu S, Sheng Y, Li Y, et al. Nevus spilus: treatment with fractional CO2 laser in combination with MedLite C6 laser: a preliminary study. Lasers Med Sci. 2017;32:1659–62. https://doi.org/10.1007/s10103-016-2128-z.
293. Gold MH, Foster TD, Bell MW. Nevus spilus successfully treated with an intense pulsed light source. Dermatol Surg. 1999;25:254–5.
294. Abrusci V, Benzecry V. Medium-sized nevus spilus of the neck treated with pulsed dye laser. Dermatol Ther. 2017;30:1–3.
295. De Almeida Jr HL, Duquia RP, Souza PRM, De Avclar Brcunig J. Prcvalcncc and charactcristics of Becker nevus in Brazilian 18-year-old males. Int J Dermatol. 2010;49:718–20. https://doi.org/10.1111/j.1365-4632.2009.04224.x.
296. Rasi A, Berenji Ardestani H, Tabaie SM. Hypertrichosis is not so prevalent in Becker's nevus: analysis of 47 cases. ISRN Dermatol. 2014;2014:1–4.
297. Nelson JS, Applebaum J. Treatment of superficial cutaneous pigmented lesions by melanin-specific selective photothermolysis using the Q-switched ruby laser. Ann Plast Surg. 1992;29:231–7.
298. Kopera D, Hohenleutner U, Landthaler M. Quality-switched ruby laser treatment of solar lentigines and Becker's nevus: a histopathological and immunohistochemical study. Dermatology. 1997;194:338–43.
299. Suh DH, Han KH, Chung JH. The use of Q-switched Nd:YAG laser in the treatment of superficial pigmented lesions in Koreans. J Dermatolog Treat. 2001;12:91–6.
300. Zhong Y, Huang L, Chen Y, Yan T, Yang B, Man MQ. 755-nm Q-switched alexandrite laser does not markedly benefit Becker's nevus: a retrospective analysis of 59 cases. Lasers Med Sci. 2021;36:699–702.
301. Liu X, Jia G, Gong X, Ding H, Wu Q, Guo L, et al. A retrospective analysis of the efficacy and safety of Q-switched and picosecond lasers for treating Becker's nevus. Dermatol Ther. 2023;2023:1–8.
302. Nanni CA, Alster TS. Treatment of a Becker's nevus using a 694-nm long-pulsed ruby laser. Dermatol Surg. 1998;24:1032–4.
303. Choi JE, Kim JW, Seo SH, Son SW, Ahn HH, Kye YC. Treatment of becker's nevi with a long-pulse alexandrite laser. Dermatol Surg. 2009;35:1105–8.
304. Wulkan AJ, McGraw T, Taylor M. Successful treatment of Becker's nevus with long-pulsed 1064-nm Nd:YAG and 755-nm alexandrite laser and review of the literature. J Cosmet Laser Ther. 2018;20:211–4.
305. Lapidoth M, Adatto M, Cohen S, Ben-Amitai D, Halachmi S. Hypertrichosis in Becker's nevus:

effective low-fluence laser hair removal. Lasers Med Sci. 2014;29:191–3.
306. Zhong Y, Huang L, Chen Y, Yan T, Yang B, Man MQ. 800 nm diode laser does not display long-term benefit for hair removal in Becker's nevus: a retrospective analysis of 24 cases. Photodermatol Photoimmunol Photomed. 2020;36:387–9.
307. Moreno Arias GA, Ferrando J. Intense pulsed light for melanocytic lesions. Dermatol Surg. 2001;27:397–400.
308. Piccolo D, Di Marcantonio D, Crisman G, Cannarozzo G, Sannino M, Chiricozzi A, et al. Unconventional use of intense pulsed light. Biomed Res Int. 2014;2014:618206.
309. Wu PR, Liu LJ, Zhang YX, Liu Y, Lin XX, Ma G. Intense pulsed light treatment for Becker's nevus. J Dermatolog Treat. 2021;32:334–9. https://doi.org/10.1080/09546634.2019.1656795.
310. Zhong Y, Huang L, Chen Y, Yan T, Yang B, Man MQ. The efficacy of intense pulsed light for Becker's nevus: a retrospective analysis of 45 cases. J Cosmet Dermatol. 2021;20:466–71.
311. Han HS, Hong JK, Yoo KH, Seo SJ. Combination of non-ablative fractional laser with Q-switched laser for the treatment of Becker's nevus: efficacy and limitations. Ann Dermatol. 2023;35:56–60.
312. Temiz SA, Arazov S, Ataseven A, Dursun R. Treatment of Becker's nevus with 577-nm pro-yellow laser: could it be a new treatment choice? J Cosmet Dermatol. 2021;20:705–6.
313. Glaich AS, Goldberg LH, Dai T, Kunishige JH, Friedman PM. Fractional resurfacing. Arch Dermatol. 2007;143:269–91. https://doi.org/10.1001/archderm.143.12.1488.
314. Balaraman B, Friedman PM. Hypertrichotic Becker's nevi treated with combination 1,550 nm non-ablative fractional photothermolysis and laser hair removal. Lasers Surg Med. 2016;48:350–3.
315. Kubicki SL, Guo EL, Sodha P, Richmond H, Friedman PM. Combination 1550 nm non-ablative fractional resurfacing and laser hair removal for treatment of Becker's nevi in skin types III–VI. Lasers Surg Med. 2023;55:99–104. https://doi.org/10.1002/lsm.23599.
316. Alajlan A, Alsuwaidan S. Efficacy of non-ablative 1927-nm fractional thulium fiber laser for the treatment of Becker's nevus: intra- and interobserver agreement study. Lasers Surg Med. 2023;55(6):547–54. https://doi.org/10.1002/lsm.23670.
317. Trelles MA, Allones I, Vélez M, Moreno-Arias GA. Becker's nevus: erbium:YAG versus Q-switched neodimium:YAG? Lasers Surg Med. 2004;34:295–7.
318. Trelles MA, Allones I, Moreno-Arias GA, Vélez M. Becker's naevus: a comparative study between erbium:YAG and Q-switched neodymium:YAG; clinical and histopathological findings. Br J Dermatol. 2005;152:308–13.
319. Meesters AA, Wind BS, Kroon MW, Wolkerstorfer A, Van Der Veen JPW, Nieuweboer-Krobotová L, et al. Ablative fractional laser therapy as treatment for Becker nevus: a randomized controlled pilot study. J Am Acad Dermatol. 2011;65:1173–9.
320. Al-Saif F, Al-Mekhadab E, Al-Saif H. Efficacy and safety of short-pulse erbium:yttrium aluminum garnet laser treatment of Becker's nevus in Saudi patients: a pilot study. Int J Heal Sci. 2017;11:14–7.

Laser Treatment of Tattoo

4

Taro Kono

Introduction

Tattooing is a permanent form of body modification that involves the insertion of ink pigments into the dermis layer of the skin. The term "tattoo" originates from the Tahitian word "ta'tau," meaning "to mark," which has been adopted into the English language. It is a cultural practice with a rich historical background spanning thousands of years and has served various purposes throughout human civilization. While tattoos were previously considered taboo, their prevalence has increased, particularly among young individuals, in recent years. According to a 2019 survey conducted in five major countries, approximately 18.5% of the population reported having tattoos [1]. However, various factors such as obtaining a new job, experiencing a change in social status, encountering medical issues, or dissatisfaction with one's appearance may prompt individuals to seek tattoo removal.

Tattoo removal treatment options include lasers, infrared light, radiofrequency, cryotherapy, surgical excision, dermabrasion, and chemical peeling with salabrasion. Apart from short-pulsed lasers, none of these procedures yield satisfactory cosmetic outcomes due to adverse effects such as scarring and dyspigmentation.

The utilization of lasers for tattoo removal originated in 1965 when Goldman et al. introduced the Q-switched (QS) ruby laser [2]. Laser treatment has since become the gold standard for tattoo removal; however, it does have certain limitations. Achieving complete removal often necessitates multiple sessions and multiple wavelengths, with outcomes frequently being only partially satisfactory. Picosecond lasers have shown superior results compared to nanosecond lasers across various aspects [3–6]. Tattoo removal in individuals with dark skin poses greater challenges, as the presence of melanin pigment can compete with the tattoo, potentially leading to dyspigmentation and scar formation.

A thorough understanding of laser principles, nature and color of the tattoo, skin type, location, amount of ink, scarring, and layering significantly enhances the likelihood of achieving satisfactory results.

Tattoo Classification

A tattoo is defined as the presence of pigment in the dermis, either intentionally applied or resulting from external trauma. Tattoos can be categorized into five types: professional tattoos, amateur tattoos, cosmetic tattoos, traumatic tattoos, and medical tattoos (Table 4.1).

T. Kono (✉)
Department of Plastic Surgery, Tokai University School of Medicine, Kanagawa, Japan
e-mail: trkono@gmail.com

S. W. N. Cheng, C. L. Goh (eds.), *Updates on Lasers in Dermatology*, Updates in Clinical Dermatology, https://doi.org/10.1007/978-3-031-71155-8_4

Table 4.1 Tattoo classification

Tattoo type	Pigment	Amount of pigment	Layering	Depth
Amateur	India ink	Spare	–	Variable
Professional	Organometallic	Variable	+/–	Variable
Cosmetic	India ink, iron oxide, titanium oxide	Spare	–	Superficial
Traumatic	Metal, carbon, dust, gunpowder	Variable	–	Variable
Medical	India ink	Spare	–	Superficial

Amateur Tattoo

Amateur tattoos typically have a less intense appearance compared to professional tattoos and are created using handheld needles or pins. They involve a smaller amount of deposited ink and exhibit color variations in contrast to professional tattoos. Common materials used include ash, charcoal, and Indian ink. Amateur tattoos often appear bluish-black or gray in color. Tattoo lightening is more achievable when carbon predominates in the pigments. In general, amateur tattoos are easier to remove than professional tattoos.

Professional Tattoo

Professional tattooing involves the intricate art of creating permanent designs on the skin using a vibrating needle and ink. This technique ensures uniform and high-density ink deposition. Tattoo ink typically consists of a mixture of organometallic dyes that produce a variety of colors. Over time, the pigment will fade through processes such as epidermal elimination, diffusion, phagocytosis by macrophages, migration deeper into the dermis, and eventually entering the lymph vessels and lymph nodes. Achieving complete tattoo removal often requires multiple sessions and multiple wavelengths, but satisfactory results are frequently not fully achieved.

Cosmetic Tattoo

Cosmetic tattoos, including eyebrow, eyelid, and lip-enhancing tattoos, are commonly performed using black, brownish, flesh-tone, and reddish pigments. These pigments often contain titanium dioxide and ferric oxide, which may cause skin darkening after laser irradiation.

Traumatic Tattoo

Traumatic tattoos occur when foreign objects, such as metals, glass, dust, and carbon-containing particles, are mechanically deposited onto the skin following explosions or surface trauma. Removing this type of tattoo can be particularly challenging if the materials are deeply implanted in the dermis and/or contain explosive substances. Traumatic tattoos can negatively impact a person's appearance not only due to pigmentation but also because of scarring resulting from the initial trauma. Pigment within fibrosed dermis is more challenging to remove due to cellular congestion.

Medical Tattoo

Medical tattoos are specialized tattoos used in the field of medicine for various purposes. These tattoos are typically gray or blue-black in color and are created using Indian ink or carbon-based materials. In general, medical tattoos are easier to remove compared to professional tattoos.

Tattoo Ink

Pigments are broadly classified into two categories: inorganic pigments and organic pigments. Inorganic pigments are derived from natural ores or oxides obtained through chemical reactions involving metals. Organic pigments, on the other hand, are derived from dyes obtained from plants and animals, such as indigo from plants and anthraquinone pigments like madder. They can also be synthesized from petroleum and other materials. Inorganic pigments can be further divided into two categories: natural mineral pigments and synthetic inorganic pigments. Natural mineral pigments are obtained from naturally occurring minerals or soil, with ochre and turquoise being common examples. Synthetic inorganic pigments are oxides or compounds resulting from chemical reactions involving metals like iron, copper, and lead. Examples include cobalt blue, lead yellow, and titanium white. Organic pigments offer several advantages over inorganic pigments, including more vibrant colors, stronger coloring power, and a wider range of hues. However, organic pigments are more commonly associated with allergies compared to inorganic pigments.

When iron oxide is heated to its melting point, it undergoes an oxidation-reduction reaction that causes a color change from brown to black. Ferric oxide (red) transforms into ferrous oxide (black), and titanium dioxide (white, $Ti4+$) converts to titanium oxide (black, $Ti3+$) [7, 8]. Paradoxical darkening of tattoos may occasionally occur after laser treatment (Fig. 4.1) [9]. Additionally, exposure to ultraviolet light can lead to secondary decomposition of tattoo pigment. Over time and with UV light exposure, tattoo pigments also gradually fade.

The Regulation on the registration, evaluation, authorization, and restriction of chemicals

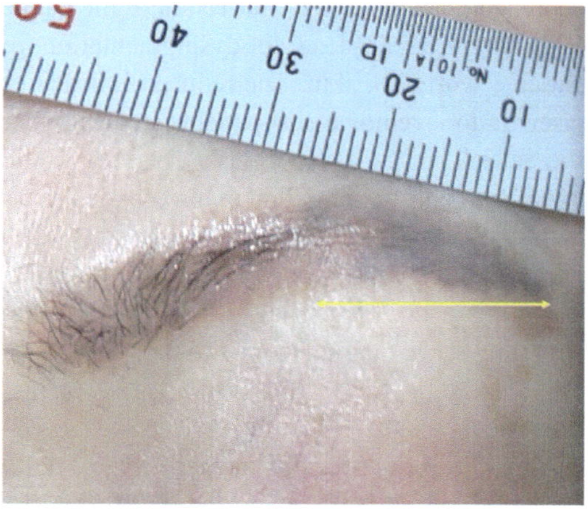

Fig. 4.1 Paradoxical darkening after 532 nm picosecond laser

(REACH) is the primary EU law aimed at safeguarding human health and the environment from chemical risks. In 2022, REACH prohibited the use of numerous tattoo pigments known to contain carcinogens. Its objective is to ban pigments that may cause cancer, genetic mutations, and reproductive disorders.

Laser Tattoo Removal

Laser Physics

Since the introduction of selective photothermolysis, short-pulsed lasers like Q-switched lasers (nanosecond lasers) have been utilized for the treatment of pigmented lesions. The thermal relaxation time (TRT) of a chromophore refers to the time required for the chromophore to dissipate 50% of the heat it absorbed during laser exposure [10]. Ideally, the pulse duration should be shorter than the thermal relaxation time of the target being treated. The diameter of tattoo particles (20–200 nm) is smaller than that of melanosomes. Q-switched lasers with their nanosecond pulse durations are not short enough to achieve optimal tattoo removal efficiency [11]. Complications such as hyper- or hypopigmentation, textural changes, and even scarring are common with nanosecond lasers. Patients with darker skin types face a higher risk of complications when undergoing tattoo removal with Q-switched lasers. In 1998, Ross et al. reported the use of Q-switched and picosecond lasers for tattoo treatment, noting the greater effectiveness of picosecond lasers [2]. This marked the first report of picosecond laser application in human tattoo treatment. Picosecond lasers primarily rely on the photomechanical effect for tattoo ink destruction. In various aspects, picosecond lasers have demonstrated superior outcomes compared to Q-switched lasers.

Laser Parameter

Wavelength

When treating tattoos, the selection of wavelength aims to optimize chromophore absorption

Table 4.2 Tattoo pigment colors and associated absorption wavelengths

Tattoo pigment color	Absorption wavelength (nm)
Black	670, 694, 730, 755, 785, 1064
Blue	670, 694, 730, 755, 785, 1064
Green	670, 694, 730, 755, 785
Purple	532, 670, 694, 730, 755, 785
Red, orange, yellow	532
White, nude	Fractional ablative laser (2790, 2940, 10,600)

and penetration depth. Multiwavelength picosecond lasers are crucial for effectively treating multicolor tattoos (Table 4.2). For black and dark blue pigments, short-pulsed lasers (Q-switched lasers, picosecond lasers) at 670, 694, 730, 755, 785, and 1064 nm can be utilized. However, it is recommended to treat dark-skinned patients with a 1064 nm short-pulsed laser to avoid targeting melanin, which could lead to dyspigmentation of the skin.

Pulse Duration

Since the thermal relaxation time of the basal layer is 1.6–2.8 ms, long-pulsed lasers, intense pulsed light (IPL), and short-pulse (nanosecond and picosecond) lasers are available for treating superficial pigmented lesions. Conversely, dermal wounds heal through collagen and extracellular matrix remodeling. It is important to avoid using long-pulsed lasers or IPLs for treating dermal melanosis and tattoos due to the high risk of scarring [7]. Short-pulsed lasers are essential in these cases. The diameter of tattoo particles is smaller than that of melanosomes, and Q-switched lasers with their pulse durations are not short enough to achieve the most efficient tattoo removal. Theoretically, picosecond lasers should outperform Q-switched lasers in terms of tattoo removal efficacy.

Fluence

Fluence adjustment is crucial in tattoo removal procedures. The clinical endpoint with picosecond lasers or Q-switched lasers is immediate dermal whitening in the tattooed skin [8]. Whitening corresponds to light scattered by small gas bubbles formed in the dermis, which gradually fades as these bubbles dissolve. This response is similar to the treatment of dermal pigmented lesions with picosecond lasers or Q-switched lasers. Low fluence is utilized for tattoos with intense color.

Spot Size

The use of a small spot size tends to result in increased photon scattering, whereas a larger spot size preserves more photons, promoting deeper dermal penetration and minimizing epidermal injury.

Preoperative Considerations (Kirby-Desai Scale)

Prior to performing laser therapy, several factors need to be considered, including Fitzpatrick skin type, tattoo location, color, ink intensity, presence of scar tissue and tissue damage, as well as layering. These factors can help predict the number of therapy sessions required and the prognosis. Kirby et al. developed the Kirby-Desai scale, a scoring system that predicts the number of sessions needed for laser-based tattoo removal [8] (Table 4.3). Higher scores indicate more frequent treatment, while lower scores indicate less frequent treatment.

Fitzpatrick Skin Types

The basal layer of the epidermis contains melanocytes that absorb laser photon energy, with decreasing absorption in the visible light range. High fluence can lead to dyspigmentation in patients with dark skin. The reduced efficacy of laser tattoo removal in patients with higher Fitzpatrick scores is due to laser operators using lower settings and longer intervals between treatment sessions to minimize side effects. The Kirby-Desai scale incorporates this variable, assigning each Fitzpatrick skin type a corresponding score ranging from 1 to 6.

Location

The head and neck regions have the largest number of regional lymph nodes and a rich vascular supply, enabling an enhanced immune response to phagocytose ink particles. The upper and lower

Table 4.3 The Kirby-Desai scale for treatment number estimation: higher scores indicate more frequent treatment, while lower scores indicate less frequent treatment

	0 point	1 point	2 points	3 points	4 points	5 points	6 points
Fitzpatrick skin type		Type I	Type II	Type III	Type IV	Type V	Type VI
		Always burns, never tans	Usually burns, tans minimally	Sometimes mild burn, tans uniformly	Burns minimally, always tans well	Very rarely burns, tans very easily	Never burns
Location		Head/neck/face	Upper trunk/shoulder	Lower trunk/upper leg	Proximal extremity	Distal extremity	
Amount of ink		Amateur	Minimal	Moderate	Significant		
Layering	None		Layering				
Scarring and tissue change	No scar	Minimal	Moderate	Significant			
Colors		Black only	Mostly black with some red	Mostly black with red and some other colors	Multiple colors		

trunk regions also have abundant vascular and lymphatic supply, albeit less than the head and neck. The proximal extremities have a greater lymphatic supply compared to the distal extremities.

Colors

Black pigment granules in tattoos range in size from 0.5 to 4.0 μm and typically consist of carbon- and iron-containing granules. Due to their small size, lack of metallic elements, and ability to absorb all wavelengths of light, black pigments are the easiest to remove. Colors other than black are often twice the size of black pigment granules. Red pigments, for example, contain a mixture of metallic and carbon elements, along with a smaller percentage of titanium dioxide, which contributes to their ease of removal. Other colors are more challenging to remove and receive higher scores on the Kirby-Desai scale.

Amount of Ink

Amateur tattoos are usually placed superficially in the dermis and tend to have less ink compared to professional tattoos. As a result, amateur tattoos typically respond more quickly to laser treatment. Conversely, professional tattoos are typically deeper in the dermis and contain a higher density of pigment. The Kirby-Desai scale categorizes the amount of ink into four categories: amateur, minimal, moderate, and significant, assigning 1 to 4 points, respectively.

Scarring and Tissue Change

Tattoo pigment within fibrosed superficial dermis is more challenging to remove due to cellular congestion. The Kirby-Desai scale incorporates scarring and tissue changes as factors.

Layered Tattoos

In some cases, patients opt to cover an undesirable tattoo by layering it with another tattoo. Layered tattoos are larger and darker, requiring more treatments for removal. The Kirby-Desai scale assigns 2 points for layered tattoos, while tattoos without layering receive 0 point.

General Approach

Prior to initiating laser therapy, particularly in patients with dark skin, it is advisable to perform a test spot to assess the risk of dyspigmentation (including paradoxical darkening) as well as the treatment's efficacy. The desired response for both Q-switched (QS) and picosecond (PS) lasers is immediate whitening.

Posttreatment Therapy

Swelling is a common observation, and in some cases, pinpoint bleeding may occur, which can be addressed by applying cold compression using an ice pack. It is recommended to avoid sun exposure, apply emollients, and use bandages for a minimum of 7–10 days after the procedure. Sun avoidance should be practiced for several months following treatment.

Technique Modifications

Multi-Pass Therapy

Tattoo removal has shown enhanced efficacy when using the R20 method, which involves multiple passes with 20-min intervals. This approach was initially reported by Kossida et al. [12]. The researchers hypothesized that the temporary increase in optical scattering caused by the immediate whitening reaction limits the penetration and efficacy of laser treatment. Thus, performing a second exposure before the fading of the immediate whitening reaction does not significantly improve effectiveness. Tattoos treated with the R20 method demonstrated superior improvement compared to those treated with conventional therapy.

Combination Therapy

The combination of ablative fractional laser and picosecond laser (or Q-switched laser) treatment has been shown to enhance the rate of pigment clearance, prevent blister formation, and reduce treatment-induced hypopigmentation. This approach was first reported by Weiss et al. [13]. Ablative fractional lasers (CO_2, Er-YAGG, Er-YSGG) facilitate trans-epidermal elimination of tattoo ink through ablated channels that are formed [14]. More recently, studies have reported the use of a combination of 1064 nm fractional picosecond laser (or Q-switched laser) and picosecond laser (or Q-switched laser) treatments [15, 16].

Adverse Effects

Complications and adverse effects are commonly observed following laser tattoo removal [17]. These complications can be categorized as immediate or delayed. Immediate complications include pain, pinpoint bleeding, edema, blisters, and crusting. Laser tattoo removal can also lead to hyper- or hypopigmentation, particularly in patients with darker skin tones. Local allergic reactions may occur after the removal of red or yellow pigment tattoos. Additionally, the use of Q-switched and/or picosecond lasers may result in darkening of the skin due to the presence of titanium dioxide and ferric oxide in brownish, flesh-tone, and reddish pigments (known as paradoxical darkening).

Conclusion

Laser therapy is considered the gold standard for tattoo removal. Factors such as Fitzpatrick skin type, tattoo location, color, ink intensity, presence of scar tissue and tissue damage, as well as presence of layered tattoos should be taken into consideration. Acquiring a comprehensive understanding of the fundamental principles of laser therapy is crucial for achieving optimal tattoo removal.

References

1. Kluger N, Seité S, Taieb C. The prevalence of tattooing and motivations in five major countries over the world. J Eur Acad Dermatol Venereol. 2019;33(12):e484–6.
2. Goldman L. Radiation from a Q-switched ruby laser, effect of repeated impacts of power output of 10 megawatts on a tattoo of man. J Invest Derm. 1965;44:69–71.
3. Ross EV, et al. Comparison of responses of tattoos to picosecond and nanosecond Q-switched neodymium: YAG lasers. Arch Dermatol. 1998;134(2):167–71.
4. Reiter O, et al. Picosecond lasers for tattoo removal: a systematic review. Lasers Med Sci. 2016;31(7):1397–405.
5. Lorgeou A, et al. Comparison of two picosecond lasers to a nanosecond laser for treating tattoos: a prospective randomized study on 49 patients. J Eur Acad Dermatol Venereol. 2018;32(2):265–70.

6. Kono T, et al. Prospective comparison study of 532/1064 nm picosecond laser vs 532/1064 nm nanosecond laser in the treatment of professional tattoos in Asians. Laser Ther. 2020;29(1):47–52.
7. Kono T, Shek SY, Chan HH, Groff WF, Imagawa K, Akamatsu T. Theoretical review of the treatment of pigmented lesions in Asian skin. Laser Ther. 2016;25(3):179–84.
8. Wanner M, Sakamoto FH, Avram MM, Chan HH, Alam M, Tannous Z, Anderson RR. Immediate skin responses to laser and light treatments: therapeutic endpoints: how to obtain efficacy. J Am Acad Dermatol. 2016;74(5):821–33.
9. Leu FJ, Huang CL, Wu YS, Wang CC. Comparison of picosecond versus nanosecond Nd:YAG lasers for the removal of cosmetic tattoos in an animal model. Lasers Med Sci. 2022;37(2):1343–50.
10. Anderson RR, Parrish JA. Selective photothermolysis: precise microsurgery by selective absorption of pulsed radiation. Science. 1983;220(4596):524–7.
11. Ho DD, London R, Zimmerman GB, Young DA. Laser-tattoo removal—a study of the mechanism and the optimal treatment strategy via computer simulations. Lasers Surg Med. 2002;30(5):389–97.
12. Kirby W, Desai A, Desai T, Kartono F, Geeta P. The Kirby-Desai scale: a proposed scale to assess tattoo-removal treatments. J Clin Aesthet Dermatol. 2009;2(3):32.
13. Kossida T, Rigopoulos D, Katsambas A, Anderson RR. T optimal tattoo removal in a single laser session based on the method of repeated exposures. J Am Acad Dermatol. 2012;66(2):271–7.
14. Weiss ET, Geronemus RG. Combining fractional resurfacing and Q-switched ruby laser for tattoo removal. Dermatol Surg. 2011;37(1):97–9.
15. Marini L, Marini S, Cutlan J. Hreljac I () Q-S laser microdrilling and multipass full-beam Q-S laser for tattoo removal—a case series. Lasers Med Sci. 2022;37(3):1763–71.
16. Sirithanabadeekul P, Vongchansathapat P, Sutthipisal N, Thanasarnaksorn W, Suwanchinda A. Outcomes of 1064-nm picosecond laser alone and in combination with fractional 1064-nm picosecond laser in tattoo removal. J Cosmet Dermatol. 2022;21(7):2832–9.
17. Hernandez L, Mohsin N, Frech FS, Dreyfuss I, Vander Does A, Nouri K. Laser tattoo removal: laser principles and an updated guide for clinicians. Lasers Med Sci. 2022;37(6):2581–7.

Fractional Photothermolysis in Skin Rejuvenation

5

Peter Wee Beng Ch'ng

Introduction

This book chapter focuses on lasers using fractional photothermolysis (FP) technology to rejuvenate and enhance the youthfulness of our skin. FP creates microscopic treatment zones (MTZs) while sparing the surrounding skin, facilitating faster re-epithelization of the treated area. This chapter discusses about the historical background and advancements in ablative fractional laser (AFL), nonablative fractional laser (NAFL), and hybrid lasers. Additionally, it discusses strategies for optimizing outcomes for patients undergoing skin rejuvenation treatments.

As we age, our skin undergoes several changes such as having more wrinkles, less elasticity, enlarged pores, thinning of skin, dyspigmentation, and sagginess. The rate of changes depends on internal as well as external factors such as solar exposure, air pollution, hormones, nutrition, and psychological factors [1].

Skin rejuvenation is a term used to describe a wide range of methods to make our skin more youthful looking by improving wrinkles, skin elasticity, sagginess, enlarged pores, scars, dyspigmentation, and prominent vessels. The methods used vary from invasive surgeries to noninvasive methods such as topical agents, medical interventions such as hormone replacement therapy, chemical peels, botulinum toxin, filler injection, energy-based devices (radiofrequency-based, micro-focused ultrasound devices) and light-emitting diode (LED) and lasers. The outcomes of the methods can range from subtle to very noticeable effects.

Laser skin rejuvenation typically offers a more subtle improvement due to its limited penetration to the dermis compared to surgery. However, it boasts shorter or even no downtime and is generally less expensive. Treatment needs to be tailored to each patient's requirements. Clearly, severe sagging skin cannot be effectively addressed with laser alone.

The concept of FP was introduced back in 2004 and remains a cornerstone in the design of modern lasers. Beyond its application in laser technology, FP principles have been adapted for use in other energy-based devices, including radiofrequency-based ones. FP creates microscopic treatment zones (MTZs) or microscopic thermal wounds while sparing the surrounding skin, which allows faster re-epithelization of the treated area [2].

As a result of dermal heating, new collagen synthesis and remodeling occur.

FP technology can be broadly categorized into ablative fractional laser (AFL), nonablative fractional laser (NAFL), and hybrid laser (Table 5.1).

P. W. B. Ch'ng (✉)
Peter Ch'ng Clinic, Gleneagles Kuala Lumpur, Kuala Lumpur, Malaysia

S. W. N. Cheng, C. L. Goh (eds.), *Updates on Lasers in Dermatology*, Updates in Clinical Dermatology, https://doi.org/10.1007/978-3-031-71155-8_5

Table 5.1 Types of fractional lasers

AFL	NAFL	Hybrid
10,600 nm fractional CO_2 laser (FCO_2)	1550 nm Erbium-doped fiber (Er:glass)	1550 nm/1927 nm Erbium-doped fiber (Er:glass)
2940 nm Erbium:yttrium aluminum garnet (Er:YAG)	1565 nm Erbium-doped fiber (Er:glass)	CO_2 with 1540 nm gallium arsenide
2790 nm Erbium:yttrium-scandium-gallium-garnet (Er-YSGG)	1540 nm Gallium arsenide	CO_2 with 1570 nm fiber
2910 nm Erbium-doped fluoride glass fiber (Er:glass)	1440 nm Nd:YAG	Er:YAG and 1470 nm
	1440 nm Diode	CO_2 with radiofrequency-based device
	1320/1440 nm Multiplex Nd:YAG	1550 nm/1927 nm Diode
	755 nm Alexandrite picosecond	
	1064 nm Nd:YAG picosecond	
	532 nm Nd:YAG picosecond	
	675 nm Diode	

Nonablative Fractional Laser (NAFL)

1550 nm Erbium glass laser was the first laser to utilize the concept of FP. Even today, newer laser systems continue to harness this wavelength for skin rejuvenation. The advantage of NAFL over AFL is the shorter downtime because of the sparing of the epidermis. However, it will require more sessions of laser treatments with less dramatic effect compared to AFL [3].

AFL also has a higher risk of postinflammatory hyperpigmentation (PIH) and more discomfort compared to NAFL in the treatment of acne scars [4].

The first study of using FP to treat melasma was published in 2005. In this study, 1550 nm erbium-doped fiber (Er:glass) laser was reported to be effective in treating melisma [5].

Four years later, another wavelength, 1927 nm fractional thulium fiber laser, was introduced. With the 1927 nm wavelength, it is able to target the epidermis with the maximum depth of penetration of 200 μm, compared with 1400–1500 μm for the 1550 nm wavelength. It was also reported to be a safe and effective treatment for melisma [6].

Caution is advised when using thulium lasers, particularly in patients with Fitzpatrick skin types V and VI who have melasma, as it could exacerbate the condition or increase the risk of PIH [7].

The mechanism in which FP helps in hyperpigmentation is thought to be the elimination of melanin together with microscopic epidermal necrotic debris (MENDs) transepidermally with an intact stratum corneum.

Picosecond laser was first used to remove tattoos and has been proven in some studies to be superior to nanosecond laser for that indication [8, 9].

Over the last few years, fractionated handpiece such as microlens arrays (MLAs) or diffractive optical elements (DOEs) has also been developed to treat facial acne scars, rejuvenation, and melasma (Figs. 5.1 and 5.2) [10, 11].

For melasma, the data has been inconsistent. In the author's opinion, the efficacy is about the same as other NAFL.

The fractionated picosecond laser is able to produce intradermal light-induced optical breakdown (LIOB) through multiphoton ionization of the skin. It has been proven to improve atrophic acne scars even in darker skin patients with good safety profile [12], but it is not superior to other NAFL such as the fractional 1550 nm erbium fiber laser and AFL [13–15].

Although picosecond laser has a relatively shorter downtime and less risk of postinflammatory hyperpigmentation compared to AFL in the treatment of acne scars, the initial downtime with petechiae may not be widely accepted (Fig. 5.3).

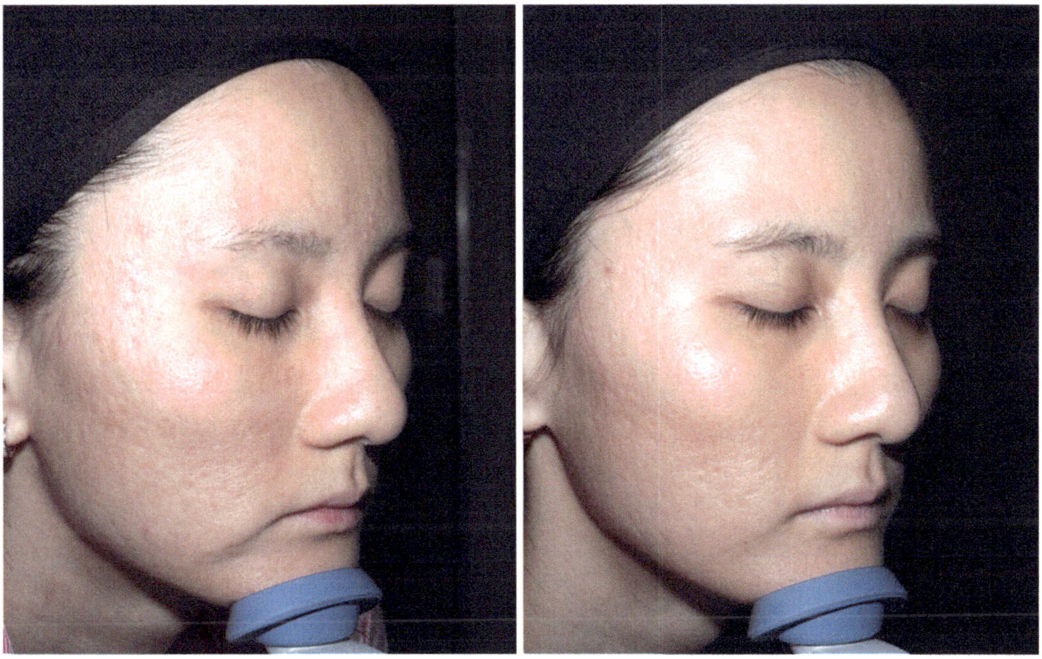

Fig. 5.1 Treatment efficacy in a patient with acne scars: left side at baseline before fractional CO_2 treatment; right side at 3-month assessment; a good result was seen on both subjective and objective assessment

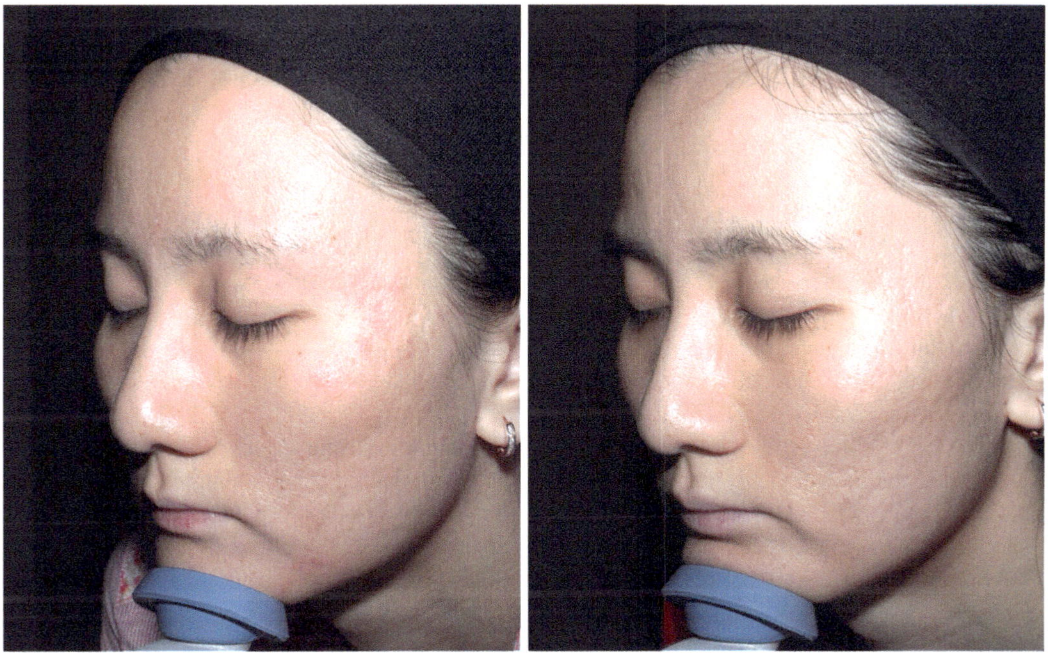

Fig. 5.2 Treatment efficacy in patient: left side at baseline before psNDYL treatment; right side at 3-month assessment; a good result was seen on both subjective and objective assessment

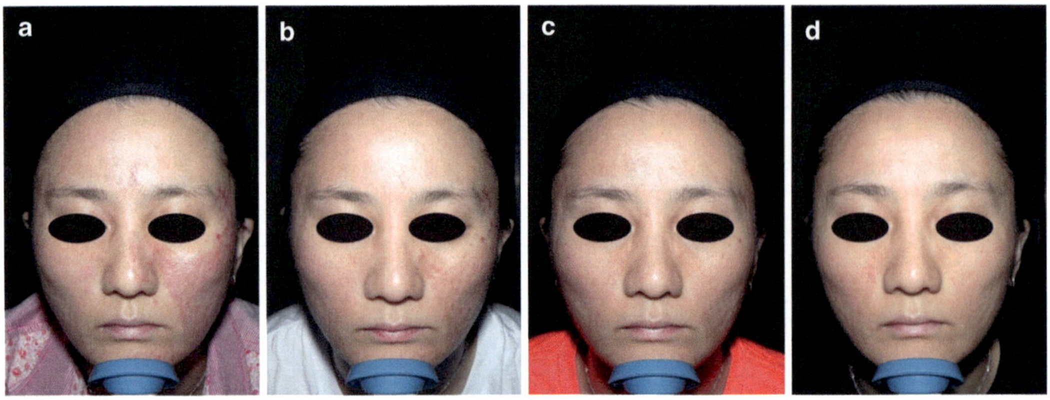

Fig. 5.3 Evolution of posttreatment sequelae. Fractional CO_2 laser on right side, psNDYL on left side. (**a**) Immediately after treatment; (**b**) 24 h after Tx; (**c**) 4 days after Tx; (**d**) 7 days after Tx

NAFL for the Treatment of Pores and Acne Scars?

Different types of acne scars respond differently to various treatment modalities, and the choice of treatment should be tailored according to the patient [16].

For deep boxcar scars, punch excision followed by resurfacing procedures like laser therapy can often yield better results compared to laser therapy alone. Furthermore, we have to understand that majority of the patients will have a combination of different types of scars. Therefore, combination treatment with different modalities such as NAFL, AFL, vascular laser, fractional radiofrequency, punch excision, chemical reconstruction of skin scar (CROSS), subcision, and filler injection tends to have better results than single modality alone.

Selecting the best modality for treating atrophic acne scars is indeed dependent on various factors including clinical presentation, patient's preference after a thorough consultation and discussion with the physician, and availability of the modalities at the particular center. Patient has to be informed that multiple sessions of lasers are required in order to achieve significant results. The final results will only be achieved at least 3 months after the last laser treatment as collagen takes time to produce.

The same principles that guide the treatment of atrophic acne scars can be applied to the treatment of enlarged pores as well.

Advancements in laser technology have indeed led to the development of newer lasers with novel wavelengths for various dermatological treatments. One such example is the 675 nm diode laser, which targets collagen, melanin, and hemoglobin. This laser not only promotes the synthesis of collagen types I and III but also enhances the expression of heat shock protein [17].

It appears to be effective and well tolerated in the treatment of melasma in patients with Fitzpatrick phototypes II–III, skin aging, and acne scars [17, 18].

AFL

The biggest advantage of AFL compared to the conventional full ablative skin resurfacing laser is the safety profile. Although full ablative skin resurfacing laser is effective for skin rejuvenation, it comes with a longer downtime and many side effects such as prolonged erythema, burning sensation, hyperpigmentation, hypopigmentation, scarring, and infection. The first AFL is fractional carbon dioxide (FCO_2) laser, which remains one of the most common lasers in dermatology practice. It can be used to treat atrophic acne scars, enlarged pores, and wrinkles.

Although it has fewer side effects compared to ablative laser skin resurfacing, there is still risk of causing PIH and scarring. Lower energy and density should be used around the neck, chest, and periocular region [19].

Studies in Asians also found high fluence with low-density fractional resurfacing effective and relatively safe [20].

Fractional erbium Yag (fractional Erb:Yag) laser was subsequently introduced after FCO_2. It targets more superficially and is therefore less effective compared to FCO_2. On top of that, side effect profile is still about the same as fractional CO_2.

The latest AFL is 2910 nm erbium-doped fluoride glass fiber (Er:glass) laser which targets water which has its peak absorption between 2900 and 3100 nm. It has been found to be effective at rejuvenating photodamaged skin and scars with minimal downtime and discomfort [21, 22].

Laser-assisted drug delivery (LADD) presents a notable advantage of AFL, enabling the delivery of various drugs such as platelet-rich plasma, tranexamic acid, kojic acid, vitamins, hyaluronic acid, poly L-lactic acid, and botulinum toxin A by applying them over the laser treatment sites immediately afterward. Additionally, some studies have shown that certain NAFLs, like fractional 1927 nm thulium fiber laser, are also capable of facilitating this drug delivery process. More details on LADD can be found in Chap. 10.

AFL treatments are typically done monthly for 3 months while the NAFL treatments are typically done monthly for four to six treatments. It is also worth noting that the 6-month delay of performing AFL or NAFL following oral isotretinoin has been disbanded. However, for full ablative skin resurfacing laser, it is still recommended to delay the procedure for 6 months following oral isotretinoin therapy [23].

Hybrid Lasers

In order to combine all the advantages of AFL and NAFL while maintaining safety, there are also lasers that can individually, simultaneously, or sequentially emit AFL with NAFL (e.g., 1550 nm/1927 nm erbium-doped fiber (Er:glass), fractional CO_2 with 1540 nm gallium arsenide, fractional CO_2 with 1570 nm fiber, fractional Er:YAG, and 1470 nm). Some lasers combine AFL with other energy-based devices, such as FCO_2 with radiofrequency-based devices. Additionally, newer laser devices, as small as a hand phone, can now fire two different wavelengths simultaneously.

Hybrid lasers, which combine multiple laser modalities into a single system, offer several advantages. By utilizing different wavelengths and technologies simultaneously or sequentially, hybrid lasers can target multiple skin concerns in a single treatment session. This not only reduces the overall procedure time but also potentially enhances treatment outcomes through synergistic effects. Furthermore, the incorporation of hybrid technology has been shown to improve patient comfort and accelerate healing [24].

Hybrid laser parameters can also be tailored according to the patient's condition. For example, if a patient has underlying melasma, physicians may want to reduce the AFL fluence and concentrate more on the NAFL parameters.

The integration of artificial intelligence (AI) into newer dermatological laser systems represents a significant advancement in personalized laser treatments. By leveraging AI algorithms, these machines can analyze individual skin characteristics and tailor the laser settings accordingly, maximizing effectiveness while minimizing risks and side effects.

Achieving the Best Outcome

To achieve optimal outcomes in skin rejuvenation, it is essential for physicians to engage in comprehensive discussions with patients regarding their concerns, expectations, various treatment modalities, downtime, and associated costs especially when multiple sessions may be required to achieve significant results.

There is no one best device for skin rejuvenation. Physicians should have a thorough understanding of the available FP devices and their indications. Knowing the past medical and surgical history, skin type, which chromophores need to be targeted, at which skin layers the treatment is focused, and the suitable laser parameters ensures optimal results. Combining FP with other modalities, such as topical treatments, botulinum toxin injection, and other energy-based devices, can enhance overall results.

Discussing the benefits and risks of laser procedures with patients is essential. If the risks outweigh the benefits, alternative rejuvenation methods should be considered. When treating the periorbital region, eye protection with metal ocular shields or wavelength-specific glasses is crucial for both patients and operating personnel [25].

FP can also be used to rejuvenate other sites such as neck, chest, and limbs. However, these areas have less sebaceous glands and are therefore more prone to photothermal injury and scar compared to the face.

Proper pre- and post-laser care including skin cooling and sun protection helps minimize the risk of adverse effects.

Obtaining informed consent and documenting baseline photographs are essential steps before initiating FP treatment. This ensures that patients understand the potential risks and benefits and allows for accurate tracking of treatment progress especially when the results of skin rejuvenation can be subtle after a single treatment.

Conclusion

Fractional photothermolysis, a groundbreaking concept introduced two decades ago, has sparked continuous innovation in laser technology for dermatological treatment. New lasers have emerged, targeting different chromophores with tailored wavelengths, aiming to minimize patient discomfort and downtime without compromising on efficacy and safety. Hybrid lasers integrate multiple lasers and energy-based devices into a single platform, allowing for comprehensive treatment of various skin concerns in one session, reducing procedure times, and enhancing outcomes through synergistic effects. AI integration further enhances personalized treatments by analyzing skin characteristics and adjusting laser settings accordingly, minimizing risks, and optimizing effectiveness. To achieve optimal outcomes in skin rejuvenation, it is essential for physicians to engage in comprehensive discussions with patients regarding their concerns, expectations, various treatment modalities, downtime, and associated costs. Additionally, physicians should possess a thorough understanding of available fractional photothermolysis (FP) devices and have ample experience in their application.

References

1. Passeron T, Krutmann J, Andersen ML, et al. Clinical and biological impact of the exposome on the skin. J Eur Acad Dermatol Venereol. 2020;34(Suppl 4):4–25.
2. Manstein D, Herron GS, Sink RK, et al. Fractional photothermolysis: a new concept for cutaneous remodeling using microscopic patterns of thermal injury. Lasers Surg Med. 2004;34:426–38.
3. Alexiades-Armenakas MR, Dover JS, Arndt KA. The spectrum of laser skin resurfacing: nonablative, fractional, and ablative laser resurfacing. J Am Acad Dermatol. 2008;58(5):719–37.
4. Ong MW, Bashir SJ. Fractional laser resurfacing for acne scars: a review. Br J Dermatol. 2012;166(6):1160–9.
5. Cohen SR, Henssler C, Horton K, Broder KW, Moise-Broder PA. Clinical experience with the Fraxel SR laser: 202 treatments in 59 consecutive patients. Plast Reconstr Surg. 2008;121(5):297e–304e.
6. Polder KD, Bruce S. Treatment of melasma using a novel 1,927-nm fractional thulium fiber laser: a pilot study. Dermatol Surg. 2012;38(2):199–206. https://doi.org/10.1111/j.1524-4725.2011.02178.x.
7. Friedman PM, Dover JS, Chapas A, Rahman Z, Ross EV, Kilmer SL, Roberts WE, Sodha P, Stimmel JB, Moncrief MBC, Waibel JS. 1,550 nm erbium-doped and 1,927 nm thulium nonablative fractional laser system: best practices and treatment setting recommendations. Dermatol Surg. 2022;48(2):195–200.
8. Kono T, et al. Prospective comparison study of 532/1034 nm picosecond laser vs 532/1034 nm nanosecond laser in the treatment of professional tattoos in Asians. Laser Ther. 2020;29(1):47–52. https://doi.org/10.5978/islsm.20-OR-07.
9. Cecchetti D, Bauer EM, Guerriero E, Sennato S, Tagliatesta P, Tagliaferri M, Cerri L, Carbone M. Comparative treatments of a green tattoo ink with Ruby, Nd:YAG nano- and picosecond lasers in normal and array mode. Sci Rep. 2022;12(1):3571. https://doi.org/10.1038/s41598-022-07021-w.

10. Chalermchai T, Rummaneethorn P. Effects of a fractional picosecond 1,064 nm laser for the treatment of dermal and mixed type melasma. J Cosmet Laser Ther. 2018;20(3):134–9.
11. Manuskiatti W, Yan C, Tantrapornpong P, Cembrano KAG, Techapichetvanich T, Wanitphakdeedecha R. A prospective, split-face, randomized study comparing a 755-nm picosecond laser with and without diffractive lens array in the treatment of melasma in Asians. Lasers Surg Med. 2021;53:95–103.
12. Manuskiatti W, Punyaratabandhu P, Tantrapornpong P, Yan C, Cembrano KAG. Objective and long-term evaluation of the efficacy and safety of a 1064-nm picosecond laser with fractionated microlens array for the treatment of atrophic acne scar in Asians. Lasers Surg Med. 2021;53(7):899–905. https://doi.org/10.1002/lsm.23368.
13. Chayavichitsilp P, Limtong P, Triyangkulsri K, Pratumchart N. Comparison of fractional neodymium-doped yttrium aluminum garnet (Nd:YAG) 1064-nm picosecond laser and fractional 1550-nm erbium fiber laser in facial acne scar treatment. Lasers Med Sci. 2020;35(3):695–700. https://doi.org/10.1007/s10103-019-02891-5.
14. Li J, Duan F, Kuang J. Fractional picosecond laser for atrophic acne scars: a meta-analysis. J Cosmet Dermatol. 2023;22(8):2205–17. https://doi.org/10.1111/jocd.15862.
15. Dai R, Cao Y, Su Y, Cai S. Comparison of 1064-nm Nd:YAG picosecond laser using fractional micro-lens array vs. ablative fractional 2940-nm Er:YAG laser for the treatment of atrophic acne scar in Asians: a 20-week prospective, randomized, split-face, controlled pilot study. Front Med (Lausanne). 2023;10:1248831. https://doi.org/10.3389/fmed.2023.1248831.
16. Bhargava S, Cunha PR, Lee J, Kroumpouzos G. Acne scarring management: systematic review and evaluation of the evidence. Am J Clin Dermatol. 2018;19(4):459–77.
17. Magni G, Pieri L, Fusco I, et al. Laser emission at 675 nm: in vitro study evidence of a promising role in skin rejuvenation. Regen Ther. 2023;22:176–80.
18. Coricciati L, Gabellone M, Donne PD, Pennati BM, Zingoni T. The 675-nm wavelength for treating facial melasma. Skin Res Technol. 2023;29(8):e13434. https://doi.org/10.1111/srt.13434.
19. Fife DJ, Fitzpatrick RE, Zachary CB. Complications of fractional CO_2 laser resurfacing: four cases. Lasers Surg Med. 2009;41(3):179–84.
20. Kono T, Chan HH, Groff WF, Manstein D, Sakurai H, Takeuchi M, Yamaki T, Soejima K, Nozaki M. Prospective direct comparison study of fractional resurfacing using different fluences and densities for skin rejuvenation in Asians. Lasers Surg Med. 2007;39(4):311–4.
21. Selim MM, Lowery JA, Maredia HS, Zelickson BD. Clinical evaluation of a new fractional ablative 2910 nm erbium laser on photodamaged skin: a pilot study. Lasers Surg Med. 2023;55(8):715–23.
22. Murray TN, Guo EL, Richmond H, Friedman PM. Single treatment scar resurfacing with a novel ablative fractional 2910 nm erbium-doped fluoride glass fiber laser. Lasers Surg Med. 2024;56:19–22.
23. McDonald KA, Shelley AJ, Pierscianowski T, Alavi A. A 2017 update: challenging the cosmetic procedural delay following oral isotretinoin therapy. J Cosmet Laser Ther. 2019;21(1):58–60.
24. Fusano M, Bencini PL, Galimberti MG. Hybrid fractional laser treatment for photodamaged facial skin rejuvenation 6 years following fractional CO_2: comparison of clinical outcome and patients' satisfaction. Lasers Surg Med. 2022;54:1045–50.
25. Huang A, Phillips A, Adar T, Hui A. Ocular injury in cosmetic laser treatments of the face. J Clin Aesthet Dermatol. 2018;11(2):15–8.

Skin Tightening and Body Contouring Devices

6

Joyce Teng Ee Lim

Introduction

Body contouring treatments are getting popular and form a significant portion of any aesthetic dermatology practice [1]. Patients prefer non-invasive body contouring to surgical treatments as they are safe, effective, with minimal downtime and without the risks of a surgical procedure. Body contouring treatments include skin tightening, non-invasive fat reduction and muscle stimulation and definition. Most devices are FDA and CE approved, and there are numerous scientific literatures on their effectiveness and safety. However, there are little comparisons between the different modalities The current body contouring devices for skin tightening use either radiofrequency, microfocused ultrasound, infrared light or lasers. Procedures for fat reduction include radiofrequency, high-intensity focused ultrasound, lasers or cryolipolysis. Electromagnetic muscle stimulation or electrical multidirectional muscle stimulation is used for muscle stimulation and definition.

J. T. E. Lim (✉)
Joyce Lim Skin and Laser Clinic, Singapore, Singapore
e-mail: drjoyce@joycelim.com

Skin Tightening

Energy-based devices (EBDs) using radiofrequency (RF), microfocused ultrasound (MFU), infrared light (IRL) and lasers can provide non-surgical skin tightening both on and off the face. They aim to improve skin laxity, even out crepiness of the skin and improve skin tone by collagen remodelling, elastogenesis and angiogenesis. While they share the same mechanisms of action, they differ in their technologies, their protocols and the assessment of their effectiveness [2, 3]. Generally, EBDs that are effective for skin tightening are RF and MFU, while lasers and IRL have not shown consistent results for skin tightening.

Mechanism of Skin Tightening

Clinical skin tightening consists of two phases—an immediate collagen contraction and secondary wound healing process [4]. When the temperature reaches 55–65 °C, the H-bond in the triple-helix collagen molecule breaks and the fibrils unbundle and get shorter and thicker, and this shortening of the collagen fibrils produces the immediate collagen shrinkage and skin tightening. Studies have shown that with multiple treatment passes, there are more shrinkage and tightening of collagen fibrils. Besides dermal contraction, some EBDs also cause contraction

S. W. N. Cheng, C. L. Goh (eds.), *Updates on Lasers in Dermatology*, Updates in Clinical Dermatology, https://doi.org/10.1007/978-3-031-71155-8_6

of the fibroseptal network and the superficial muscular aponeurosis, and this results in body contouring.

A few months after the procedures, the thermal injury stimulates a wound healing response that generates new collagen, elastin and angiogenesis. There are improved collagen density and additional tightening over time. Clinical and animal studies have both shown that after 10 min of exposure to temperatures of 39–43 °C, the amount of collagen increases from approximately 15% to 20% after a 3-month follow-up period. The skin tightening is seen clinically. Studies had demonstrated the skin tightening objectively in various histological, immunohistochemical and electron microscope analyses [5].

Selection of Patients

Three groups of patients will benefit from skin tightening [6]. The first group are those with mild to moderate skin laxity or those with wrinkled and creepy skin and who are not keen on surgery. Patients between the ages of 35 and 60 years and who have realistic and appropriate expectation are good candidates. The second group are those who have recurrent laxity, who had undergone surgical procedures and who are looking at improvement of their skin laxity without going through another surgical procedure. The third group are those looking for pre-rejuvenation or who want to maintain their skin rejuvenation.

Patients for skin tightening include those with mild-moderate nasolabial fold, skin laxity at the cheeks and jaw line, submental laxity, hooding of upper eyelids and creepiness of the neck skin. Patients for body skin tightening must have mild to moderate skin laxity, be in good physical shape and be at a stable weight. They should be within 4–6 kg of their ideal weight. Patients who have skin laxity post-pregnancy and those who have weight loss are good candidates. "Creepy" skin at the knees and inner upper arm can benefit from skin tightening devices.

Unsuitable patients are those with unrealistic expectations, those with poor general and mental health and those with obesity. Those with poor skin quality such as severe elastosis and severe photodamage are not ideal patients. Skin tightening is avoided in the presence of active skin infection or inflammation.

Treatment Plan and Assessment for Skin Tightening

A detailed history and physical examination must be performed to assess patients' suitability and whether there are any contraindications. Skin tightening is delayed in the presence of active infection, skin wounds, immunocompromised state, delayed wound healing and pregnancy.

The area to be treated is cleaned, and make-up and lotions are removed. If there are excessive hairs, the treatment area is shaved to allow the device handpiece to have full contact with the skin. Jewellery, metal buckles, ornaments and body piercing near the treatment must be removed.

Standardised photographs of the treatment areas should be taken in an upright position.

Topical anaesthesia is applied before the procedure, and this must be thoroughly removed to ensure that there is good contact with the treatment device and the skin. Oral analgesics and in some cases oral antianxiety medication can be given, depending on the device and energy used, the treatment depths and the pain threshold of the patient. Nerve blocks and sedation are not recommended as the patient needs to provide feedback on the heat sensation so that the optimal temperature for skin tightening can be achieved and to avoid excessive heat and burns. Local infiltration is also not recommended as this will alter tissue impedance resulting in increased adverse events or decreased efficacy.

During assessment, identify and discuss the areas of concern and treatment goals with the patient and choose the areas of treatment for optimal skin tightening and contouring. The skin is palpated and assessed for mobility, firmness and thickness. The skin must be palpated and manipulated in different directions to help determine the direction of the desired tissue tightening. Mark the vectors in the direction of desired tissue contraction, and mark the problem areas where more passes or energy is required. In some devices, a treatment grid pattern is applied.

Managing Patients' Expectation

All patients will receive the benefit of increased collagen density. However, not all patients will achieve the same visible results. Some may not see any appreciable change, while others may have subtle, good or dramatic improvement. Results are affected by patients' factors (such as individual wound healing response, degree of skin laxity and photodamage, differences in skin thickness and underlying tissue) or by treatment technique or by the device used (RF or MFU).

Radiofrequency Skin Tightening

Radiofrequency (RF) devices for skin tightening include monopolar, bipolar, multipolar, multisource and fractional RF with or without microneedling. Monopolar RF utilises one "active" electrode and a "passive" return electrode. The current runs from the active electrode, through the body, and is returned at the return pad location. A bipolar RF device typically has two active electrodes, and no passive electrode. In a bipolar arrangement, the current flows back and forth between the two electrodes, and tissue is heated between and beneath the electrodes. The depth of heating is calculated as half the distance between the two electrodes. Multipolar RF utilises multiple electrodes to emit energy at various changing directions to allow for deeper as well as more superficial penetration of energy.

Fractional RF, similar to fractional laser, treats segments of the skin and soft tissue, leaving islands of untreated skin to increase safety and reduce recovery time. RF can be delivered through microneedles (RFMN), and this allows for heating at controlled depths and can be targeted to heat the subcutaneous fat, the reticular dermis and the surrounding tissue. The needles can be of various lengths to target different depths, can be insulated (to protect the epidermis) or non-insulated and vary in the numbers of pins per RF pulse [7, 8].

Newer RF devices are introduced recently. One has real-time impedance intelligence monitoring [9]. A "hands-free" bipolar RF device for face and neck contouring was introduced recently [10]. Another device treats large areas like the abdomen using multisource RF energy delivered through six electrodes arranged either in a linear or in a concentric pattern with each electrode connected to an independently controlled RF generator [11, 12]. New bipolar RF devices can be used for subdermal heating where one electrode is inserted into the subdermal plane and the other electrode held above the skin. The two electrodes are at a set distance with a current flowing between them [13]. A recent device combines RFMN with ultrasound imaging and mapping. This device offers a variety of frequency options along with insulated and non-insulated needles and the ability to treat to a depth of 4.0 mm (0.1 mm step) deep. The ultrasound imaging visualises the optimal needle depth and allows for personalised depth measurements.

Contraindications for RF Skin Tightening

Contraindications include patients with implanted devices such as pacemakers, internal defibrillators, cardio converters, prosthetic metal implants and electronic implanted device.

Mechanism of Action of RF

RF devices generate "resistive" heating for skin tightening as a result of tissue resistance to the movement of electrons within an RF field (Ohm's law). The RF electrode creates an electric field deep within the tissue which changes polarity or charge many times per second. The polarised electrons and negatively charged ions within the electric field are attracted and repelled at that same frequency. The tissue's natural resistance to this movement generates heat, the so-called resistive heating. RF devices do not depend on chromophores and hence are safe for use in all skin types. Skin tightening is modest, and there may be some contouring [14]. RFMN is able to penetrate deeper and gives better result than RF without microneedling.

RF Treatment

After assessing the treatment plan, the skin on the upper back is cleaned with alcohol and dried, and the entire return pad is placed in contact with the patient's skin. The upper back is chosen as this position delivers the optimal energy and also helps keep the pad in place. If RF treatment is needed around the eyelids, plastic eye shields must be inserted.

During treatment, ensure that there is an adequate layer of coupling gel. More gel is placed over bony areas. The handpiece is applied firmly and perpendicular to the treatment area, ensuring that there is full tip-to-skin contact, with all four corners of the tip in contact with the skin surface. Apply enough downward pressure to maintain full contact with the skin. In some devices where there is vibration, do not press too hard to impede the vibration. A footswitch or hand switch is used to deliver the RF energy. The handpiece is then moved to the adjacent area with no or some overlap depending on the RF device. Always re-position the skin, and pull in the direction of desired tissue contraction during the treatment passes. Usually, two passes are delivered over the entire treatment to ensure even heating of the skin. Additional passes are delivered along the vectors and on the problem areas. Multiple passes show better results than single pass, and multiple sessions give better results than a single session [15, 16].

During treatment, monitor the patient's response to heat and calibrate the temperature settings accordingly. Look for optimal endpoints like mild erythema and subtle oedema. Watch for persistent erythema, swelling or hives, and if they occur, reduce the RF energy.

RFMN Treatment

RFMN can be delivered in three modes: cycle mode, fixed mode and repetition mode. The cycle mode is when the needles penetrate the skin and retract from the skin with every pulse. The fixed mode is when the needles are inserted into the skin and energy is delivered when the footswitch is activated. The needles retract from the skin and energy stops once the footswitch is released. This can be employed for stacking of pulses when desired. The repetition mode can be a single pulse mode or auto repeated mode when pulses are delivered automatically with predetermined pulse repetition rate. In some machine as the needle is retracted, it can deliver RF energy at different depths with each pulse. RFMN is combined with bipolar RF to get better results without increased complications [8]. The RFMN allows for subdermal adipose remodelling and skin tightening, and the addition of bipolar RF tightens the skin by contraction of the underlying fibroseptal network.

The handpiece is applied firmly and perpendicular to the treatment area, and RF energy is delivered in single pulse. The handpiece is moved to the adjacent area usually with 20–50% overlap depending on the device. The handpiece should be completely released from the skin rather than sliding the needles to avoid abrasions. One to two additional pulses may be applied at the same site (stacking) in fixed mode. However, pulses should not be stacked over bony areas such as the forehead, periorbital or jawline. Minor pinpoint bleeding may be seen.

RFMN treatment may be applied to all skin types. It is important to start at a lower energy when treating dark Fitzpatrick skin types and increasing the energy gradually with each treatment. Higher RF energy can be applied to deeper treatment areas, and the energy is reduced by 20% when treating over bone or in off-face areas. Avoid pulse stacking when treating thin skin and over bony areas. Usually for the face treatment, needle depth may be 1–2 mm, while for the body treatment, the needle depth is usually 3–4 mm.

Post-treatment

Remove any coupling gel, and cool the skin immediately. A moisturiser and sunscreen are applied after the treatment. For RFMN, a topical antibiotic may be applied. Patient should avoid make-up for a week. The microneedle tracks usually close in 2–3 days.

Complications of RF Skin Tightening

Transient erythema is seen, and this usually resolves within a few hours. Localised heating may occur if the handpiece is held too long in contact with the skin for devices in motion. Superficial crusting is common after RFMN. Rare complications include burns, blisters, pigmentary changes and scarring. Post-treatment surface irregularities such as nodules or lumps are rare and are seen when treating over thin skin. They are felt rather than seen and usually resolve spontaneously. Post-treatment changes in skin sensation such as itchiness or numbness can occur when treating over the forehead, temple, preauricular region and jawline. They usually resolve in days or weeks. Indentations may occur due to overheating of fat lobules or fibrous septa or due to the incomplete removal of the topical anaesthetic.

Microfocused Ultrasound (MFU) for Skin Tightening

Microfocused ultrasound (MFU) devices for skin tightening use 0.4–1.2 J/mm^2 of energy. This energy can be focused on the skin and subcutaneous tissue producing small thermal coagulation points (TCPs) within the mid- and deep dermis, the superficial musculoaponeurotic system (SMAS) and the subcutaneous tissue [17, 18]. The TCPs are small (<1 mm^3) and discrete and are laid along a linear pattern. Most devices have transducers at 10.0 MHz, 7.0 MHz and 4.0 MHz with focal depths of 1.5 mm, 3.0 mm and 4.5 mm, respectively. The transducers deliver TCP which tighten skin and subcutaneous tissue at different depths. A study showed that using a single transducer at a single depth (10.0 MHz, 1.5 mm) is effective for superficial skin rejuvenation [19].

Most transducers deliver a single line of TCP. There is one device where several lines of TCP are laid down simultaneously at a single depth. Some transducers can deliver MFU beyond 5 mm to target the deeper abdominal fascia. There is one MFU device that combines MFU with high-resolution ultrasound imaging (MFU-V), which enables visualisation of tissue planes to a depth of 8 mm and allows the operator to visualise the depth of the TCP [20].

Mechanism of Action of MFU

MFU creates TCP which heats targeted tissues to 60–70 °C in discrete areas while sparing the adjacent non-target tissues [21, 22]. MFU-V devices allow for accurate localisation and the correct placement of the TCP on the SMAS, leading to contraction of the SMAS and skin tightening and lifting [23]. The heat causes localised denaturation and contraction of collagen. Over the next few months, there are neocollagenesis, elastogenesis and angiogenesis, which result in skin tightening and lifting of lax tissues. A systemic review on the efficacy of MFU on skin tightening showed that a single treatment improved skin tightening of various degrees in more than 90% of patients [24]. There is a long-term skin improvement up to 6–12 months. Numerous studies show that MFU can tighten lax skin in the lower face and neck [25, 26], infraorbital lax skin [27, 28], arms, thighs and knees [29]. Another study showed that MFU can improve the appearance of fine wrinkles [30].

MFU Treatment

An adequate layer of ultrasound gel is applied, and the selected transducer is placed upright on the skin. In MFU-V, there is accurate visualisation of the treatment depth and the presence of non-target tissues like the bone and blood vessel, allowing for more precise placement of the TCP. Ultrasound imaging also ensures proper coupling between the gel and the transducer. Multiple passes of TCP are applied per treatment to give better results [31]. A large prospective study showed that there were benefits in treating at two different depths using two different transducers [26] and varying the vector direction of the treatment lines and varying the energy levels [32]. The total number of TCP lines will depend on the severity of the skin laxity with 500–600 lines for mild laxity, 600–700 for moderate laxity and over 800 for more advanced laxity. Various protocols are available based on the devices and degree of skin laxity [32]. After the procedure, the coupling gel is removed, and the skin is checked for any welts, erythema or burns.

Complications of MFU

MFU is a safe treatment for skin laxity. The most common complaint is the pain during the procedure. This can be minimised by applying topical anaesthesia or taking analgesics or anti-inflammatory agents before the procedure. Some patients may require concomitant application of a cold air or a vibratory device during treatment. Less common side effects include transient erythema, oedema, bruising, an arching sensation at the treatment region and welts. Welts are uncommon and are often seen with the use of the superficial 1.5 mm transducers and with ineffective coupling of the ultrasound gel with the transducer. Normally, welts will subside spontaneously and do not require specific treatments. Rare complications had been reported, and they include post-inflammatory hyperpigmentation, muscle weakness and numbness [33–35].

Non-invasive Fat Reduction

Non-invasive fat reduction is a popular body contouring treatment. Four different technologies are used for fat reduction, and they are cryolipolysis, radiofrequency (RF), high-intensity ultrasound (HIFU) and lasers (infrared laser and low-level laser therapy LLLT). Most devices use either cooling or heating technology to induce adipose cell apoptosis. Other devices use non-thermal cavitation of adipose tissue and electroporation of fat cell membrane leading to apoptosis.

It is difficult to compare the effectiveness of the different technologies as the studies use different treatment protocols, treat different body locations and have different follow-up times and different outcome measures. In a review comparing the different studies and devices, evidence suggested that the different devices are safe and effective and the treatments have a high patients' satisfaction [36]. One difference between the devices is the time to achieve peak reduction of fat. This varies from immediately after treatment with LLLT (from immediate emptying of targeted adipocytes) to 4–8 weeks after cryolipolysis or HIFU (from apoptosis). Recurrence of fat deposition is greater after LLLT compared to cryolipolysis or HIFU as LLLT does not cause necrosis or apoptosis of adipocytes. LLLT requires multiple treatments, whereas the other devices can achieve fat reduction after a single treatment. Patients treated with cryolipolysis and RF have reported 70–100% satisfaction, while those treated with HIFU reported a lower satisfaction rate of below 60%.

Selection of Patients

Patients who will benefit from non-invasive fat reduction are those with localised pockets of subcutaneous fat. Patients should be in good health with a BMI of 22–28. Areas that can be treated include the submental area, abdomen, lumbar rolls, hip rolls/flanks, inner and outer thigh, inner arms, subaxillary area, brassiere rolls and male breast [37].

Treatment Plan and Assessment

On the day of the procedure, the patient's weight and baseline photographs in a 360-degree position are taken. When taking photos of the abdomen, patient's hand should be at 90-degree angle to the body with the hands resting on the elbows. When taking photos of the arms, the arms should be stretched out at right angles to the body.

In a standing position, the body is assessed globally, and all potential treatment areas identified. Identify areas for debulking or for sculpting. Debulking is ideal for large-volume reduction. Assess and create a customised treatment plan ensuring full coverage of treatable fat.

Management of Patient's Expectation

Results vary from patient to patient and from device to device. Generally, 23–27% fat reduction has been reported with each treatment. However, they do not give surgical results, and careful selection of patients is needed to avoid disappointment. Patients who are obese, patients with skin laxity or poor skin quality and those with cellulite will not benefit from these treatments. The treatments are for fat reduction and are not for customised body contouring.

Cryolipolysis for Fat Reduction

The development behind cryolipolysis arose from the clinical observation of cold-induced panniculitis in infants (popsicle panniculitis) and in adults (equestrian panniculitis) [38, 39]. These observations suggest that lipid-rich tissues are more susceptible to cold injury than the surrounding water-rich tissue. From these observations, in 2007, Manstein et al. introduced cryolipolysis, a non-invasive method for fat reduction with cooling [40]. In cryolipolysis, an applicator is applied with suction to the targeted fat area and is set at a specific cooling temperature for a preset period of time. This targets adipocytes while sparing the skin, nerves, vessels and muscles.

Cryolipolysis is shown to be safe and effective for non-invasive fat reduction [41, 42]. There is no significant impact on lipid levels or liver function tests [37, 43]. A systemic review of 19 studies with over 1500 patients reported significant fat reduction in multiple body areas ranging from 10.3% to 28.5% [37]. In two case studies, results were reported to be persistent and visible at 6 and 9 years post-treatment [44]. In a post-treatment patient satisfaction survey, cryolipolysis provided a high degree of patient satisfaction and recommendation rate [45]. Recent evidence suggests that cryolipolysis may stimulate collagen remodelling and tightens skin [46]. Other studies document visceral fat reduction by 16.2 cm^2 [47] and reduction of the cross-sectional area of visceral adipose tissue by 15.6% [48].

New applicators, treatment protocols, colder temperatures (−15 °C) and shorter treatment times (30 and 45 min) have improved the treatment efficacy [49, 50]. The new applicators have better shape to conform to the natural body curvatures, improve vacuum seal, increase the volume of tissue drawn, improve tissue contact as well as reduce pain for the patient [45]. Applicator cooling panels are equipped with thermistors to measure the temperature of the treated tissue. New devices are equipped with two arms to treat two areas simultaneously [45, 51].

Mechanism of Action of Cryolipolysis

Adipose cells are more susceptible to cold-induced injury compared to cells which are water-rich such as the skin, nerve and muscles. Crystallisation of adipose cells will occur at a higher temperature than the freezing point of water; hence, adipose cells are affected while the other cells are not. In cryolipolysis, heat is extracted from the tissue at the surface of the skin, cooling the fat to just above freezing. Within adipose cells, crystals are formed, and the fat cells undergo apoptosis within the first few days following treatment. As adipose cells die, they collapse, and macrophages digest and consume the dead cells and lipids. The natural inflammatory process clears the apoptotic cells and their contents through the lymphatic system, peaking at around 4 weeks. This removal process can take up to 3–4 months resulting in fat layer reduction [50].

Contraindication to Cryolipolysis

Cryolipolysis is contraindicated in people with cryoglobulinemia and paroxysmal cold haemoglobinuria [52]. It should be used with caution in people with cold-sensitive conditions such as Raynaud's syndrome, cold urticaria, severe varicose veins, dermatitis or loss of skin continuity due to prolonged exposure to the localised cold. It is not indicated for patients who are too obese or too thin, in people with loose skin and also in the presence of abdominal hernia.

Cryolipolysis Treatment

The treatment area is cleaned with alcohol and the gel pad applied. The correct applicator is placed on the treatment area followed by suction and cooling. As the cooling begins, the patient will feel intense cold, tingling, stinging, aching and cramping. These sensations will subside as the area becomes numb. Treatment time and protocol vary with the different devices. After the treatment, the applicator and gel pad are removed. The area is massaged for 2 min to manipulate the crystallised fat, and this improves treatment efficacy. Shock waves may be applied for a synergistic effect [53].

Post-treatment

In the days and weeks after treatment, the patient may experience redness, bruising, swelling tenderness, cramping and aching. Sensation of itching, skin sensitivity or numbness can last for a few weeks. These sensations are normal. Patients will see results between 1 and 3 months.

Side Effects of Cryolipolysis

In a systemic review of over 3300 patients, side effects of cryolipolysis are mild and transient. This includes erythema, bruising, oedema and paraesthesia [54]. Erythema is noted immediately after treatment and subsides within a week. This is likely due to the strength of the vacuum and the temperature at which the skin is kept for extended durations [55]. Vaso-vagal symptoms like dizziness, light-headedness, nausea, flushing, sweating and fainting may occur during or immediately after treatment [56]. A nerve biopsy taken at 3 months after treatment showed no long-term changes to nerve fibres, concluding that temperature and duration of cryolipolysis have no permanent effect on nervous tissue [57].

Incorrect assessment and placement of applicators may lead to demarcation, a visual step-off, unnatural results and a rippled look. First- or second-degree freeze burn may occur during treatment due to improper placement of the gel pad. It usually resolves without sequelae with proper care.

Subcutaneous induration, generalised hardness and/or discrete nodules have been reported, and this resolves spontaneously within 3–6 months. Late-onset pain typically begins 3–4 days after the treatment and resolves naturally, on average within several weeks.

Paradoxical adipose hyperplasia (PAH) is a rare and serious side effect, with an incidence estimated to be of 0.0051%, or approximately 1 in 20,000 [58]. It generally develops 4–5 months after treatment but may be seen as early as 2 months. The incidence has decreased by more than 75% with the use of newer applicators [59].

Radiofrequency for Fat Reduction

RF technology induces fat reduction by selective apoptosis of fat cells with minimal risk to the skin and dermal tissues [60]. The efficacy of these treatments depends on two factors: temperature achieved in the subcutaneous tissue and the length of time the tissue is exposed to the RF energy. Adipocytes heated to 42–45 °C and maintained at that temperature for a minimum of 15 min are forced into apoptosis and programmed cell death, leading to gentle denaturation of the membrane, release of contained lipids and reduction of fat volume.

Radiofrequency devices differ in frequencies (1–27 MHz) and voltages and also in their mode of delivery (contact or non-contact RF). Contact RF devices can be monopolar or bipolar/multipolar and operated hands free or hands held [60, 61]. Non-contact RF uses an RF applicator held 1 cm above the skin [62–64]. Some devices require a number of treatment sessions [62–64], while others require just one treatment to get the expected desired results [61]. Treatment time varies from 15 to 45 min to achieve apoptotic adipose threshold. Some devices have lower RF frequencies, which can stimulate collagen and tighten skin as well [61].

Newer devices combine RF with ultrasound technology for fat reduction. Others are multifunctional combining RF fat reduction with other body contouring capabilities like muscle toning.

Mechanism of Action of RF Fat Reduction

Radiofrequency (RF) utilises the resistance (impedance) of tissue to generate heat rather than directly transfer heat to the adipose tissue. In contact RF devices, the rapidly alternating RF current causes oscillation of cellular molecules that are in its path. This intermolecular motion and collisions in turn create thermal energy (Joule heating) caused by tissue reactivity [60, 65, 66]. Adipocytes have high tissue resistance and relatively low heat transfer coefficients. This allows adipocytes tissue to generate significant heat when the RF energy passes through and at the same time do not transfer significant heat to the surrounding tissues. The heat disrupts the adipocyte cell membrane and eventually leads to apoptosis of the adipocytes.

In non-contact RF devices, panels above the target tissue generate a rapidly oscillating and powerful electromagnetic field, known as RF field [62, 67]. The frequency of RF field devices is much higher at 27 MHz. At this frequency, Joule heating does not occur but dipole heating does; it is not tissue resistivity that is important, but tissue permittivity. Tissues with poor permittivity are selectively targeted by the RF field. Adipose tissue has poor permittivity compared with other tissues including the skin, nerves, blood vessels and muscles. The rapidly changing electromagnetic field causes vibrational and rotational changes within the adipocytes, generating kinetic energy and selectively heating them up to over the apoptotic threshold of 43 °C. This induces apoptosis and eventually programmed cell death.

Subsurface RF device is designed to heat adipose tissue and tighten the overlying skin. The subcutaneous tissue is heated to 65 °C while limiting the skin temperature to 40 °C. This device is aimed to fill the gap between patients who are not severe enough for liposuction but not mild enough for non-surgical skin tightening.

Contraindication

Patients with implanted devices such as pacemakers, defibrillators, cardio converters, cochlear implants and prosthetic metal implants are contraindicated. RF treatment should be deferred in patients with a recent history of abdominal cosmetic or surgical treatments, patients with skin infection or skin inflammation and in pregnant or lactating women.

Radiofrequency Fat Reduction Treatment

Patient is treated in the supine or prone position. The treatment area is identified and cleaned. This can be the abdomen, flanks, thighs, buttocks, arms or submental region. The return pads are placed on the back. The treatment procedure is different for contact or non-contact RF devices or subsurface RF treatment.

In **contact handheld devices**, the single RF applicator (with or without suction) is glided over the treatment area until the desired temperature and treatment duration are completed. It is then moved to the next area. The skin temperature is raised to 42–45 °C within a short time and is kept at between 43 and 44 °C, while the subcutaneous tissue temperature is at least 3–4 °C higher. This allows for deep volumetric heating of the tissue without damaging the epidermis. During treatment, the patient will rate the degree of heat and pain sensation. The temperature is raised and kept at the highest level that the patient can tolerate and must be at apoptotic level (43–44 °C skin temperature). Treatment time varies from 15 to 45 min depending on the different devices.

In **contact hand-free devices**, the temperature-controlled RF applicators are arranged and placed on the treatment areas, and multiple areas are treated simultaneously. Paired applicators are placed in parallel with up to a 1.0 cm separation gap between the applicators to ensure that the therapeutic temperature is maintained within the entire distance of the gap. Up to six RF applicators can be used at one time, arranged to match the patients' fat pocket distribution. The applicators are held in place by plastic wraps or a belt. In one device, the treatment time is 15 min, 4 min to reach the desired temperature and 10 min keeping the skin temperature at 42–45 °C. Most devices use continuous real-time monitoring to keep the skin temperature constant.

In **contactless RF devices**, the applicator has a slightly curved and large central fixed panel with two adjustable hinged wings at either end. This applicator is placed over the treatment area (usually 1 cm above), without touching the overlying skin, and the wings are adjusted to fit the contour of the abdomen, the flanks, the thighs or the arms. The skin temperature is raised and maintained between 42 and 45 °C. The skin must be kept dry during the procedure.

Post-treatment

After the treatment, the skin is examined for erythema and burns. The skin may feel warm for a short duration. A moisturiser is applied. Extracorporeal shock-wave therapy may be performed after the RF treatment to improve waist circumferential reduction in non-contact RF devices [68]. However, this has not been shown to be effective in contact RF devices. Fat reduction is seen after 6–8 weeks. Depending on the RF devices, treatments may be repeated at 3–4 weekly intervals for up to four to six sessions.

Side Effects

Side effects are mild and transient and include mild redness and temporary oedema. Thermal burns, bruises and cutaneous sensory changes or painful dysesthesia may occur [62]. Pain score varies from 2 to 4 out of 10 [69]. Paradoxical fat hyperplasia is uncommon but has been reported [70]. A systemic review of 30 publications on subsurface RF [71] showed that most patients experienced seromas, prolonged swelling and numbness. The most frequent complications were induration and nodules with several studies reporting marginal mandibular neuropraxia.

High-Intensity Focused Ultrasound for Fat Reduction

High-intensity focused ultrasound (HIFU) heats up adipose tissue in a focused mode without energy dispersion in the treated area. The temperature of adipose tissues is raised above 56 °C to cause apoptosis of adipocytes, without affecting the adjacent tissue [72]. The adipocyte membrane is broken, and triglycerides are released into the intercellular space, where free fatty acids are oxidised in the tissues that require energy or transported to the liver, where they are metabolised. There are numerous studies that investigate the clinical efficacy of HIFU for fat reduction [72–77]. However, the devices are different, the study protocols are different and not standardised and the study numbers are small. A literature review to investigate evidence-based efficacy of HIFU in aesthetic body contouring assigned the studies to level of evidence IV [78].

Mechanism of Action

Mechanism of action depends on whether it is a low-frequency or a high-frequency ultrasound device. Low-frequency devices cause non-thermal effect (cavitation), while high-frequency devices cause thermal necrosis of adipose tissue [79, 80].

Non-thermal focused ultrasound device induces cavitation and mechanical disruption of adipocytes. Pressure waves create vapour cavities in adipocytes, disrupting their cellular membranes to cause them to rupture. This is an acoustic, non-thermal mechanical effect, with no significant heating of tissues. The surrounding tissue, blood vessels and nerves are unharmed. Lower frequency ultrasound devices create cavitation more easily.

In **thermal necrosis of adipocytes**, ultrasound energy is focused at a controlled depth to induce vibrations of adipose tissue. This creates a localised temperature spike in adipose tissue above 56 °C, the thermal necrosis threshold with minimal cavitation. Irreversible fat death occurs after 1 second at 56 °C or higher. Adjacent adipose tissue not treated remains below the 56 °C threshold and is unaffected.

Both effects occur without causing damage to adjacent tissues. Most lipids and cellular debris are removed within 12 weeks after the procedure, with 95% removed within 18 weeks.

Contraindication

HIFU is contraindicated if the fat cannot be pinched or the amount pinched is less than 1 inch or 2.5 cm. It is also contraindicated if the fat layer is less than 1 cm beyond the focal depth of 1.3 cm. Patients with redundant skin folds or skin that folds or cannot lie flat during treatment are excluded from HIFU. Patient should have a body mass index of less than 30.

Treatment Procedure

The patient lies in the supine position. The treatment area is identified, cleaned and marked. For high-frequency devices, there must be adequate adipose tissue with 1.0 cm of fat tissue beyond the focal depth and at least 2.5 cm of pinchable fat. The ultrasound liquid is sprayed onto the treatment area. The ultrasound transducer is then placed on the treatment area and activated. This is then moved to the next adjacent area, and the process is continued till the whole area is treated.

Post-treatment

The treated area may have bruises and mild skin sensitivity, and these resolve within 2 weeks. There is a consistent reduction in abdominal circumference of at least 2 cm after a single treatment [80].

Side effects

Side effects are mild and transient and include ecchymosis, erythema, skin sensitivity and burns [81, 82]. Long-term follow-up safety data did not reveal dimpling, indurations, burns or scars.

Lasers for Fat Reduction

There are two groups of lasers for non-invasive fat reduction. The low-level laser therapy (LLLT) was approved by the FDA for fat reduction in 2010 [83], and the 1060 nm diode laser was approved in 2015 [84]. LLLT uses a single wavelength (635 nm) or a range of wavelengths to target fat cells through a non-thermal or photochemical (biostimulatory) reaction [85]. Results from LLLT vary depending on the devices used; some are reported as not effective under ultrasound assessment, while others have demonstrated good results [86–88]. The diode laser light at 1060 nm penetrates to the level of adipose tissue and is preferentially absorbed by adipocytes [89]. Results after the diode laser are seen after a single treatment and demonstrate equivalent reduction in fat thickness compared with cryolipolysis [89].

Contraindications

Generally, there are no specific contraindications to laser fat reduction. It can be done in the absence of pinchable fat. It has been used to treat post-liposuction deformities [90]. Fat deposition has a tendency to recur after LLLT, and hence it is not for someone who is looking for a more permanent result.

Mechanism of Action

LLLT creates pores in the adipocyte cell membrane, allowing for lipid leakage and without inducing lipolysis or cell lysis. Transitory micropores were visualised on scanning electron microscopy. It was proposed that up to 99% of fat could be released from the adipocytes when treated with a 635–680 nm LLLT for a period of 6 min [87]. However, this mechanism of action remains somewhat controversial as other authors fail to demonstrate any transitory micropores [91, 92].

A more recent study suggests that LLLT targets the mitochondrion, specifically, cytochrome c oxidase, a photo acceptor. There is photoexcitation of cytochrome c oxidase through a series of reactions called the photo signal transduction. This results in a transient pore in the bi-lipid membrane of adipose cell allowing triglycerides and fatty acids to move into the interstitial space. The excess fat is then eliminated through the body.

The 1060 nm laser preferentially targets adipose tissue, heating cells to a controlled temperature between 42 and 45 °C and, along with surface cooling, protects the overlying skin and other surrounding cells. Within 5 min of heat application, there is structural damage to the adipocytes. Histologic studies showed inflammatory response gradually progressing up to a month and lasting up to 6 months. The body's immune response eliminates the cellular debris over the course of 6–8 weeks.

Treatment Procedure

Patient lies supine or prone with the treatment area exposed. Eyes are protected by safety goggles.

Using **LLLT**, the laser head is placed on the treatment area. Usually, each head will have multiple diode lasers which emit red light. The laser is activated for 10 min for each treatment position. Patient will need multiple treatments, usually 2–3 times a week over 2–3 weeks.

Using **the 1060 nm laser**, a belt with frames that hold the laser diodes in place is affixed to the treatment area with straps and clips. The belt can hold four diodes at a time. In smaller patients, only two diodes are utilised. The diode energy is distributed over the surface of the applicator's treatment window, keeping the energy density uniform. There is an immediate cooling and gradual warming in the treatment area for the first 4 min and then an interchange between heating and cooling sensations for the next 21 min. Active treatment time is 25 min, and the procedure is well tolerated with no downtime.

In another device, each applicator contains a water-cooled window for contact tissue cooling to prevent the skin from overheating and four touch sensors to ensure proper placement and contact during laser emission.

Post-treatment

After laser treatment, the skin is examined for bruises, burn, erythema, oedema, purpura and nodules. Rarely, nodules may be felt or seen, and these can be improved with massages. LLLT shows the earliest peak results, sometimes immediately after treatment. However, as LLLT causes neither necrosis nor apoptosis of the adipocytes, fat deposition has a tendency to recur [93].

Side Effects

Side effects are mild and related to the heat from the laser [94, 95]. The most commonly reported side effect is transient tenderness. Nodules have been reported, and they are self-limiting [96].

Muscle Stimulation and Definition

Body sculpting is becoming increasingly popular as a non-invasive body contouring procedure. Neuromuscular electrical stimulation has been used for therapeutic indications during muscle injury to prevent muscle atrophy and to strengthen skeletal muscles. It has been shown to increase the strength of athletes by 30–40% when used as an adjunct to traditional exercise [97]. Recently, these muscle stimulation technologies have been applied for aesthetic use.

Muscle stimulating devices use either electromagnetic muscle stimulation (EMMS) or electrical multidirectional muscle stimulation (EMDS). In 2018, the FDA approved the high-intensity focused electromagnetic field (HIFEM) for buttock and abdomen remodelling. Since then, newer devices have been FDA-cleared for strengthening, toning and firming the muscles of the abdomen, buttocks and thighs. These devices induce supramaximal involuntary contractions that cause muscle hypertrophy, increase in muscle strength and improvement in muscle tone [98–100]. Data suggested that there is a reduction of subcutaneous fat [101] and also visceral adipose tissue [102]. A further advantage of muscle stimulation is a reduction in the distance between the large abdominal muscles. One prospective study in ten HIFEM-treated postpartum women found an average 16.7%, 22.7% and 23.2% reduction in abdominal separation at 1, 3 and 6 months and a 46% reduction 1 year after HIFEM treatments [103, 104].

EMMS devices are used together with other fat reduction devices, or targeted pressure or microwave energy for fat reduction and improving skin laxity leading to a significant improvement in muscle tissue thickness and tone [105–109]. The simultaneous use of HIFEM and RF not only treats muscle and subcutaneous fat [100] but has been shown to be more effective for muscle contouring than HIFEM alone, level of evidence 2 [111].

Selection of Patients

Studies show that muscle stimulating devices will benefit all patients regardless of BMI. Patients reported high satisfaction rate and good experience [100, 112]. However, those with a normal BMI have shown better response in adipose tissue reduction and improvement in diastasis recti [113]. Patients with an overweight BMI might have reduced efficacy due to the intervening adipose tissue, which increases the distance between the machine and the muscles. Despite this, patients with a greater BMI still report high treatment satisfaction. A cohort of 22 patients with an overweight BMI (25–30 kg/m^2) reported the largest improvement in body satisfaction scores after abdominal EMMS treatment [100].

Mechanism of Action

EMMS induces alternating low-frequency (3–5 Hz) magnetic waves that directly depolarise skeletal muscle motor neurons. This stimulates high-intensity involuntary muscle contractions (supramaximal muscle contraction) that far exceed capabilities of voluntary muscle contraction, resulting in muscle fibre hypertrophy. HIFEM has also been shown to reduce adipose tissue despite the electromagnetic waves having no direct effect on fat. Recent data suggests that fat reduction may be metabolically driven, due to endoplasmic reticulum (ER) stress-mediated apoptosis of adipocytes because of the increased metabolic demand state that HIFEM induces [113]. This increased energy demand depletes existing glycogen stores; thus, the body switches to adipose tissue as the energy source.

The effect on muscle hypertrophy may be further promoted when heated with RF up to 40 °C [110]. The RF increases blood circulation within the targeted muscle tissue and enhances muscle tissue regeneration. There is no dissipation of thermal energy to surrounding tissue.

EMDS generates electrical impulses leading to depolarisation and initiation of the action potential at the skeletal muscle level. This triggers rapid and sustained supramaximal contractions, resulting in muscle hypertrophy.

Treatment Procedure

The patient is treated in the supine or prone position. The applicator or applicators are positioned over the targeted muscles and fixated by a belt or plastic wrap. In **MMS device**, the initial stimulation intensity is set according to the patient's tolerance threshold and was further increased during the treatment based on the patient's feedback. In **EMDS device**, three operation modes (Prep, Tone and Sculpt) are applied sequentially, with the intensity being independently adjusted for each operational mode. No anaesthesia is required. Four treatment sessions are required over a 2-week period, with no consecutive treatment days.

Post-treatment

There is no post-treatment protocol. Muscle hypertrophy and fat reduction are seen as early as 1 month post-treatment, and peak efficacy extends beyond the treatment period. Improvements beyond baseline extend up to 6 months, with a small decrease in efficacy at 1 year [103, 104].

Side Effects

The most commonly reported side effects included mild muscle fatigue and soreness after treatment that resolved within 48 h of treatment [114, 115]. There were no reported instances of rhabdomyolysis or kidney injury. Most procedures have minimal or no pain.

Summary

Non-invasive body contouring procedures have increased dramatically in recent years. The common procedures include skin tightening, non-invasive fat reduction and muscle stimulation and definition. Most patients will undergo combination treatments rather than stand-alone treatments. To date, large blinded randomised controlled studies are lacking. However, current studies suggest that these procedures are effective and safe.

References

1. Mazzoni D, Lin MJ, Dubin DP, et al. Review of non-invasive body contouring devices for fat reduction, skin tightening and muscle definition. Australas J Dermatol. 2019;60:278–83.
2. Pritzker RN, Hamilton HK, Dover JS. Comparison of different technologies for noninvasive skin tightening. J Cosmet Dermatol. 2014;13:315–23.
3. Kwan KR, Kolansky Z, Abittan BJ. Skin tightening. Cutis. 2020;106:134–7.
4. Bonjorno AR, Gomes TB, Pereira MC, et al. Radiofrequency therapy in esthetic dermatology: a review of clinical evidences. J Cosmet Dermatol. 2020;19(2):278–81.
5. Boen M, Vanaman Wilson MJ, Fabi S, et al. Skin tightening- does it really exist? Semin Cutan Med Surg. 2017;36(4):202–6.
6. Northington M. Patient selection for skin-tightening procedures. J Cosmet Dermatol. 2014;13(3):208–11.
7. McDaniel D, Weiss R, Weiss M, et al. Two-treatment protocol for skin laxity using 90-watt dynamic monopolar radiofrequency device with real-time impedance intelligence monitoring. J Drugs Dermatol. 2014;13(9):1112–7.
8. Kauvar ANB, Gershonowitz A. Clinical and histologic evaluation of a fractional radiofrequency treatment of wrinkles and skin texture with novel 1-mm long ultra-thin electrode pins. Lasers Surg Med. 2022;54(1):54–61.
9. Dayan E, Chia C, Burns AJ, et al. Adjustable depth fractional radiofrequency combined with bipolar radiofrequency: a minimally invasive combination treatment for skin laxity. Aesthet Surg J. 2019;39(Suppl 3):S112–9.
10. Labadie JG, Chilukuri S, Cohen J, et al. Noninvasive hands-free bipolar radiofrequency facial remodeling device for the improvement of skin appearance. Dermatologic Surg. 2023;49(1):54–9.
11. Tanaka Y. Skin tightening following multisource, phase controlled radiofrequency treatments with novel unique concentric electrodes in Asian patients. J Clin Aesthet Dermatol. 2019;12:E58–63.
12. Rousseaux I, Robson S. Body contouring and skin tightening using a unique novel multisource radiofrequency energy delivery method. J Clin Aesthet Dermatol. 2017;10(4):24–9.
13. Dayan E, Chapas A, Marte J, et al. A prospective trial: handsfree thermoregulated bipolar radiofrequency for face and neck contouring. Plast Reconstr Surg Glob Open. 2022;10:e4194.
14. El-Domyati M, El-Ammawi TS, Medhat W, et al. Radiofrequency facial rejuvenation: evidence-based effect. J Am Acad Dermatol. 2011;64(3):524–35.
15. Jacobson LG, Alexiades-Armenakas M, Bernstein L, et al. Treatment of nasolabial folds and jowls with a noninvasive radiofrequency device. Arch Dermatol. 2003;139:1371–2.
16. Sukal SA, Geronemus RG. Thermage: the nonablative radio-frequency for rejuvenation. Clin Dermatol. 2008;26:602–7.
17. Minkis K, Alam M. Ultrasound skin tightening. Dermatol Clin. 2014;32(1):71–7.
18. Gliklich RE, White WM, Slayton MH, Barthe PG, Makin IR. Clinical pilot study of intense ultrasound

therapy to deep dermal facial skin and subcutaneous tissues. Arch Facial Plast Surg. 2007;9:88–95.
19. Lowe S. Single treatment, single depth superficial micro focused ultrasound with visualisation for rhytid improvement. Plast Reconstr Surg Global Open. 2021;9(7):e3662.
20. Fabi SG. Non-invasive skin tightening: focus on new ultrasound techniques. Clin Cosmet Investig Dermatol. 2015;8:47–52.
21. White WM, Makin IR, Barthe PG, Slayton MH, Gliklich RE. Selective creation of thermal injury zones in the superficial musculoaponeurotic system using intense ultrasound therapy: a new target for noninvasive facial rejuvenation. Arch Facial Plast Surg. 2007;9:22–9.
22. Laubach HJ, Makin IR, Barthe PG, Slayton MH, Manstein D. Intense focused ultrasound: evaluation of a new treatment modality for precise microcoagulation within the skin. Dermatol Surg. 2008;34:727–34.
23. Fabi SG. Microfocused ultrasound with visualization for skin tightening and lifting: my experience and a review of the literature. Dermatol Surg. 2014;40:S164–7.
24. Contini M, Hollander MHJ, Vissink A, et al. A systemic review of the efficacy of microfocused ultrasound for facial skin tightening. Int J Environ Res Public Health. 2033;20(2):1522.
25. Fabi SG, Goldman MP. Retrospective evaluation of micro-focused ultrasound for lifting and tightening the face and neck. Dermatol Surg. 2014;40(5):569–75.
26. Oni G, Hoxworth R, Teotia S, Brown S, Kenkel JM. Evaluation of a microfocused ultrasound system for improving skin laxity and tightening in the lower face. Aesthet Surg J. 2014;34(7):1099–110.
27. Suh DH, Oh YJ, Lee SJ, et al. A intense-focused ultrasound tightening for the treatment of infraorbital laxity. J Cosmet Laser Ther. 2012;14:290–5.
28. Pak CS, Lee YK, Jeong JH, Kim JH, Seo JD, Heo CY. Safety and efficacy of ulthera in the rejuvenation of aging lower eyelids: a pivotal clinical trial. Aesthet Plast Surg. 2014;38(5):861–8.
29. Alster TS, Tanzi EL. Noninvasive lifting of arm, thigh, and knee skin with transcutaneous intense focused ultrasound. Dermatol Surg. 2012;38:754–9.
30. Dayan SH, Fabi SG, Goldman MP, Kilmer SL, Gold MH. Prospective, multi-center, pivotal trial evaluating the safety and effectiveness of micro-focused ultrasound with visualization (MFU-V) for improvement in lines and wrinkles of the dĕcolletage. Plast Reconstr Surg. 2014;134(4 Suppl 1):123–4.
31. Lee HS, Jang WS, Cha YJ, et al. Multiple pass ultrasound tightening of skin laxity of the lower face and neck. Dermatol Surg. 2012;38:20–7.
32. Park JY, Lin F, Suwanchinda A, et al. Customised treatment using microfocused ultrasound with visualisation for optimised patient outcomes: a review of skin tightening energy technologies and a pan-Asian adaptation of the experts' panel's gold standard consensus. J Clin Aesthet Dermatol. 2021;14(5):E70–9.
33. Sasaki GH, Tevez A. Clinical efficacy and safety of focused-image ultrasonography: a 2-year experience. Aesthet Surg J. 2012;32:601–12.
34. Suh DH, Shin MK, Lee SJ, et al. Intense focused ultrasound tightening in Asian skin: clinical and pathologic results. Dermatol Surg. 2011;37:1595–602.
35. Jeong KH, Suh DH, Shin MK, Lee SJ. Neurologic complication associated with intense focused ultrasound. J Cosmet Laser Ther. 2013;16:43–4.
36. Kennedy J, Verne S, Griffith R, et al. Non-invasive subcutaneous fat reduction: a review. J Eur Acad Dermatol Venereol. 2015;29(9):1679–88.
37. Ingargiola MJ, Motakef S, Chung MT, et al. Cryolipolysis for fat reduction and body contouring: safety and efficacy of current treatment paradigms. Plast Reconstr Surg. 2015;135(6):1581–90.
38. Duncan WC, Freeman RG, Heaton CL. Cold panniculitis. Arch Dermatol. 1966;94:722–4.
39. Epstein EH Jr, Oren ME. Popsicle panniculitis. N Engl J Med. 1970;282:966–7.
40. Manstein D, Laubach H, Watanabe K, et al. Selective cryolysis: a novel method of non-invasive fat removal. Lasers Surg Med. 2008;40:595–604.
41. Avram MM, Harry RS. Cryolipolyis for subcutaneous fat layer reduction. Lasers Surg Med. 2009;41:703–8.
42. Kim J, Kim DH, Ryu HJ. Clinical effectiveness of non-invasive selective cryolipolysis. Cosmet Laser Ther. 2014;16(5):209–13.
43. Klein KB, Zelickson B, Riopelle JG, et al. Non-invasive cryolipolysis for subcutaneous fat reduction does not affect serum lipid levels or liver function tests. Lasers Surg Med. 2009;41:785–90.
44. Bernstein EF. Long term efficacy follow-up on two cryolipolysis case studies 6 and 9 years post treatment. J Cos Dermatol. 2016;15(4):561–4.
45. Altmann J, Jehle F, Mang W Patient satisfaction, recommendation rate and patient comfort with an FDA-Cleared cryolipolysis system, Aesthetic Surg J Open Forum 2022;4:ojac067.
46. Stevens WG, Gould DJ, Pham LD, et al. Molecular and histological evidence detailing clinically observed skin improvement following cryolipolysis. Aesthet Surg J. 2022;42(1):56–67.
47. Lee D, Lee K. Abdominal fat reduction through cryolipolysis. J Biosci Med. 2018;6(1):44–52.
48. Hwang IC, Kim KK, Lee KR. Cryolipolysis-induced abdominal fat change: split-body trails. PLoS One. 2020;120:e0242782.
49. Bernstein EF, Bloom JD, Basilavecchio LD, et al. Non-invasive fat reduction of the flanks using a new cryolipolysis applicator and overlapping two-cycle treatments. Lasers Surg Med. 2014;46(10):731–5.
50. Silva HL, Hernandez EC, Vazquez MG, et al. Non-invasive submental fat reduction using colder cryolipolysis. J Cosmet Dermatol. 2017;16:460–5.
51. Urdiales CF, Ruiz LC, Soria JM, et al. Assessing the efficacy of cryoadipolysis with the cooltech system: case study. EJMI. 2020;4(1):126–33.

52. Meyer PF, Costa e Silva JD, de Vasconcellos LS, et al. Cryolipolysis: patient selection and special consideration. Clin Cos Invest Dermatol. 2018;11:499–503.
53. Ferraro GA, De Francesco F, Cataldo C, et al. Synergistic effects of cryolipolysis and shock waves for non-invasive body contouring. Aesthet Plast Surg. 2012;36:666–79.
54. Hedayati B, Juhasz M, Chu M, et al. Adverse events associated with cryolypolysis: a systemic review of the literature. Dermatol Surg. 2020;46(Suppl 1):S8–S13.
55. Dierickx CC, Mazer JM, Sand M, et al. Safety, tolerance, and patient satisfaction with non-invasive cryolipolysis. Dermatol Surg. 2013;39:1209–16.
56. Garibyan L, Cornelissen L, Sipprell W, et al. Transient alterations of cutaneous sensory nerve function by non-invasive cryolipolysis. J Invest Dermatol. 2015;135(11):2623–31.
57. Coleman SR, Sachdeva K, Egbert BM, et al. Clinical efficacy of non-invasive cryolipolysis and its effects on peripheral nerves. Aesthet Plast Surg. 2009;33:482–8.
58. Jalian HR, Avram MM, Garibyan L, et al. Paradoxical adipose hyperplasia after cryolipolysis. JAMA Dermatol. 2014;150:317–9.
59. Nikolis A, Enright KM. A multicentre evaluation of paradoxical adipose hyperplasia following cryolipolysis for fat reduction and body contouring. A review of 8658 cycles in 2114 patients. Aesthet Surg J. 2021;41(8):932–41.
60. Boisnic S, Divaris M, Nelson AA, et al. A clinical and biological evaluation of a novel, non-invasive radiofrequency device for the long-term reduction of adipose tissue. Lasers Surg Med. 2014;46:94–103.
61. Somenek MT, Ronan SJ, Pittman TA. A multisite single-blinded, prospective pilot trial for non-invasive fat reduction of the abdomen and flanks using a monopolar 2 MHz radiofrequency device. Lasers Surg Med. 2021;53(3):337–43.
62. Choi SY, Kim YJ, Kim SY, et al. Improvement in abdominal and flank contouring by a novel adipocyte-selective non-contact radiofrequency device. Lasers Surg Med. 2018;50:738–44.
63. Qin J, Guo ME, Xu XG, et al. A clinical evaluation of non-invasive and contactless radiofrequency technique in the treatment of abdominal fat. J Cosmet Dermatol. 2021;20(9):2765–8.
64. Moradi A, Palm M. Selective non-contact field radiofrequency extended treatment protocol: evaluation of safety and efficacy. J Drugs Dermatol. 2015;14(90):982–5.
65. Weiss R, Weiss M, Beasley K, et al. Operator independent focused high frequency ISM band for fat reduction: porcine model. Lasers Surg Med. 2013;45(4):235–9.
66. Franco W, Kothare A, Ronan SJ, et al. Hyperthermic injury to adipocyte cells by selective heating of subcutaneous fat with a novel radiofrequency device: feasibility studies. Lasers Surg Med. 2010;42(5):361–70.
67. Goo B, Kim DS. Impact of contactless apoptosis-inducing RF on temperature of human skin surface and subcutaneous layer as well as porcine histology: a pilot study. Med Laser. 2016;5(1):29–31.
68. Kim H. The combination of extracorporeal shock wave therapy and noncontact apoptosis-inducing radiofrequency achieved significant waist circumferential reduction: a pilot study. Laser Ther. 2017;26(2):129–36.
69. Taub A, Bartholomeusz J. Ultrasound evaluation of a single treatment with a temperature controlled multifrequency monopolar radio frequency device for the improvement of localized adiposity on the abdomen and flanks. J Drugs Dermatol. 2020;19(1):28–34.
70. Agochukwu-Nwubah N, Mentz H. Paradoxical adipose hyperplasia after non-invasive radiofrequency treatment: a novel report and review. J Cosmet Dermatol. 2020;19:866–8.
71. Swanson E. A systemic review of subsurface radiofrequency treatments in plastic surgery. Ann Plast Surg. 2022;89(3):274–85.
72. Haar GT, Coussios C. High intensity focused ultrasound: physical principles and devices. Int J Hyperth. 2007;23:89–104.
73. Fatemi A, Kane MA. High-intensity focused ultrasound effectively reduces waist circumference by ablating adipose tissue from the abdomen and flanks: a retrospective case series. Aesthet Plast Surg. 2010;34:577–82.
74. Jewell ML, Solish NJ, Desilets CS. Non-invasive body sculpting technologies with an emphasis on high-intensity focused ultrasound. Aesthet Plast Surg. 2011;35(5):901–12.
75. Wilkerson EC, Bloom BS, Goldberg DJ. Clinical study to evaluate the performance of a non-invasive focused ultrasound device for thigh fat and circumference reduction compared to control. J Cosmet Dermatol. 2018;17:157–61.
76. Coleman WP 3rd, Coleman W 4th, Weiss RA, et al. A multicenter controlled study to evaluate multiple treatments with nonthermal focused ultrasound for non-invasive fat reduction. Dermatol Surg. 2017;43:50–7.
77. Gold MH, Coleman WP IV, Coleman W II, et al. A randomized, controlled multicenter study evaluating focused ultrasound treatment for fat reduction in the flanks. J Cosmet Laser Ther. 2019;21(1):44–8.
78. Atiyeh BS, Chahine F. Evidence-based efficacy of high-intensity focused ultrasound (HIFU) in aesthetic body contouring. Aesthetic Plast Surg. 2021;45(2):570–8.
79. Jewell ML, Desilets C, Smoller BR. Evaluation of a novel high-intensity focused ultrasound device: preclinical studies in a porcine model. Aesthet Surg J. 2011;31:429–34.
80. Kyriakou Z, Corral-Baques MI, Amat A, et al. HIFU-induced cavitation and heating in ex vivo porcine subcutaneous fat. Ultrasound Med Biol. 2011;37:568–79.

81. Gadsden E, Aguilar MT, Smoller BR, et al. Evaluation of a novel high-intensity focused ultrasound device for ablating subcutaneous adipose tissue for non-invasive body contouring: safety studies in human volunteers. Aesthet Surg J. 2011;31(4):401–10.
82. Guth F, Bitencourt S, Bedinot C, et al. Immediate effect and safety of HIFU single treatment for male subcutaneous fat reduction. J Cosmet Dermatol. 2017;17:385–9.
83. Jackson RF, Dedo DD, Roche GC, et al. Low-level laser therapy as a non-invasive approach for body contouring: a randomized, controlled study. Lasers Surg Med. 2009;41:799–809.
84. Schilling L, Saedi N, Weiss R. 1060 nm diode hyperthermic laser lipolysis: the latest in non-invasive body contouring. J Drugs Dermatol. 2017;16(1):48–52.
85. Karu T. Photobiological fundamentals of low power laser therapy. IEEE J Quantum Electron. 1987;23:1703–18.
86. Courtney ML, Elm BS, Irmina D, et al. Efficacy of a multiple diode laser system for body contouring. Lasers Surg Med. 2011;43:114–21.
87. Caruso-Davis MK, Guillot TS, Podichetty VK, et al. Efficacy of low-level laser therapy for body contouring and spot fat reduction. Obes Surg. 2011;21(6):722–9.
88. Nestor MS, Zarraga MB, Park H. Effect of 635 nm low-level laser therapy on upper arm circumference reduction: a double-blind, randomized, sham-controlled trial. J Clin Aesthet Dermatol. 2012;5(2):42–8.
89. Decorato JW, Chen B, Sierra R. Subcutaneous adipose tissue response to a non-invasive hyperthermic treatment using a 1060 nm laser. Lasers Surg Med. 2017;49(5):480–9.
90. Petti C, Stoneburner J. Clinical study to assess the 1,060 nm diode laser for the treatment of post-liposuction deformities. Lasers Surg Med. 2019;51(9):785–9.
91. Neira R, Arroyave J, Ramirez H, et al. Fat liquefaction: effect of low-level laser energy on adipose tissue. Plast Reconstr Surg. 2002;110:912–22.
92. Brown SA, Rohrich RJ, Kenkel J, et al. Effect of low-level laser therapy on abdominal adipocytes before lipoplasty procedures. Plast Reconstr Surg. 2004;113(6):1796–804.
93. Avci P, Nyame TT, Gupta GK, Sadasiyam M, et al. Low-level laser therapy for fat layer reduction: a comprehensive review. Lasers Surg Med. 2013;45(6):349–57.
94. Bass LS, Doherty ST. Safety and efficacy of a non-invasive 1060 nm diode laser for fat reduction of the abdomen. Drugs Dermatol. 2018;17(1):106–12.
95. Katz B, Doherty S. Safety and efficacy of a non-invasive 1,060-nm diode laser for fat reduction of the flanks. Dermatol Surg. 2018;44(3):388–96.
96. Kislevitz M, Wamsley C, Kang A, et al. Clinical evaluation of the safety and efficacy of a 1060-nm diode laser for non-invasive fat reduction of the abdomen. Aesthet Surg J. 2021;41(10):1155–65.
97. Porcari J, Ryskey A, Foster C. The effects of high intensity neuromuscular electrical stimulation on abdominal strength and endurance, core strength, abdominal girth, and perceived body shape and satisfaction. Int J Kinesiol Sports Sci. 2018;6(1):19.
98. Rambhia PH, Turner L, Ugonabo N, et al. Muscle stimulation for aesthetic body shaping: a comprehensive and critical review. Dermatol Surg. 2022;48(10):1076–82.
99. Laughman RK, Youdas JW, Garrett TR, et al. Strength changes in the normal quadriceps femoris muscle as a result of electrical stimulation. Phys Ther. 1983;63:494–9.
100. Fabi S, Dover JS, Tanzi E, Bowes LE, Tsai FUF, Odusan A. A 12-week, prospective, non-comparative, non-randomized study of magnetic muscle stimulation for improvement of body satisfaction with the abdomen and buttocks. Lasers Surg Med. 2020;53(1):79–88.
101. Katz B, Bard R, Goldfarb R, Shiloh A, Kenolova D. Ultrasound assessment of subcutaneous abdominal fat thickness after treatments with a high-intensity focused electromagnetic field device: a multicenter study. Dermatol Surg. 2019;45(12):1542–8.
102. Kent DE, Kinney BM. The effect of high-intensity focused electromagnetic procedure on visceral adipose tissue: retrospective assessment of computed tomography scans. J Cosmet Dermatol. 2021;20:757–62.
103. Kinney BM, Kent DE. MRI and CT assessment of abdominal tissue composition in patients after high-intensity focused electromagnetic therapy treatments: one-year follow-up. Aesthet Surg J. 2020;40(12):NP686–93.
104. Jacob CI, Rank B. Abdominal remodeling in postpartum women by using a high-intensity focused electromagnetic (HIFEM) procedure: an investigational magnetic resonance imaging (MRI) pilot study. J Clin Aesthet Dermatol. 2020;13:S16–20.
105. Kilmer SL, Cox SE, Zelickson BD, et al. Feasibility study of electromagnetic muscle stimulation and cryolipolysis for abdominal contouring. Dermatol Surg. 2020;46(Suppl 1):S14–21.
106. Jacob C, Kent D, Ibrahim O. Efficacy and safety of simultaneous application of HIFEM and synchronized radiofrequency for abdominal fat reduction and muscle toning: a multicenter magnetic resonance imaging evaluation study. Dermatol Surg. 2021;47:969–73.
107. Nistico SP, Bonan P, Coli F, et al. A new protocol to treat abdominal subcutaneous fat combining microwaves and flat magnetic stimulation. Bioengineering. 2022;9(5):182.
108. Duncan DI, Busso M. Effectiveness of combined use of targeted pressure energy, radiofrequency, and high-intensity focused electromagnetic fields to improve skin quality and appearance of fat and

muscle tissue in different body parts. J Cosmetic Dermatol. 2023;22:200–5.
109. Manuskiatti W, Nanchaipruek Y, Gervasio M, et al. Combination of monopolar 2 MHZ radiofrequency and electrical multidirectional stimulation for reducing abdominal circumference and enhancing the muscle definition in subjects with overweight range body mass index. Lasers Surg Med. 2022;54:1198–206.
110. Jacob C, Weiss R. Simultaneous HIFEM and synchronised RF procedure can be effectively used for increasing muscle mass and decreasing fat in the upper arm. J Clin Aesthet Dermatol. 2023;16(2):50–4.
111. DiBernardo B, Chilukuri S, McCoy JD, et al. High-intensity focused electromagnetic filed with synchronised radiofrequency achieves superior gluteal muscle contouring than high-intensity focused electromagnetic filed procedure alone. Aesthet Surg J Open Forum. 2023;5:ojac087.
112. Moradi A, Fabi S, Rapaport D, et al. Electromagnetic muscle stimulation: a retrospective study of patient experience. J Cosmet Dermatol. 2022;21(10):271–8.
113. Halaas Y, Bernardy J. Mechanism of nonthermal induction of apoptosis by high-intensity focused electromagnetic procedure: biochemical investigation in a porcine model. J Cosmet Dermatol. 2020;19:605–11.
114. Kinney BM, Lozanova P. High intensity focused electromagnetic therapy evaluated by magnetic resonance imaging: safety and efficacy study of a dual tissue effect based non-invasive abdominal body shaping. Lasers Surg Med. 2019;51:40–6.
115. Jacob C, Kinney B, Busso M, et al. High intensity focused electromagnetic technology (HIFEM) non-invasive buttock lifting and toning of gluteal muscles: a multi-center efficacy and safety study. J Drugs Dermatol. 2018;17(11):1229–32.

7 Laser- and IPL-Assisted Hair Reduction

Shi Yu Derek Lim and Suzanne Wei Na Cheng

Introduction

The presence of excessive, unwanted hair can be seen across a spectrum of disorders, as well as in physiologically normal individuals. Women with unwanted facial hair find it psychologically distressing, and the condition imposes a significant drain on their time and emotions [1]. Methods of removing undesired hair include laser-assisted hair reduction, electrolysis, waxing, threading, and depilatory creams.

Laser hair reduction functions based on the extended theory of selective photothermolysis [2]. Irradiation by the laser targets eumelanin within the hair bulb. Heat is subsequently transferred to the follicular stem cells in the bulge of the outer root sheath, destroying the stem cells and thus leading to hair reduction. The highest amount of the target chromophore, melanin, is found in hair follicles in anagen. As such, they are most prone to thermal damage during laser hair reduction [3].

The concept of laser hair "removal" is a misnomer, as no laser is able to permanently remove all unwanted hairs, but only results in a reduction in the number of hairs. Repeated treatment sessions are required for satisfactory hair reduction as only a proportion of hairs are in anagen at any timepoint—this ranges from 42–51% in the limbs to 85% in the scalp [4]. Light-coloured hairs and darker skin phototypes pose the main challenges to laser hair reduction, as lighter hairs contain less melanin to be targeted during the process, and darker skin contains more melanin which is prone to absorbing thermal energy during treatments, leading to undesirable erythema, burns, blisters, and pigmentary changes.

Indications

The indications for laser hair reduction may be categorized as such:

- Aesthetically undesirable hair
- Becker's naevus and other naevoid conditions with excess hair
- Hirsutism
- Hypertrichosis
- Reduction of hair on skin grafts, flaps, and peristomal areas [5, 6]
- Gender-affirming interventions [7]
- Treatment of conditions due to inflammation or occlusion of hair follicles, including dissecting cellulitis, folliculitis decalvans, acne keloidalis nuchae, pseudofolliculitis barbae,

S. Y. D. Lim (✉) · S. W. N. Cheng
National Skin Centre, Singapore, Singapore
e-mail: dereklimsy@nsc.com.sg; suzannecheng@nsc.com.sg

S. W. N. Cheng, C. L. Goh (eds.), *Updates on Lasers in Dermatology*, Updates in Clinical Dermatology, https://doi.org/10.1007/978-3-031-71155-8_7

hidradenitis suppurativa, pilonidal sinus, keratosis pilaris, and trichostasis spinulosa [8, 9]

Contraindications

Laser hair reduction is generally a safe procedure. However, clinicians should be aware of the contraindications and discuss deferring the procedure or alternative methods of hair reduction when present.

Absolute contraindications to laser hair reduction are as follows:

- Photosensitizing disorders and photodermatoses
- Presence of infection or other active skin diseases at intended sites of treatment
- Intended reduction of grey or white hairs (will not respond to treatment)
- Patient unable to co-operate

We recommend deferring the procedure in the following scenarios:

- Pregnancy and lactation
- Recent skin tanning in the last 6 weeks
- Recent hair removal (waxing, threading, epilation) in the last 2 weeks
- Use of isotretinoin or other photosensitizing medications in the last 6 months
- Skin breaks at intended sites of treatment

We recommend adequate preoperative counselling and discussion of the risks, benefits, and alternatives to laser hair reduction in patients with the following:

- Skin disease with Koebnerization or pathergy
- Tattoos at intended sites of treatment
- History of keloids or hypertrophic scars
- History of herpes simplex virus (HSV) infection at intended sites of treatment
- Photosensitive epilepsy
- Coagulopathies
- Current or past gold therapy
- Patients with unrealistic expectations

Other important counselling points before treatment are vital to manage patients' expectations:

- Hairs may take up to 3 weeks to fall out after treatment.
- Multiple sessions will be required to achieve a satisfactory cosmetic result, with subsequent hair regrowth to be expected with time. Follow-up treatments are often required to maintain hair reduction.

Energy-Based Devices Used in Hair Reduction

A wide range of laser and other energy-based device systems have been employed, either singly or in combination, for hair reduction. These include the long-pulsed ruby laser (694 nm), alexandrite laser (755 nm), diode laser (810 nm), and neodymium-doped yttrium-aluminium-garnet (Nd:YAG) laser (1064 nm), as well as intense pulsed light (IPL) therapy.

Ruby Laser

The long-pulsed ruby laser (694 nm) was the device first employed for hair reduction. In a single-arm study involving 51 patients of skin phototypes II–IV undergoing one to six treatments with a spot size of 7 mm and fluence ranging from 10 to 70 J/cm^2, the majority of patients were found only to have sparse regrowth at a median follow-up of 8 months after the last treatment. Transient pigmentary changes were noted in 30% of subjects, but no long-lasting sequelae occurred [10]. However, darker skin phototypes experience a higher frequency of adverse events such as blistering, scabbing, and pigmentary changes taking months to resolve, as the shorter wavelengths emitted by the ruby laser are absorbed by melanin in the epidermis, which is increased in darker skin [11].

Alexandrite Laser

The long-pulsed alexandrite laser (755 nm) penetrates deeper than the ruby laser, resulting in less epidermal melanin absorption. In a large retrospective analysis of 2359 patients of skin phototypes II–V, those who underwent an average of five treatments with the alexandrite laser at an initial fluence of 16 J/cm^2 experienced a mean hair reduction of 80%. Darker skin phototypes, who received treatments utilizing lower fluences, had lower rates of hair reduction. No scarring or long-term permanent pigmentary alterations resulted, and complications were more frequently observed in darker skin phototypes. Hair induction adjacent to the areas of treatment occurred in a small minority of patients [12].

Comparison of varying pulse durations in split-face studies did not reveal any significant difference in efficacy and the incidence of adverse events [13, 14]. In a split-body study comparing the multipass low-fluence (5–8 J/cm^2), high-frequency (5 Hz) alexandrite laser and the high-fluence (15–20 J/cm^2), low-frequency (1.5 Hz) long-pulsed Nd:YAG laser for axillary hair reduction in 30 women of skin phototypes IV–VI, there was greater mean hair reduction and lower pain in the side treated with the alexandrite laser [15].

Diode Laser

The diode laser (810 nm) penetrates deeper into the skin than the ruby and alexandrite lasers. In an observational study involving 40 women of skin phototypes III–V undergoing four to eight sessions of laser hair reduction with the 810 nm diode laser, good-to-excellent improvement was observed in 51.8% of treatment sites. No major adverse effects were observed. However, paradoxical hypertrichosis was observed in five patients [16]. The use of a low fluence (maximal fluence of 20 J/cm^2) and high repetition rate (up to 10 Hz) in 71 female patients of skin phototypes IV–VI resulted in general excellent hair reduction, with poorer results in the bikini area. No pigmentary sequelae were reported in any of the patients [17].

Other studies also demonstrate that lower fluences appear to be better tolerated, with no difference in efficacy outcomes. In a non-blinded study comparing females with hirsutism undergoing diode laser treatment with low (mean 30.83 J/cm^2) and high (42.10 J/cm^2) fluences, the low-fluence group required slightly more treatment sessions to reach their desired goal (5.47 sessions vs. 4.50 sessions in the high-fluence group), but showed higher satisfaction at 6 months after treatment [18]. A split-body design involving 96 female volunteers of skin phototypes III–V compared low fluence and high repetition rate (10 J/cm^2, 10 Hz) versus high fluence and low repetition rate (34–38 J/cm^2, 1 Hz) of diode laser modes for axillary hair reduction and found that while hair reduction rates were similar across both groups, higher fluences resulted in increased pain scores and transient post-procedural pigmentary changes [19]. A larger 10 × 30 mm spot size was also found to be more effective than a 10 × 10 mm spot size in a split-body study involving ten women undergoing axillary hair reduction, with patients receiving treatment with the spot size reporting slightly more pain, without other adverse events noted [20].

A novel blend diode laser incorporating three wavelengths (810, 940, and 1064 nm) was tested for axillary hair reduction against the conventional 810 nm diode laser in a split-body study involving 14 patients who underwent three treatment sessions. With the blend laser using an average of 40% more fluence per session, the blend laser produced slightly more pain but resulted in 12% more hair removed at 6 months after treatment [21].

Neodymium-Doped Yttrium Aluminium Garnet (Nd:YAG) Laser

The long-pulsed Nd:YAG laser (1064 nm) has been employed in laser hair removal and has a better safety profile in darker skin phototypes due to its longer wavelength, helping to target dark hairs, while minimizing its absorption by epidermal melanin. Its adjustable pulse duration also enables heat dissipation and epidermal cooling

[22]. A systematic review including 13 studies assessing the Nd:YAG laser for hair removal reported long-lasting hair reduction, in excess of 70%, persisting up to 18 months after the last treatment session. The most common adverse effects were transient erythema, pain, perifollicular oedema, post-inflammatory hyperpigmentation, and peeling. No long-lasting adverse effects were reported up to 24 months post-treatment [23].

Though higher fluences (60–80 J/cm^2) are more effective, adequate cooling is paramount in reducing pain and epidermal injury [24, 25]. Larger spot sizes (>7 mm) and longer pulse durations (≥50 ms) were found more effective compared to the converse, with a similar incidence of adverse events [26]. Comparison between submillisecond short (0.6–1.6 ms) and conventional long (20–30 ms) pulse durations in a split-face design did not reveal any difference in efficacy, with no serious adverse effects observed with both modes [27]. The use of an "in motion" technique, involving continuous slow movement of the handpiece in a linear or circular fashion and executing multiple back-and-forth passes, was found to result in less pain and incidence of burns [28].

Blended Wavelengths

The use of simultaneous multiple blended wavelengths has also been employed. A prospective split-body study compared the use of a blended diode laser (incorporating 810, 960, and 1060 nm) and the 810 nm diode laser for axillary hair reduction in 14 adult females of skin phototypes III and IV. Three treatment sessions were performed. The blended laser utilized an average of 40% more influence per session, with a tendency towards greater hair reduction in the participants of skin phototype IV at 6-month follow-up, though this was not statistically significant. No long-lasting adverse effects were reported in both groups. Greater pinprick and heat sensation were reported with the blended laser [21].

Another retrospective study involving 36 patients evaluated the use of a blended alexandrite 755 nm and Nd:YAG 1064 nm emitting laser in 149 patients (males and females) of skin phototypes I–V. Mean hair reduction at 12–14 months of follow-up, after four to five laser sessions, ranged from 74% to 83% across different sites. No permanent adverse events were reported [29].

Intense Pulsed Light

Though both laser and IPL treatments release light energy to be absorbed by the hair follicle, IPL releases broad-spectrum visible light, unlike laser systems which emit monochromatic coherent energy of a single wavelength. Cut-off filters are used to select for specific energy ranges. In a retrospective analysis involving 650 female patients of skin phototypes IV and V who underwent IPL treatment for facial hair reduction, around 90% of patients demonstrated a good-to-excellent response, across different treatment areas. All patients reported mild pain, erythema, and follicular oedema, but no pigmentary changes were observed in any of the patients [30]. The elimination of shorter wavelengths at the 600–645 nm range by using a 645–950 nm filter results in improved efficacy, less pain, and reduced pigmentary sequelae [31]. Studies comparing IPL against lasers show that IPL is generally less effective than laser for hair reduction [32].

Treatment Settings

In our practice, because of darker skin type in our Asian patients, we most frequently utilize the 1064 nm long-pulsed Nd:YAG laser for assisted hair reduction, and we will base further discussion of laser settings on this.

Pulse Duration

The pulse duration should be decided based on hair shaft thickness and skin phototype.

We calibrate pulse duration to hair shaft thickness, with shorter pulse durations (20 ms) for

Table 7.1 Starting fluences for different skin phototypes

Site	Skin phototype IV (J/cm^2)	Skin phototypes V and VI (J/cm^2)
Face and neck	40	34–36
Axillary, pubic, and gluteal fold	45–48	40–45
Limbs	48–50	42–45

thinner hairs and longer pulse durations (25 ms) for thicker hairs.

For skin phototypes III–IV, shorter pulse durations (20 ms) are employed. Longer pulse durations (25 ms) are safer for darker skin phototypes V and VI.

Spot Size

Larger spot sizes allow for deeper penetration and more efficient hair reduction. We usually employ a spot size of 10 mm.

Fluence

While higher fluences help to achieve greater permanent hair reduction, they also come with a higher risk of adverse effects. The ideal fluence would be the maximal tolerated fluence, which yields the desired endpoint of perifollicular erythema and oedema without adverse effects.

Our usual starting fluences are as outlined below in Table 7.1, with an increase of 5–10% for subsequent treatments if well tolerated.

Preoperative Preparation

The treatment area should be cleaned with normal saline and demarcated with the use of skin tape. Long hair should be clipped or ideally shaved 2–3 days prior. A eutectic mixture of local anaesthetics (EMLA) containing topical lidocaine 2.5% and prilocaine 2.5% should be applied under occlusion for 60 min, before treatment is started. The total area that can be treated per session is limited by the maximum amount of EMLA that can be safely applied.

Intraoperative

Cooling should be employed, with the use of a cooling handpiece, cool air, or both. A gliding motion is used, with pulses overlapped by 10%. For contoured areas where gliding is challenging, we recommend a single-shot technique. The endpoint of treatment is singeing of the hair, with perifollicular erythema and oedema (Fig. 7.1).

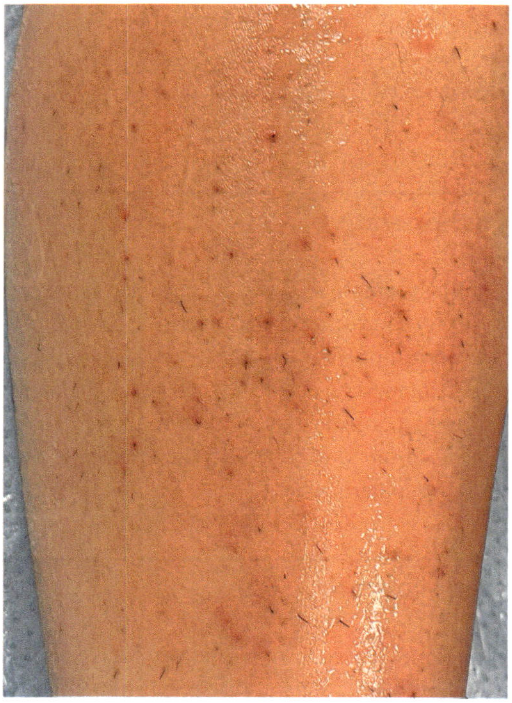

Fig. 7.1 Singeing of the hairs and perifollicular erythema signify the endpoint of laser-assisted hair reduction

Table 7.2 Reported complications of laser and IPL hair reduction

	Duration		
Complication	Transient	Short term	Permanent
Pain	✓		
Erythema	✓		
Oedema	✓		
Blisters and erosions	✓		
Burns	✓		
Infection, e.g., HSV reactivation [33]	✓		
Bruising	✓		
Extrusion of hair shafts	✓		
Urticaria [34]	✓		
Cutaneous vasculitis [35]	✓		
Eye injury	✓	✓	✓
Pigmentary changes		✓	✓
Leukotrichia		✓	✓
Paradoxical hypertrichosis		✓	✓
Darkening of tattoos		✓	✓
Sweat gland dysfunction (hyperhidrosis, bromhidrosis, Fox-Fordyce disease) [36, 37]		✓	✓
Reticulate erythema		✓	
Koebnerization or pathergy [38]		✓	
Skin atrophy			✓
Scarring			✓
Changes in naevi [39]			✓

Post-operative

Cooling is employed with ice packs immediately post-procedure, to reduce pain and oedema. Strict sun protection for at least 2 weeks after each treatment must be enforced. Other than the application of a moisturizer, we do not encourage the use of cosmetic products to the treatment area until the epidermis has healed.

Complications

While laser hair reduction is a safe procedure, it is important for physicians to be cognizant of potential complications. Pain, erythema, and perifollicular oedema are commonly experienced by patients immediately after the procedure. Post-inflammatory hyperpigmentation, lasting up to months, may also result, especially in darker skin phototypes. The use of longer wavelengths and pulse durations, coupled with appropriate cooling measures, can help to enhance the safety profile of laser hair reduction. Table 7.2 outlines the complications reported in laser hair reduction.

Conclusion

Laser hair reduction is effective and safe, with largely transient adverse effects to be expected. Preoperative counselling is vital to communicate to patients the need for repeated treatments and to emphasize that hair reduction, rather than total hair removal, is to be expected. Care should be exercised in darker skin phototypes, who may require more sessions to achieve desirable results.

References

1. Lipton MG, Sherr L, Elford J, Rustin MH, Clayton WJ. Women living with facial hair: the psychological and behavioral burden. J Psychosom Res. 2006;61(2):161–8.
2. Altshuler GB, Anderson RR, Manstein D, Zenzie HH, Smirnov MZ. Extended theory of selective photothermolysis. Lasers Surg Med. 2001;29(5):416–32.
3. O'Sullivan JDB, Nicu C, Picard M, et al. The biology of human hair greying. Biol Rev Camb Philos Soc. 2021;96(1):107–28.
4. Casey AS, Goldberg D. Guidelines for laser hair removal. J Cosmet Laser Ther. 2008;10(1):24–33.
5. Lumley C. Intraoral hair removal on skin graft using Nd:YAG laser. Br Dent J. 2007;203(3):141–2.
6. Royston SL, Cole RP, Wright PA. Peristomal hair removal with an Alexandrite laser. Color Dis. 2013;15(8):1043–4.
7. Yuan N, Feldman AT, Chin P, Zaliznyak M, Rabizadeh S, Garcia MM. Comparison of permanent hair removal procedures before gender-affirming vaginoplasty: why we should consider laser hair removal as a first-line treatment for patients who meet criteria. Sex Med. 2022;10(5):100545.
8. Aleem S, Majid I. Unconventional uses of laser hair removal: a review. J Cutan Aesthet Surg. 2019;12(1):8–16.
9. Toosi S, Ehsani AH, Noormohammadpoor P, Esmaili N, Mirshams-Shahshahani M, Moineddin F. Treatment of trichostasis spinulosa with a 755-nm long-pulsed alexandrite laser. J Eur Acad Dermatol Venereol. 2010;24(4):470–3.
10. Campos VB, Dierickx CC, Farinelli WA, Lin TY, Manuskiatti W, Anderson RR. Ruby laser hair removal: evaluation of long-term efficacy and side effects. Lasers Surg Med. 2000;26(2):177–85.
11. Chana JS, Grobbelaar AO. The long-term results of ruby laser depilation in a consecutive series of 346 patients. Plast Reconstr Surg. 2002;110(1):254–60.
12. Kutlubay Z. Alexandrite laser hair removal results in 2359 patients: a Turkish experience. J Cosmet Laser Ther. 2009;11(2):85–93.
13. Noormohammadpour P, Ehsani AH, Farnaghi F, et al. Effect of different pulse durations on the efficacy of long-pulsed alexandrite-assisted hair removal; a split-face comparison study. J Lasers Med Sci. 2021;12:e21.
14. Boss WK Jr, Usal H, Thompson RC, Fiorillo MA. A comparison of the long-pulse and short-pulse Alexandrite laser hair removal systems. Ann Plast Surg. 1999;42(4):381–4.
15. Moftah N, Tymour M, Ibrahim SMA. Multipass low fluence, high-frequency 755-nm alexandrite laser versus high fluence, low-frequency 1064-nm long-pulsed Nd: YAG laser in axillary hair reduction of dark skin phototypes: an intra-individual randomized comparative study. J Dermatolog Treat. 2022;33(4):2079–84.
16. Pai SB, Suvarna P, Shetty VM, Pathan S. Efficacy of 810 nm diode laser in hair reduction in Indian subpopulation using a novel Gabor filter-based detection software and hair algorithm. J Cosmet Dermatol. 2022;21(3):1004–12.
17. Agarwal M, Velaskar S, Gold MH. Efficacy of a low fluence, high repetition rate 810nm diode laser for permanent hair reduction in Indian patients with skin types IV-VI. J Clin Aesthet Dermatol. 2016;9(11):29–33.
18. Ebrahimzadeh Ardakani M, Azad M, Ghanei N, Etaee F, Naguib T, Daveluy S. Comparison of patient satisfaction with diode laser treatment of female hirsutism: low fluence or high fluence? J Cosmet Laser Ther. 2021;23(5-6):113–5.
19. Li W, Liu C, Chen Z, et al. Safety and efficacy of low fluence, high repetition rate versus high fluence, low repetition rate 810-nm diode laser for axillary hair removal in Chinese women. J Cosmet Laser Ther. 2016;18(7):393–6.
20. Jo SJ, Kim JY, Ban J, Lee Y, Kwon O, Koh W. Efficacy and safety of hair removal with a long-pulsed diode laser depending on the spot size: a randomized, evaluators-blinded, left-right study. Ann Dermatol. 2015;27(5):517–22.
21. Gold MH, Biron J, Wilson A, et al. Safety and efficacy for hair removal in dark skin types III and IV with a high-powered, combined wavelength (810, 940 and 1060 nm) diode laser: a single-site pilot study. J Cosmet Dermatol. 2022;21(5):1979–85.
22. Nabi N, Bhat YJ, Dar UK, et al. Comparative study of the clinico-trichoscopic response to treatment of hirsutism with long pulsed (1064 nm) Nd:YAG laser in idiopathic hirsutism and polycystic ovarian syndrome patients. Lasers Med Sci. 2022;37(1):545–53.
23. Modena DAO, Miranda ACG, Grecco C, Liebano RE, Cordeiro RCT, Guidi RM. Efficacy and safety of ND:YAG 1064 nm lasers for photoepilation: a systematic review. Lasers Med Sci. 2020;35(4):797–806.
24. Nanda S, Bansal S. Long pulsed Nd:YAG laser with inbuilt cool sapphire tip for long term hair reduction on type- IV and V skin: a prospective analysis of 200 patients. Indian J Dermatol Venereol Leprol. 2010;76(6):677–81.
25. Rogachefsky AS, Becker K, Weiss G, Goldberg DJ. Evaluation of a long-pulsed Nd:YAG laser at different parameters: an analysis of both fluence and pulse duration. Dermatol Surg. 2002;28(10):932–5; discussion 936.
26. Raff K, Landthaler M, Hohenleutner U. Optimizing treatment parameters for hair removal using long-pulsed Nd:YAG-lasers. Lasers Med Sci. 2004;18(4):219–22.
27. Byalakere Shivanna C, Shenoy C, Lalitha S, Jaju P, Zorman A. Comparison of submillisecond pulse (FRAC3) and long-pulse 1064 nm Nd:YAG laser hair removal. J Cosmet Dermatol. 2022;21(8):3393–7.
28. Nistico SP, Bennardo L, Bennardo S, et al. Comparing traditional and in motion Nd:YAG laser in hair removal: a prospective study. Medicina (Kaunas). 2022;58(9):1205.

29. Zerbinati N, Protasoni M, Dalla Gasperina D, et al. Combined laser assisted treatment for permanent hair removal for skin types I-V with Alexandrite 755 nm and ND:YAG 1064 nm lasers. Dermatol Ther. 2021;34(1):e14599.
30. Deshpande A. Efficacy & safety of intense pulsed light therapy for unwanted facial hair: a retrospective analysis in skin of color. J Cosmet Laser Ther. 2021;23(5–6):116–21.
31. Hee Lee J, Huh CH, Yoon HJ, Cho KH, Chung JH. Photo-epilation results of axillary hair in dark-skinned patients by intense pulsed light: comparison between different wavelengths and pulse width. Dermatol Surg. 2006;32(2):234–40.
32. Kao YC, Lin DZ, Kang YN, Chang CJ, Chiu WK, Chen C. Efficacy of laser in hair removal: a network meta-analysis. J Cosmet Laser Ther. 2023;25(1-4):7–19.
33. Reis J, Santos FV. Perianal reactivation of herpes simplex virus type 2 after laser-assisted hair removal. Sex Transm Dis. 2021;48(2):e30–1.
34. Landa N, Corrons N, Zabalza I, Azpiazu JL. Urticaria induced by laser epilation: a clinical and histopathological study with extended follow-up in 36 patients. Lasers Surg Med. 2012;44(5):384–9.
35. Moreno-Arias GA, Tiffon T, Marti T, Camps-Fresneda A. Urticaria vasculitis induced by diode laser photo-epilation. Dermatol Surg. 2000;26(11):1082–3.
36. Byth LA, Byth J. Fox-Fordyce disease: insights from cases induced by laser hair removal. Australas J Dermatol. 2020;61(2):188–9.
37. Helou J, Haber R, Kechichian E, Tomb R. A case of generalized bromhidrosis following whole-body depilatory laser. J Cosmet Laser Ther. 2015;17(6):318–20.
38. Alkhalifah A. A case report of vitiligo induced by Alexandrite hair removal laser. Case Rep Dermatol. 2021;13(3):521–4.
39. Dessinioti C, Tsiakou A, Christodoulou A, Stratigos AJ. Clinical and dermoscopic findings of nevi after photoepilation: a review. Life (Basel). 2023;13(9):1832.

8 Lasers in Paediatric Dermatology

Lee Hwee Chyen

Introduction

Since the advent of lasers in dermatology by Dr. Leon Goldman in 1963, laser surgery has revolutionized how we treat multiple skin conditions, including that of paediatric dermatoses. Unlike in adults, performing procedures in the paediatric population of varying age groups does carry a different set of challenges. In this chapter, we discuss common indications for dermatologic lasers in our Asian paediatric population and focus on special considerations and tips for treating this particular group of patients.

Common Lasers in Paediatric Patients and Their Indications

Vascular Lesions (PWS, Haemangiomas)

Vascular lesions are amongst the most common indications for use of lasers in paediatric procedural dermatology, with haemoglobin as the target chromophore to achieve the desired clinical endpoint. Pulsed dye laser (PDL) at 585 or 595 nm is the mainstay of laser treatment for vascular lesions in paediatric dermatology. More details on vascular lasers can be found in Chap. 2.

Port Wine Stains and Capillary Malformations

Port wine stains (PWSs) are congenital capillary malformations (CMs) that occur in about 0.3–0.5% of newborns with no gender predilection [1]. They can occur on their own or rarely, in association with syndromes such as Sturge-Weber syndrome (SWS) or PIIK3CA-related overgrowth syndrome (PROS). They can rarely be acquired later in life. The head and neck region is the most commonly involved location. Initially presenting as flat erythematous patches, they will grow proportionately with the child and may become darker and/or more hypertrophic with time if left untreated.

Treatment

PDL therapy remains the gold standard for PWS treatment [2]. Treatment parameters depend on the thickness, location of the PWS, Fitzpatrick skin type and patient age. Settings and parameters are adjusted based on clinical response, with the clinical endpoint being that of purpura, which may last for a few days to a week. Optimal treatment intervals are 2–4 weeks; shorter treatment intervals lead to more rapid clearance (Fig. 8.1). Larger spot sizes also allow deeper penetration and faster clearance too.

Recommended settings with the 595 nm PDL based on our experience: 7–10 mm spot size, flu-

L. H. Chyen (✉)
Epi Dermatology & Laser Specialist Clinic, Singapore, Singapore

S. W. N. Cheng, C. L. Goh (eds.), *Updates on Lasers in Dermatology*, Updates in Clinical Dermatology, https://doi.org/10.1007/978-3-031-71155-8_8

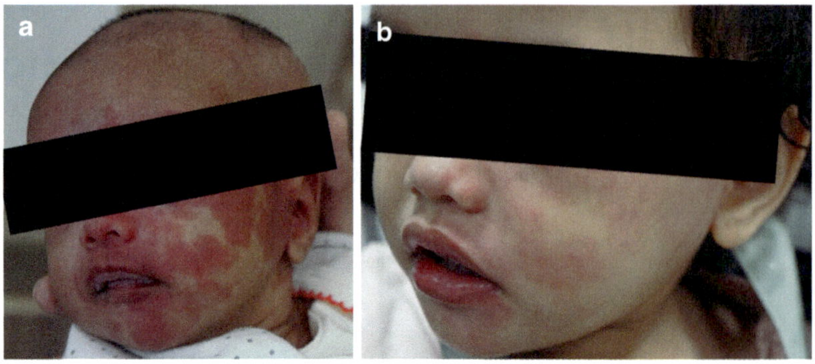

Fig. 8.1 (**a**) An extensive port wine stain on a child at 4 months of age. (**b**) Significant clinical response is seen after eight sessions of PDL treatment at 4-week intervals

ence of 7–9 J/cm^2 and 0.45–1.5 ms pulse duration. Pulses may overlap about 10–20% with treatment intervals 2–4 weeks apart.

Common side effects are discomfort, blistering, purpura, erythema, oedema and post-inflammatory dyspigmentation (either hypo- or hyperpigmentation, depending on the skin type).

Earlier treatment results in better clinical outcomes; infants who started laser treatment before 6 months of age had an average clearance of 89% after 1 year of treatment [3, 4]. This is because younger patients have thinner skin, allowing better laser penetration. The total treatment area is also smaller. Furthermore, there is less melanin with more haemoglobin F present as an additional target for the PDL. Lesions in younger patients also have thinner and more superficial vessels and lack a nodular component, thus making them more amenable to PDL therapy.

Other factors affecting the treatment outcomes include the anatomical location and size of the PWS [5–8]. For facial lesions, those on the mid-forehead have the best treatment response, followed by periorbital and neck lesions. The ones on the centro-facial region tend to be the most resistant. While lesions on the limbs are more resistant than those of the face, those on the proximal extremities are more responsive than those of the distal extremities. PDL treatment also tends to be more effective at the peripheral borders of lesions, and thus, those lesions which are larger in circumference seem to have better response rates.

Another reason why treatment is best done earlier is that as PWSs mature, they can become more nodular and hypertrophic. These resistant PWSs may require lasers of longer wavelengths with multiple passes.

Lastly, treating children in the first year of life is also easier, as smaller children can be swaddled or restrained and risks of general anaesthesia (GA) may be avoided.

Treatment response varies, depending on the characteristics of the PWS. Fading by 80% is usually observed after eight to ten treatments [3]. However, the clinical improvement post-laser may slow down with successive laser treatments. This is likely due to destruction of smaller, more superficial capillaries. The residual component comprises deeper, larger capillaries that are more resistant to laser treatment.

Even in the event of superior response rates following laser treatment as discussed above, PWS may still recur years after completion of therapy [9].

Considerations in Asian Skin

Darker skin types may result in post-inflammatory hyperpigmentation. Lower fluence, longer pulse durations and longer treatment intervals may be recommended in this case. Epidermal cooling, by way of the cooling system attached to the PDL, is also crucial to prevent epidermal damage and subsequent dyspigmentation. It is also advised to do test spots at the first visit to assess treatment response and determine the ideal treatment parameters before proceeding to treat the entire lesion.

Haemangiomas

Infantile haemangiomas (IHs) are benign, high-flow vascular tumours present during infancy.

They typically have a rapidly proliferative phase followed by a quiescent and then finally an involuting phase.

PDL has been used in IH, though this is controversial. This is because the depth of PDL is limited [10]. If effective in proliferative haemangiomas, it is usually due to its role in targeting the superficial component of the IH, with no effect on the proliferation of the deep or subcutaneous component.

In recent years, the use of PDL in the treatment of ulcerated haemangiomas in combination with dressings and oral propranolol has been reported [11] (Fig. 8.2). The PDL treatment is believed to decrease pain with subsequent healing of the ulceration. However, if not performed properly with the right settings and technique, PDL may also cause iatrogenic ulceration [12]. PDL therapy is also pivotal in the treatment of partially involuted or residual haemangiomas following systemic therapy, especially in older children who may find these cosmetically bothersome (Fig. 8.3).

Recommended settings with the 595 nm PDL based on our experience:

(a) For IH (superficial): 7–10 mm spot size, fluence of 7–12 J/cm^2 and 0.45–1.5 ms pulse duration. Pulses may overlap about 10–20%. While not the first-line treatment for superficial haemangiomas in the proliferative phase, if ever used, lower fluences and shorter pulse durations should be employed due to the potential risk of iatrogenic ulceration.

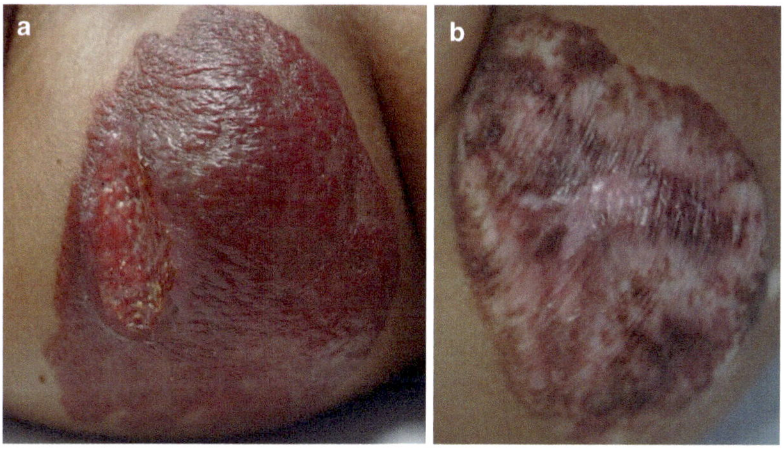

Fig. 8.2 (**a**) Ulcerated haemangioma on the left buttock of a 2-month-old baby. (**b**) Clinical response after combined PDL treatment and oral propranolol

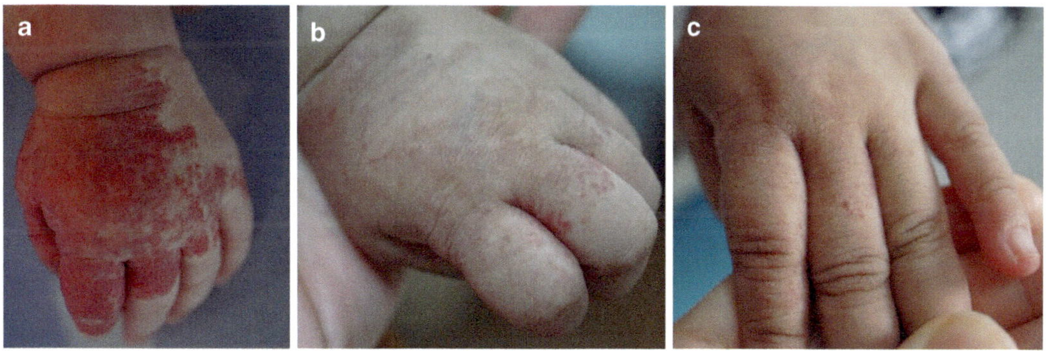

Fig. 8.3 (**a**) Extensive infantile haemangioma on the left hand of a 2-month-old child. (**b**) Residual haemangioma noted after completing oral propranolol therapy of about 6 months' duration. (**c**) Treatment outcome after two sessions of PDL treatment for the residual haemangioma while the child is no longer on systemic therapy

(b) Ulcerated haemangioma: 7–10 mm spot size, fluence 5–8 J/cm^2 with 0.45–1.5 ms pulse duration. Minimize overlapping of pulses, and treatment can be repeated judiciously and more frequently at 2–3 weeks, with frequent reviews and dressings.

As the case with PWS, epidermal cooling with the attached cryogen cooling spray is mandatory in all cases to prevent epidermal damage.

Other Vascular Lesions

PDL has also been effectively used in other common vascular conditions in the paediatric population such as telangiectasias, angiokeratomas and angioma serpiginosum (Fig. 8.4).

Pigmented Lesions

Naevus of Ota and Naevus of Ito

Naevus of Ota (NOO) is a form of dermal melanocytosis that is more common in Asians and more frequently in females. NOO usually presents at birth in about half of the patients, with the remainder presenting around puberty. The initial presentation is that of unilateral, blue-grey or slate-brown pigmentation over the eye, ear and nose, often following the first and second branches of the trigeminal nerve. Scleral involvement on the same side is common and warrants ophthalmological evaluation to exclude concomitant glaucoma.

Naevus of Ito (NOI) is another form of dermal melanocytosis that occurs not on the face but along the posterior supraclavicular and lateral cutaneous brachial nerves.

While benign, NOO and NOI do not fade over time and persist beyond childhood, potentially having cosmetic implications on the child. They are amenable to laser treatment, and given the dermal depth of pigmentation, pigment lasers with longer wavelengths are recommended. These include the Q-switched (QS) alexandrite and ND:YAG lasers and, more recently, picosecond (PS) lasers (Fig. 8.5). Potential side effects include texture changes, hypo- or hyperpigmentation, incomplete clearance and scarring [13, 14].

Both the 755 nm PS alexandrite and 1064 nm PS Nd:YAG lasers have been found to be effective and well tolerated for the treatment of NOO. When comparing 755 nm QS alexandrite with that of 755 nm PS laser, the latter was found

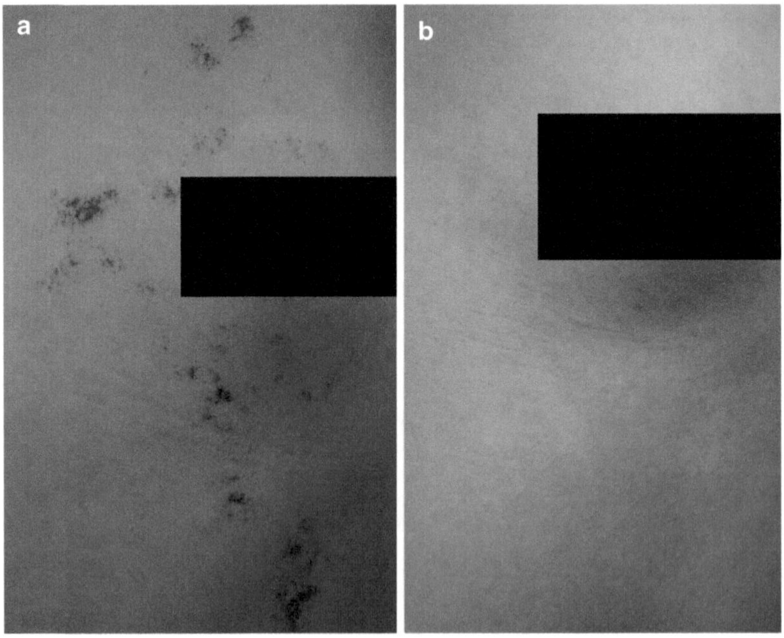

Fig. 8.4 (**a**) Angioma serpiginosum on the left chest of a 10-year-old girl approaching puberty. (**b**) Treatment outcome after two sessions of PDL therapy

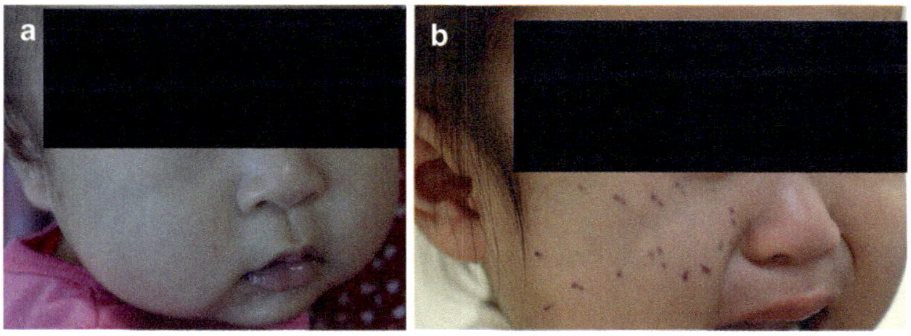

Fig. 8.5 (**a**) Naevus of Ota on the right cheek of a 5-month-old baby. (**b**) Treatment response after three sessions of picosecond 1064 nm laser, at 2-month intervals

to be superior in terms of overall clinical response rates and side effects [15].

It is recommended to start treatment earlier in life for a few reasons. Firstly, as the child grows, the lesion may become darker due to the influence of sex hormones in puberty and cumulative ultraviolet light exposure with time. The lesion becomes less amenable to laser treatment, and more sessions are required. The histologic depth of the lesion can change with age, making it harder to treat. Lesions with depths of 1 mm or less have been found to demonstrate excellent clearance with the QS alexandrite laser. Conversely, deeper and older lesions are believed to be more resistant to treatment and more prone to recurrence. Patients younger than 10 years of age have been demonstrated to need fewer sessions and lower mean fluence for successful treatment than that of older counterparts [16].

For darker skin types, a test spot is recommended before committing to treatment over the whole area. The clinical endpoint is variable. When using QS lasers, the ideal recommended endpoint is that of immediate dermal whitening as it indicates melanosome destruction. However, this has been associated with post-inflammatory hyperpigmentation, especially in darker skin types.

Based on anecdotal experience and reports, the use of PS lasers on these lesions in children has shown optimal clinical responses without necessarily having to reach this clinical endpoint.

Café Au Lait Macules (CALMs)

Café au lait macules (CALMs) are common light brown patches found in infancy or early childhood. Often present in about 10–20% of the population, they may be associated with several genodermatoses such as neurofibromatosis and McCune-Albright syndrome. Solitary lesions are not uncommon and are benign, in which case treatment is purely for cosmetic reasons. In general, the response of CALMs to pigment laser therapy is quite variable; incomplete clearance and high recurrence rates of up to 50% have been reported [16].

There is no definite association between the age of the patient and treatment response. However, the morphological appearance of CALMs has been reported to be linked to treatment response. Lesions with irregular, jagged borders like that of "*Coast of Maine*" have been observed to respond better to pigment lasers than that of "*Coast of California*" lesions with smooth and well-demarcated borders.

More details on lasers for NOO, NOI and CALM can be found in Chap. 3.

Tattoos

Tattoo removal appears to be increasingly relevant in paediatric dermatology. In counselling paediatric patients to undergo tattoo removal, we must first assess the reason behind the tattoo. In the past, tattoos were generally associated with secret societies and gangs, especially amongst the youth in Southeast Asia. However, tattoos are fast becoming popular amongst teenagers and adolescents for other reasons. In recent years, tattoos represent a form of self-expression and/or body art. Tattoos are now becoming "trendy" amongst the paediatric population.

In our clinical practice, it is observed that tattoo removal in the paediatric population is usually requested by schools or parents and caregivers. The removal is less commonly requested by patients themselves who regret the tattoo. As the procedure is costly, tedious and potentially painful and multiple sessions are required, persuading paediatric patients to undergo tattoo removal poses a new challenge for paediatric dermatologists.

Tattoo removal in this age group is encouraged for a few reasons. Firstly, students with tattoos are subject to disciplinary measures at school, including suspension. Secondly, tattoos can potentially affect further employment and career prospects for youths. Bekhor et al. reported significant bias against employment of persons with visible tattoos in certain industries such as hospitality, beauty, retail and office sectors [17].

In order to help these paediatric patients complete their education and improve their career prospects in future, various outreach programs have been established to assist in this. These include subsidized tattoo removal programmes for youths. This generally requires a multidisciplinary approach, mainly for the laser practitioners to work with not just the patient undergoing tattoo removal, but also the parents/caregivers, social workers, student welfare officers, counsellors and psychologists, to encourage and motivate them to start and persist with tattoo removal. National Skin Centre of Singapore runs a tattoo removal programme in collaboration with the Ministry of Education for at-risk youths and young offenders under 21 years of age [18, 19]. The laser sessions for tattoo removal for eligible paediatric patients under this programme are fully subsidized, with the aim to help them avoid disciplinary measures at school so they can continue pursuing their education and look for gainful employment.

The treatment process and clinic response in tattoo removal depend on various factors. In general, amateur tattoos are easier to remove than professional tattoos because they have less ink deposited and are usually less complex to remove [20] (Fig. 8.6). Professional tattoos tend to be deeper; hence, more treatment sessions are required.

The pigment colour, quality of ink and age and size of tattoo will also affect the treatment and clinical response. Older tattoos require fewer

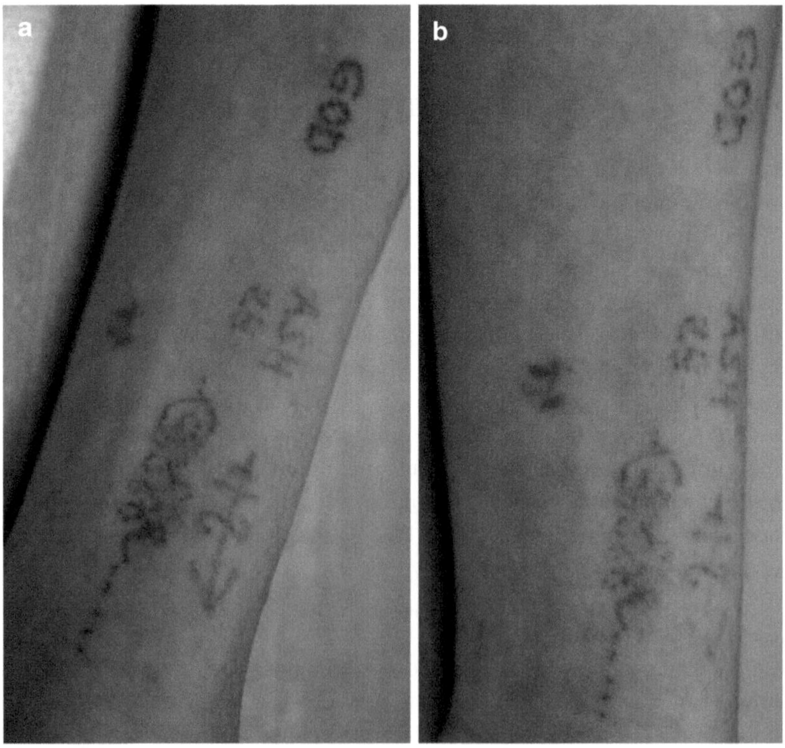

Fig. 8.6 (**a**) Amateur tattoos in a 14-year-old boy. (**b**) Treatment response after one session with the picosecond laser

treatments as the ink migrates into the deep dermis and are cleared away by lymphatics.

Like in adults, PS lasers have become the treatment of choice for tattoo removal.

The 532 nm wavelength is best for targeting red, yellow and orange pigments. The 755 and 785 nm wavelengths are used for green, blue and purple pigments. Lastly, black pigments are amenable to 755 and 1064 nm wavelengths.

Multiple sessions are usually required with treatment intervals of about 6–8 weeks. Risks include pain, blistering, oedema, dyspigmentation, textural changes and scarring.

More details on lasers for tattoo removal can be found in Chap. 4.

Hypertrichosis and Hirsutism

Hypertrichosis is defined as an increase in body hair beyond the normal range for the patient's reference group. This is independent of androgens and can occur in either gender and over any part of the body. Hirsutism, on the other hand, is when females develop an increase in growth of terminal hairs in androgen-dependent areas (e.g. upper lip, chin, chest, medial thighs).

Either way, the excessive growth of unwanted hair can cause a negative impact on the self-esteem and psychosocial health of children and adolescents [21, 22].

Laser hair removal is a common non-surgical cosmetic procedure amongst the paediatric population with unwanted hair. It can also help with hidradenitis suppurativa and recurrent pilonidal abscesses by way of hair follicular destruction. However, compared to that of adults, there is limited data on the efficacy and safety of laser hair removal in the paediatric population (i.e. under 18 years of age). In a systematic review, the youngest patient undergoing intense pulse light (IPL) or laser hair removal was 9 months, with the oldest, 17 years old [22]. Diagnoses ranged from localized lumbosacral to generalized hypertrichosis. Generally, the studies reported significant hair reduction, and the treatment was well tolerated with no complications such as scarring or dyspigmentation.

It is important for patients and caregivers to understand that laser hair removal, while long lasting, may not always be permanent. Multiple sessions are required, and patients with dark terminal hairs on fair skin usually achieve the best clinical response rate.

A variety of lasers can be used, including the long-pulsed Nd:YAG (1064 nm), long-pulsed alexandrite (755 nm) and diode (800–810 nm) lasers.

The ideal wavelength to treat patients of darker skin types is that of 1064 nm long-pulsed Nd:YAG, in view of the lower risk of epidermal damage with this wavelength. Aggressive cooling is important to prevent any complications.

Pain management is particularly crucial in paediatric patients. This can be managed with cooling in the form of ice packs, topical anaesthesia or, less commonly, general anaesthesia.

The desired clinical endpoint is that of perifollicular erythema and oedema without epidermal damage (i.e. no greying, crusting or blistering). Test spots with different fluences are suggested to find the ideal fluence that can achieve this desired endpoint before treating the entire area.

Risks include pain, discomfort, erythema, perifollicular oedema, dyspigmentation, blistering and scarring. Paradoxical hypertrichosis has been reported in darker skin types, usually on the face and neck [22]. This is believed to be due to subtherapeutic fluences during treatment, and the treatment includes repeated laser hair removal at optimal settings.

More details on laser-assisted hair removal can be found in Chap. 7.

Special Considerations in Paediatric Patients Before the Procedure

In general, complications of lasers in children include pain, blistering, swelling, scarring and dyspigmentation (post-inflammatory hypo- or hyperpigmentation). These effects can be mitigated by first ensuring that the laser is performed by physicians with expertise in paediatric procedural dermatology. Prior to the procedure, the laser practitioner should also assess the patient's suitability for the procedure carefully, perform a thorough review and conduct a preoperative assessment. The following are some important factors that need to be considered during patient selection and before the paediatric patient is deemed suitable for the procedure.

Age, Maturity and Cognitive Development of the Child

Paediatric patients range from 0 to 18 years of age, and each different stage of childhood carries a different set of considerations. For instance, unlike infants, children beyond the age of 3 may be less cooperative, and swaddling may be challenging. Conversely, adolescents are more likely to be cooperative during the procedure compared to that of an infant.

Psychosocial Factors

While most birthmarks are benign, depending on their nature, extent and anatomical location, their cosmetic appearance may have a negative impact on the child psychosocially.

This is therefore an important factor to consider when deciding the age at which the child should undergo a procedure. Early treatment of potentially stigmatizing birthmarks, where possible, is therefore advisable.

Decision-Making

Unlike that of adult dermatology, decision-making in paediatric dermatologic procedures involves a third party. While the consent is formally obtained from the parent or legal guardian of the child, it is also important to assess the age, maturity and cognitive development of the patient. If the child is able to understand, it is important to include him or her in the discussion and to also respect the child's right to assent to any procedures. Parents should also be aware of the indications for laser therapy, the nature of the laser and expected outcomes and course of treatment before making an informed choice.

Analgesia and Anaesthesia

Poor pain control can have negative implications on the child. Many procedures require more than one session and if pain is not managed well on the first session, it would be difficult to continue repeated sessions.

Topical Anaesthesia

Topical anaesthetic agents are used in most cases. EMLA (eutectic mixture of 2.5% lidocaine and 2.5% prilocaine) cream is often used in small amounts under occlusion. It is generally effective and well tolerated, but the dose should not exceed 1 g/10 cm^2 and must be adjusted according to the application area. Table 8.1 demonstrates the recommended maximum doses, application area and application times for paediatric patients.

When applying EMLA cream to the skin of paediatric patients, special care must be taken to limit the dose and area of application, as well as to prevent accidental ingestion of the cream or the occlusive dressing. Sometimes, a secondary protective covering (e.g. bandage, gauze) to pre-

Table 8.1 Recommended maximum dosage, application area and application time of EMLA based on age and body weight of paediatric patients

Age and body weight requirements	Maximum total dose of EMLA cream (g)	Maximum application area (cm^2)	Maximum application time (h)
0 to 3 months or <5 kg	1	10	1
3 to 12 months and >5 kg	2	20	4
1 to 6 years and >10 kg	10	100	4
7 to 12 years and >20 kg	20	200	4

If a patient greater than 3 months old does not meet the minimum weight requirement of >5 kg, the maximum total dose of EMLA cream should be restricted to that which corresponds to the patient's weight

The above table was adapted from https://www.accessdata.fda.gov/drugsatfda_docs/label/2000/19941s11lbl.pdf

vent inadvertent disruption of the application site may be useful.

While well tolerated, EMLA may have common side effects such as erythema, pallor and oedema. Rarely, systemic complications such as methaemoglobinaemia and systemic toxicity may occur [23].

The systemic absorption of lidocaine and prilocaine in EMLA is an adverse effect; the amount absorbed and the complications depend on surface area and duration of application. Factors such as excessive use, broken skin, prolonged duration of application and large treatment area may result in high blood levels of the drug.

Systemic adverse reactions of lidocaine toxicity include central nervous system (CNS) and cardiovascular (CVS) toxicity [23, 24]. CNS toxicity may present with CNS excitation and/or depression. At low serum lidocaine levels, the initial symptoms include light-headedness, circumoral numbness and tinnitus. Higher levels can cause seizures, coma and respiratory depression. CVS toxicity presents with arrhythmias and/or myocardial depression. These include bradycardia, hypotension and cardiovascular arrest.

In addition, cases of methaemoglobinaemia in children have been reported after EMLA application for dermatological procedures and other procedures such as lumbar puncture, circumcision and central vein insertion [25]. These occur when vulnerable patients are exposed to large amounts of prilocaine. Risk factors for developing methaemoglobinaemia include age (younger than 3 months), prematurity, excessive amounts of EMLA, prolonged durations of application and skin inflammation or impaired skin barrier function (e.g. in atopic dermatitis). The high methaemoglobin (MetHb) impairs oxygenation. Patients may present with varying degrees of hypoxia; the higher the MetHb levels, the greater the severity of symptoms. At MetHb levels between 15% and 30%, patients present with cyanosis. At levels 30–50%, dyspnoea, tachycardia and headache develop. Levels exceeding 50%, while rare, will present with altered mental state, respiratory depression, seizures, coma, arrhythmias and even mortality.

The diagnosis should be suspected when the paediatric patient presents with sudden onset of cyanosis and persistent hypoxia, which are refractory to increased supplemental oxygen [26]. The treatment depends on the severity of the condition. Firstly, the culprit agent (i.e. EMLA cream) should be removed immediately, and the patient should be given supplemental oxygen. When MetHb levels are <20% and the patient is asymptomatic, no further action is required. This is because normally metabolizing red blood cells in a healthy individual will reduce the MetHb in a few hours. When the patient is symptomatic and intervention is required, the gold standard treatment for infant methaemoglobinaemia is that of intravenous methylene blue 1–2 mg/kg over 5 min. Clinical response is fast, and the dose may be repeated in 1 h as required.

While we have discussed various signs and symptoms of local anaesthesia systemic toxicity, these may be challenging to elicit in very young children. As such, persistent crying post-procedure may be the first and only warning sign [27].

As soon as the diagnosis of any of the above is suspected, an urgent referral to a paediatric intensivist should be made, as the patient will require close monitoring and sometimes management in an intensive care unit, in severe cases.

Others

When the child is restless and unable to cooperate or there are extensive treatment areas, sedation or general anaesthesia (GA) may be required. In general, the use of GA in children under 3 years of age is controversial and not recommended due to the risk of affecting brain development [28, 29]. The risks versus benefits of the procedure under GA should therefore be discussed between the physician and parents and/or caregivers.

Common Complications and Mitigating Factors

Aside from careful patient selection, there are other mitigating factors for these common complications which are associated with lasers in the paediatric population:

Pain

Children generally have a lower pain threshold than adults. Other than anaesthesia (as discussed above), other pain management techniques such as cooling packs and vibrating devices can be employed to soothe the area and minimize discomfort. Distraction techniques can also be employed by an assistant to calm the patient.

Epidermal Damage

This may manifest as blistering, swelling and potential scarring. Appropriate laser settings and techniques must be employed based on the patient's skin type and condition. Especially for patients of darker skin types and treatment-naïve patients, a test spot on a small area is highly recommended to determine the minimal settings required to achieve the desired clinical endpoint. Epidermal cooling during and immediately after the procedure is also important to reduce the chance of permanent epidermal damage, particularly in darker skin types.

Dyspigmentation (Hyper- or Hypopigmentation)

Again, employing the right laser techniques and settings is crucial to minimize the risk of undesired pigmentary changes. Understanding the indications for the laser, patient's skin type and desired clinical endpoint required is important. Post-laser care is also crucial to reduce the chance of post-inflammatory pigmentary changes. Post-laser care in the form of bland emollients, topical steroids and/or topical antibiotic formulations may be prescribed, depending on the condition. Sun avoidance and sun protection should also be strictly reinforced after the procedure till the next review.

Risk of Infection

Laser treatment may temporarily impair the skin barrier, thereby resulting in a risk of infections. Viral infections in the form of herpes simplex virus (HSV) infections have been reported post-laser, especially with perioral and/or facial procedures. HSV reactivation may also present with secondary bacterial infection or impetiginization, which can also increase the risk of pigmentary changes and scarring. It is therefore important to screen all patients for a prior history of HSV infection. HSV prophylaxis can thus be administered prior to the procedure in the form of oral antiviral agents.

Ocular Damage

Laser therapy may potentially cause ocular damage. It is thus important to prepare the patient and administer the necessary protection. If the child is unable to cooperate, it is best not to proceed with the procedure unless under GA/sedation, during which the appropriate eye protection can be administered. We will elaborate on eye protection in children in further detail under the following section "*Optimizing the Environment for the Procedure*".

Optimizing the Environment for the Procedure

Parental Presence

Unless otherwise specified, presence of one parent or caregiver during the procedure is preferred. This helps to calm the patient in unfamiliar surroundings and alleviate any potential separation anxiety [30]. Overall, this can also increase parental satisfaction and help them understand what the procedure is like.

Positioning of the Patient

In any procedure, starting out with optimal positioning of the patient is crucial. For most infants, swaddling is highly recommended. Some have also adopted a "parent-child tent" at the head of the treatment table [31].

Nursing Support

Good nursing support is also required. The assisting staff can help to distract, coax, swaddle or help with eye protection. In some cases, they may also help to alleviate anxiety of not just the patient, but also the accompanying parent.

Distraction Techniques

Depending on the age of the patient, there are many ways to distract a child during procedures. This ranges from singing to the use of devices. Modern technology and devices can be very useful tools in distracting a child during the procedure. For instance, playing a child's favourite show or game on a mobile device or allowing him or her to listen to music with headphones are all potential distracting techniques to calm a child.

Patient Consent and Cooperation

For older children, it is also highly recommended that the clinician attempts to discuss the procedure with the child, not just the parent or caregiver. The child's comfort is paramount to achieve good results, so it is highly recommended to "communicate" and "negotiate" what the procedure will be like and reassuring them that the treatment will not start until they are ready [30].

Laser and Ocular Safety

Direct ocular exposure to lasers can cause permanent ocular damage. Standard protective eye equipment or goggles may be too large or uncomfortable for children of younger age groups. Alternative methods for young children include that of laser-safe adhesive eye pads or shields in smaller sizes, or, simply, overlapping patches of white gauze, during the procedure. When working around the eyelids, corneal shields must be used. If the patient is awake, the shields can be inserted after quick administration of anaesthetic eye drops. To minimize the risk of corneal abrasion with corneal shields, lubricant eye gels are applied during insertion.

Skin Cooling

Epidermal cooling during laser therapy can reduce pain as well as reduce the risk of epidermal damage. Some laser devices come with their own dynamic cooling devices and cryogen sprays; post-procedure cooling can also be done with the gentle application of ice packs or water-cooled handheld tools.

Conclusion

Laser surgery remains a very useful tool in the treatment of skin conditions in paediatric dermatology. Children are not just "little adults". Each age and condition requires specific considerations. Aside from understanding laser techniques, laser treatment in the paediatric population poses unique challenges that are different from that of adult dermatology. As discussed, it is important to recognize the necessity for early treatment in some paediatric conditions and the need for adjustments of settings in different skin types and safety measures, along with the emotional needs and concerns that paediatric patients (and their caregivers) may have.

References

1. Jacobs AH, Walton RG. The incidence of birthmarks in the neonate. Paediatrics. 1976;58(2):218–22.
2. Chapas AM, Geronemus RG. Our approach to pediatric dermatologic laser surgery. Lasers Surg Med. 2005;37(4):255–63.
3. Shahriari M, Makkar H, Finch J. Laser therapy in dermatology: kids are not just little people. Clin Dermatol. 2015;33(6):681–6.
4. Chapas AM, Eickhorst K, Geronemus RG. Efficacy of early treatment of facial port wine stains in newborns: a review of 49 cases. Lasers Surg Med. 2007;39(7):563–8.
5. Renfro L, Geronemus RG. Anatomical differences of port-wine stains in response to treatment with the pulsed dye laser. Arch Dermatol. 1993;129(2):182–8.
6. Lanigan SW. Port wine stains on the lower limb: response to pulsed dye laser therapy. Clin Exp Dermatol. 1996;21(2):88–92.
7. Nguyen CM, Yohn JJ, Huff C, Weston WL, Morelli JG. Facial port wine stains in childhood: prediction of the rate of improvement as a function of the age of the patient, size and location of the port wine stain and the number of treatments with the pulsed dye (585 nm) laser. Br J Dermatol. 1998;138(5):821–5.
8. Cantatore JL, Kriegel DA. Laser surgery: an approach to the pediatric patient. J Am Acad Dermatol. 2004;50(2):165–84.
9. Cunningham BB. Laser therapy and dermatologic surgery. Curr Opin Pediatr. 1998;10(4):405–10.
10. Ziad K, Badi J, Roaa Z, Emily AH. Laser treatment of infantile hemangioma. J Cosmet Dermatol. 2023;22(Suppl 2):1–7.

11. McCuaig CC, Cohen L, Powell J, Hatami A, Marcoux D, Maari C, Caouette-Laberge L, Bortoluzzi P, Ondrejchak S, Dubois J. Therapy of ulcerated hemangiomas. J Cutan Med Surg. 2013;17(4):233–42.
12. Frieden IJ. Which hemangiomas to treat—and how? Arch Dermatol. 1997;133(12):1593–5.
13. Chan HH, King WW, Chan ES, Mok CO, Ho WS, Van Krevel C, Lau WY. In vivo trial comparing patients' tolerance of Q-switched Alexandrite (QS Alex) and Q-switched neodymium:yttrium-aluminum-garnet (QS Nd:YAG) lasers in the treatment of nevus of Ota. Lasers Surg Med. 1999;24(1):24–8.
14. Kang W, Lee E, Choi GS. Treatment of Ota's nevus by Q-switched alexandrite laser: therapeutic outcome in relation to clinical and histopathological findings. Eur J Dermatol. 1999;9(8):639–43.
15. Osborn LP, Nieman EL. Update on lasers in pediatric dermatology: how primary care providers can help patients and families navigate appropriate treatment options and timelines. Curr Opin Pediatr. 2023;35(4):436–44.
16. Patel PD, Mohan GC, Bhattacharya T, Patel RA, Tsoukas M. Pediatric laser therapy in pigmented conditions. Am J Clin Dermatol. 2019;20(5):647–55.
17. Bekhor PS, Bekhor L, Gandrabur M. Employer attitudes toward persons with visible tattoos. Australas J Dermatol. 1995;36(2):75–7.
18. Tattoo removals subsidised for young people finding work or trying to stay in school. https://www.straitstimes.com/singapore/tattoo-removals-subsidised-for-young-people-finding-work-or-trying-to-stay-in-school.
19. NSC health fund. https://www.nsc.com.sg/about-nsc/Pages/NSC-Health-Fund.aspx.
20. Alster TS, Lupton JR. Lasers in dermatology. An overview of types and indications. Am J Clin Dermatol. 2001;2(5):291–303.
21. Cordisco MR. An update on lasers in children. Curr Opin Pediatr. 2009;21(4):499–504.
22. Sharon E, Levi A, Lapidoth M, Snast I. Laser and light therapy for pediatric hair removal: a systematic review. Lasers Med Sci. 2023;38(1):156.
23. Tran AN, Koo JY. Risk of systemic toxicity with topical lidocaine/prilocaine: a review. J Drugs Dermatol. 2014;13(9):1118–22.
24. Rincon E, Baker RL, Iglesias AJ, Duarte AM. CNS toxicity after topical application of EMLA cream on a toddler with molluscum contagiosum. Pediatr Emerg Care. 2000;16(4):252–4.
25. Shamriz O, Cohen-Glickman I, Reif S, Shteyer E. Methemoglobinemia induced by lidocaine-prilocaine cream. Isr Med Assoc J. 2014;16(4):250–4.
26. Friedman N, Scolnik D, McMurray L, Bryan J. Acquired methemoglobinemia presenting to the pediatric emergency department: a clinical challenge. CJEM. 2020;22(5):673–7.
27. Schweitzer-Chaput A, Callot D, Bouazza N, Lesage F, Oualha M, Paret N, Boyer-Gervoise M, Treluyer JM, Chouchana L. Local anesthetics systemic toxicity in children: analysis of the French pharmacovigilance database. BMC Pediatr. 2023;23(1):321.
28. Chen BK, Eichenfield LF. Advances in pediatric dermatologic surgery. Adv Dermatol. 2000;16:477–500; discussion 501. +5.
29. Rappaport B, Mellon RD, Simone A, Woodcock J. Defining safe use of anesthesia in children. N Engl J Med. 2011;364(15):1387–90.
30. Alegre-Sánchez A, Pérez-García B, Boixeda P. Pulsed-dye laser treatment of port-wine stains in children: useful tips to avoid general anaesthesia. Pediatr Dermatol. 2017;34(5):619–21.
31. Yoo SS, Liggett J, Cohen BA. Use of parent-child tents in pediatric laser surgery. Dermatol Surg. 2003;29(4):399–401.

Use of Lasers in Acne Vulgaris

9

Jae Yoon Jung and Dae Hun Suh

Abbreviations

ALA	Aminolevulinic acid
DCD	Dynamic cooling device
GEA	Global evaluation acne
ICG	Indocyanine green
IGA	Investigator's global assessment
IPL	Intense pulsed light
IRB	Institutional Review Board
KTP	Potassium-titanyl-phosphate
LED	Light-emitting diode
LPDLs	Long-pulse dye lasers
MAL	Methyl aminolevulinate
MAL	Methyl aminolevulinic acid
MASS	Michaëlsson acne severity score
PAE	Post-acne erythema
PDL	Pulsed dye laser
PDT	Photodynamic therapy
PIH	Post-inflammatory hyperpigmentation
PpIX	Protoporphyrin IX
RCT	Randomized controlled trials
SA	Salicylic acid
TGF	Transforming growth factor
UV-A	Ultraviolet A

J. Y. Jung
Oaro Dermatology Clinic, Seoul, South Korea

D. H. Suh (✉)
Department of Dermatology, Seoul National University College of Medicine, Acne, Rosacea, Seborrheic Dermatitis and Hidradenitis Suppurativa Research Laboratory, Seoul National University Hospital, Seoul, South Korea
e-mail: daehun@snu.ac.kr

Lasers Therapies

532 nm Potassium-Titanyl-Phosphate (KTP) Laser

The 532 nm potassium-titanyl-phosphate (KTP) laser is a broad-spectrum green light and commonly used as a vascular laser for the treatment of vascular diseases such as telangiectasia and rosacea. Hemoglobin and melanin are the major chromophores targeted by this laser.

There have been several reports suggesting its effectiveness in treating acne [1, 2]. Although the exact treatment mechanism for acne is not clear, it is hypothesized to involve selective photothermolysis of blood vessels and photoactivation of porphyrins in *Cutibacterium acnes* (*C. acnes*) bacteria and to produce limited nonspecific thermal injury to sebaceous glands and, thus, a photodynamic effect.

In one split-face study, 38 patients with mild to moderate acne received once- or twice-weekly treatments in one half of their face, while the other half remained as untreated [1]. Treatment was performed with 4 mm spot size, 20–40 ms pulse duration, and 5–12 J/cm^2 fluence according

S. W. N. Cheng, C. L. Goh (eds.), *Updates on Lasers in Dermatology*, Updates in Clinical Dermatology, https://doi.org/10.1007/978-3-031-71155-8_9

to skin type. After 4 weeks of treatment, they achieved 31% ($p = 0.005$) and 40% ($p < 0.001$) improvement of Michaëlsson acne severity score (MASS), respectively. For both groups, changes of MASS were insignificant for untreated sites.

Baugh and Kucaba conducted a randomized split-face study of 26 patients to evaluate the 532 nm KTP laser for the treatment of mild-to-moderate acne. Laser treatment fluence was 12 J/cm^2 with a 30–40 ms pulse width and a 1–5 Hz frequency. Results showed a mean 34.9% ($p = 0.011$) and 20.7% ($p = 0.25$) reduction of MASS at the 1-week and 4-week post-final treatments, respectively [2].

Side effects observed with the 532 nm KTP treatment are mild erythema, edema, and transient crusting [1, 2]. However, pigmentary side effects should be considered especially in dark-skinned patients because of its high absorption by melanin.

585 and 595 nm Pulsed Dye Laser (PDL)

Similar to the KTP laser, the pulsed dye laser (PDL) has been primarily used for the treatment of vascular lesions. PDL targets oxyhemoglobin within vessels and decreases dermal vessels associated with inflammation [3]. It improves inflammation and inhibits keratinocyte proliferation by elevating transforming growth factor (TGF)-β [4]. It can kill *C. acnes* by photochemical effects of red light on porphyrin [5]. These mechanisms contribute to the effectiveness of PDL in the treatment of inflammatory acne (Fig. 9.1). The PDL wavelength is also believed to destroy the sebaceous glands [6, 7], which accounts for the efficacy of PDL in treating noninflammatory acne.

There have been conflicting reports regarding the efficacy of PDL for acne treatment. Seaton and colleagues [8] reported a 53% reduction in total lesion counts in PDL-treated patients compared to 9% and 10% reduction in controls, respectively, after one treatment. However, subsequent two randomized controlled trials (RCTs) could not replicate this result [9, 10]. Vries and colleagues [11] proposed that this discrepancy could be due to different laser devices and settings, especially the pulse duration used.

Recent results of the meta-analysis demonstrated that only one or two PDL sessions are not superior to the control group in treating acne vulgaris [12]. However, four or more PDL sessions or using longer pulse duration (10 or 40 ms) could significantly decrease acne severity score [12].

Leheta and colleagues [13] compared fortnightly PDL with topical treatment (tretinoin, benzoyl peroxide) and chemical peeling (trichloroacetic acid 25%) in treating acne. All three groups demonstrated a significant improvement, with no significant difference among the three groups [13].

PDL is the most common laser used for the treatment of post-acne erythema (PAE) as it

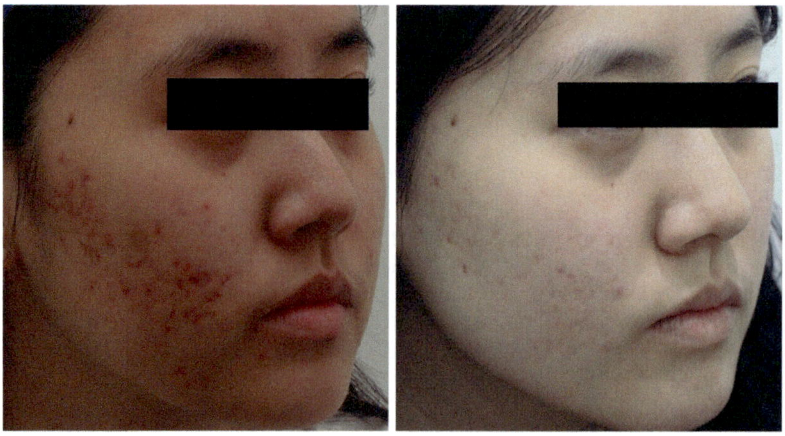

Fig. 9.1 A 20-year-old acne patient. Before acne treatment (left), after treatment (right). Improvement of active acne and acne red marks is observed simultaneously after three sessions of treatment with 595 nm pulsed dye laser at 3-week intervals

coagulates microvessels in the dermis. A pilot study using two sessions of 595 nm PDL for 20 acne patients with skin Fitzpatrick types III and IV showed significant improvement of PAE and improvement in skin elasticity [14]. A case study also reported significant improvement of PAE in two patients following 595 nm PDL [15].

Additionally, PDL is known to promote remodeling of the epidermis and collagen synthesis by the significant increase in TGF-β, a potent stimulator of neocollagenesis [4, 10, 14, 16]. This finding makes it useful for the treatment of atrophic scars and keloids.

Combination treatment of the PDL with other therapies shows promising results. Adjunctive PDL (three PDL treatments at 3-week intervals) with 30% salicylic acid chemical peel achieved statistically significant greater improvement in acne based on Global Evaluation Acne (GEA) scale score compared with the peel-only group ($p = 0.003$) [17]. Glaich and colleagues [18] reported an 84% reduction in mean acne lesion count and effective treatment of acne scarring and PAE by using a 595 nm PDL and a 1450 nm diode laser in combination. Both 585 nm PDL and combined 585/1064 nm laser treatment were found to be effective at treating inflammatory and noninflammatory acne lesions, although the 585/1064 nm laser was significantly better than PDL treatment at treating noninflammatory acne [4]. Adding of PDL to oral isotretinoin (0.25 mg/kg/day) resulted in a statistically significant greater improvement than the standard higher dose isotretinoin (0.5 mg/kg/day) as monotherapy at 3 and 6 months [19].

PDL is usually recommended in lighter skin types to reduce the risk of adverse effects such as PIH and hypopigmentation due to its relatively high absorption rate by melanin.

800 nm Diode Laser with Gold-Coated Microparticles

Gold-coated microparticles can be transported by the trans-appendageal route; they are less likely to be absorbed by the epidermis and are more selectively absorbed by the sebaceous glands. Since the gold-coated microparticles have a large-size nanoshell, minimal systemic uptake is expected [20]. They have a maximal optical absorption in the 800 nm range. Gold-coated microparticles in combination with 800 nm diode laser were associated with selective thermal injury in the sebaceous follicles of swine and human skin [21]. This results in a decrease in sebum production.

Fuchs and colleagues [22] evaluated 28 patients with moderate-to-severe facial acne who received three weekly facial treatments with topically applied gold microparticles and 800 nm diode laser pulses (30 ms of pulse duration, 25–35 J/cm^2 of fluence). Seventy-six percent of patients achieved 40% or more reduction in weighted lesion count (score of 0.5 for open/closed comedones, 1 for papule, 2 for pustule, and 3 for nodule) at 12-week follow-up, with a mean reduction of 63%.

Park and colleagues [23] conducted three treatments for two Korean patients with recalcitrant acne using the 805 nm diode laser followed by the transdermal delivery of gold nanoshells. The number of acne lesions was decreased, and new acne lesions were prevented up to 4 months posttreatment.

Suh and colleagues [24] performed three successive treatments at 1–2-week intervals for 12 patients with moderate-to-severe acne vulgaris. Significant reductions in acne lesions were observed after the use of gold photothermal therapy (papules, $p = .001$; pustules, $p < .001$; and comedones, $p = .001$) without serious adverse effects.

1064 nm Nd:YAG Laser

The 1064 nm Nd:YAG laser can penetrate the deep dermis and cause diffuse heating of dermal tissues without damaging the epidermis. The main chromophores targeted are water and melanin, and it is known to have effects on scars, wrinkles, and photorejuvenation [25–27]. For this reason, it has primarily been researched for scar treatment in acne [27]. While its use is less common for active acne, there have been reports of its effectiveness in reducing sebum production and inflammation [4, 28].

Jung and colleagues [4] treated 16 Korean acne patients using a long-pulsed 1064 nm laser (pulse duration 40 ms, 7 mm spot size, and 40–50 J/cm^2) in combination with a 585 nm PDL (7 mm spot size and 7–9 J/cm^2). Improvement in inflammatory acne was observed in 58.6% of cases, along with a decrease in IL-8 and an increase in TGF-β on a histological level. No significant adverse effects were reported.

Jung and colleagues [28] reported treatment of acne in 22 patients using a dual-mode (quasi-long-pulse 300 μs and Q-switched mode) 1064 nm Nd:YAG laser assisted with a topically applied carbon suspension. Patients received three treatment sessions at 2-week intervals in a randomized split-face manner. The carbon lotion distributes within the stratum corneum and partially penetrates the hair follicles, acting as an exogenous chromophore. The first pass is performed using the quasi-long-pulse mode with low fluence (7 mm spot size handpiece, 1.8–2.0 J/cm^2). This treatment does not break down the carbon particles but allows them to be absorbed and converted into heat energy, leading to nonselective photothermolysis of the epidermis, upper dermis, and pilosebaceous units. It is believed to regulate the inactivation of *C. acnes* and inflammation. Heat damage to the sebaceous glands reduces sebum production, decreasing noninflammatory acne. It also influences the dermal vasculature, inducing various proteins such as HSP-70, IL-6, TGF-β, and procollagen, leading to fibroblastic proliferation and dermal matrix rearrangement [28]. The second pass with low fluence (7 mm spot size, 1.8–2.3 J/cm^2) in Q-switched mode ablates part of the stratum corneum and epidermis, providing a peeling effect on the skin surface and plugged pores, improving comedones, and offering skin rejuvenation effects. Similar to the first pass, it also promotes collagen synthesis. At the final visit, the inflammatory acne lesions were reduced on the laser-treated side by 58.6% ($p < .001$), but increased on the untreated side by 5%. The noninflammatory acne lesions were reduced on the laser-treated side by 52.4% ($p < .001$), demonstrating that this treatment method is safe and effective for skin rejuvenation, pore treatment, and active acne [28] (Fig. 9.2).

The efficacy of long-pulsed 1064 nm Nd:YAG laser and IPL in inflammatory and noninflammatory acne lesions was compared in one study [29]. Thirty patients of skin phototypes III–V with facial acne were randomly assigned to receive three sessions of either Nd:YAG or IPL at 2-week intervals. The Nd:YAG group showed significantly reduced noninflammatory lesion count by 65.7% (vs. 30.8% in the IPL group). One month after the last session, the difference in improvement between noninflammatory and inflammatory lesions showed a significant difference in the Nd:YAG group and a nonsignificant difference in the IPL group. Nd:YAG showed a significant difference in the improvement score in noninflammatory lesions and a nonsignificant difference in inflammatory lesions, compared to IPL [29]. In another split-face study on 34 participants with mild-to-moderate facial acne, clinical efficacy of 1064 nm Nd:YAG (spot 7 mm, pulse duration 5 ms, and fluence 30 J/cm^2) was compared with 595 nm PDL [30] (three sessions at 2-week interval) (spot size 7 mm, pulse duration 10 ms, and fluence of 8.5 J/cm^2). As compared with baseline, mean inflammatory acne lesion counts, acne erythema grading, and erythema index were significantly reduced on both sides. However, there were no significant differences between the two [30].

1320 nm Nd:YAG Laser

The 1320 nm Nd:YAG laser operates at a mid-infrared wavelength and is known to have a thermolytic effect on the sebaceous glands. Another theoretical advantage of using 1320 nm Nd:YAG laser to treat active acne is the potential to concurrently improve atrophic acne scarring [31–33]. Previous studies have demonstrated the clinical efficacy of 1320 nm Nd:YAG laser therapy in the treatment of acne scarring, and the mechanism of action is by collagen remodeling and increased collagen production [31–33]. However, research

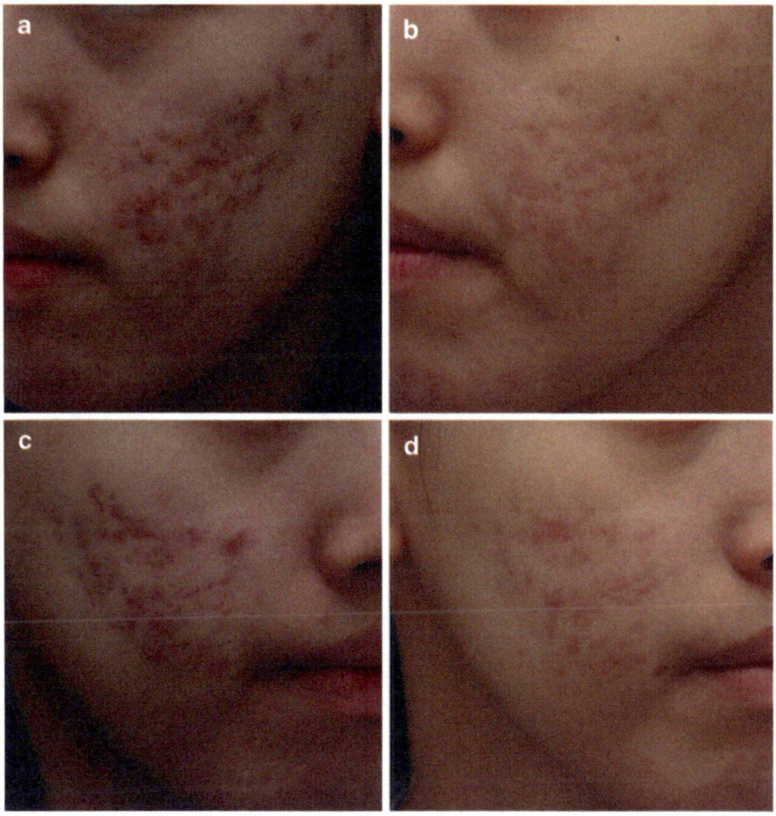

Fig. 9.2 A 29-year-old patient with acne. Before acne treatment (**a, c**), after local application of carbon lotion, treated with 1064 nm Nd:YAG laser using two different pulse durations, quasi-long pulse and Q-switched, in a continuous treatment method for three sessions at 2-week intervals. Two weeks after treatment (**b, d**): improvement of inflammatory acne lesions can be observed

on the use of this wavelength laser for active acne lesion treatment is limited.

Deng and colleagues [34] performed six treatments at 2-week intervals using fractional 1320 nm Nd:YAG laser (fluencies of 10–15 J/cm^2, densities of 25 MTZ/cm^2, five to six passes on acne lesions) on 41 acne patients. The authors reported statistically significant reductions in inflammatory and noninflammatory lesions by 57% and 30%, respectively. Additionally, sebum levels as assessed using a Sebumeter were significantly decreased in the treated group by 30% ($p < 0.05$). Side effects documented in this study were 3 days of erythema without pigmentary complications.

However, another study involving 46 subjects using a split-face approach reported a temporary and significant reduction in the number of open comedones after three treatments with the 1320 nm laser, but there was no statistically significant difference in the number of inflammatory acne lesions [35]. Therefore, further research is needed to determine the efficacy of using this wavelength for the treatment of active acne.

1450 nm Diode Laser

The 1450 nm diode laser is one of the most commonly used and popular devices for active acne lesions (Fig. 9.3). Anatomically, the sebaceous glands are distributed in the upper dermis, located at depths of 200–1000 μm from the skin surface, with higher density in areas such as the face, chest, and back. Increased sebum production is one of the major causes of acne and has a significant impact on enlarged pores. Since water is the main chromophore in sebaceous glands, wavelengths that have a high absorption in water and can reach the depth where sebaceous glands are distributed are considered effective for sebaceous gland treatment. The penetration depth according to wavelength is defined as the depth at which 36.8% of the surface fluence rate reaches.

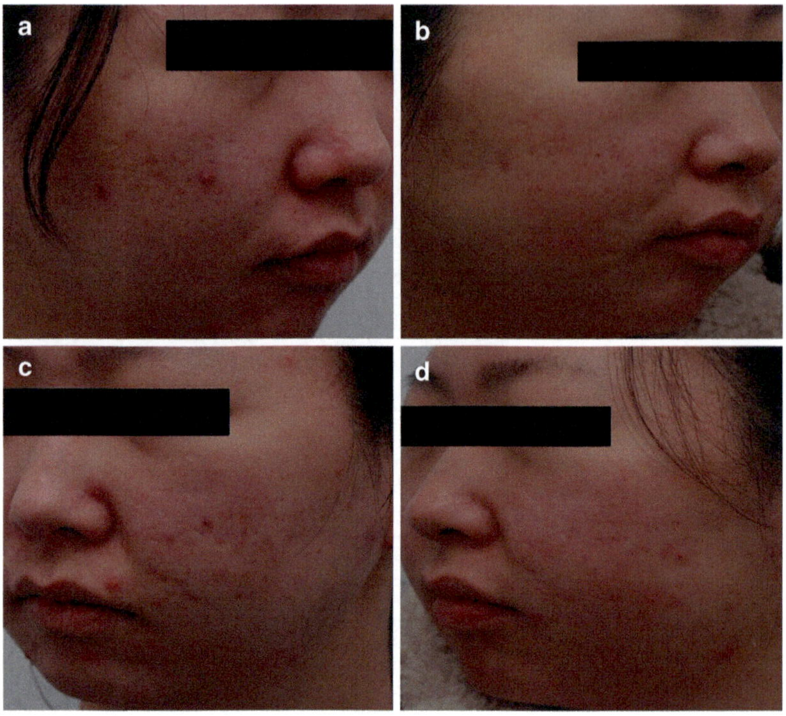

Fig. 9.3 A 24-year-old acne patient. Before acne treatment (**a, c**), after treatment (**b, d**). Improvement of active acne is observed after three sessions of treatment with 1450 nm diode laser at 2-week intervals

According to Monte Carlo simulations based on light transmission and heat transfer calculations, the penetration depth of the 1450 nm wavelength is 439 μm, which aligns with the upper dermis where sebaceous glands are predominantly distributed [36]. In animal experiments and investigations on human skin using 1450 nm laser, a thermal damage zone was observed in the upper epidermis, demonstrating the destruction of sebaceous glands [36].

Typically, the treatment fluence ranges from 12 to 14 J/cm^2, as high as 16 J/cm^2, in previous 1450 nm diode laser therapy. The conventional high-fluence 1450 nm diode laser treatment can reduce facial acne lesions effectively. However, even with the application of topical anesthetic cream and using dynamic cooling device, the treatment is often very painful for many patients to tolerate [37–39].

In a few studies, using lower energy (8–11 J/cm^2) with a double-pass technique was as effective, less painful, and better tolerated [40–42]. In addition to conventional stamp-mode treatment, the novel moving mode with multiple passes of lower energies to lengthen laser exposure time around the whole face was successfully used in one Korean study [43]. In a 20-week, randomized, split-face study, the patients were treated with three consecutive sessions at 4-week intervals. One half of the face received a dual regimen consisting of low-fluence stamping mode (5–6 J/cm^2) for inflammatory acne lesions only, followed by 4–5 passes of moving mode for the full face. The other side received a single-pass treatment of conventional high-fluence stamp mode (14–15 J/cm^2). At the final 12-week follow-up evaluations, the dual-mode side demonstrated improvements in both inflammatory and noninflammatory lesion counts, better acne severity assessments, and reduction in sebum secretion compared with stamp-only side [43].

The most concerning complication using 1450 nm laser treatment is post-inflammatory hyperpigmentation (PIH), primarily seen in dark skin type. Reported PIH occurrence rates ranged up to 39% depending on the study [44]. Two factors that caused side effects were the use of high fluence and long cooling times. The side effect of PIH is significant due to the sensitivity of dark skin type to cryogen-induced injury. PIH could subsequently be minimized by decreasing the dynamic cooling device (DCD) spray duration in a few studies [41, 43, 44]. Decreasing the laser fluence to minimize epidermal damage may also potentially reduce the incidence of PIH [42, 43].

1540 and 1550 nm Erbium Glass Laser

The 1540 nm and 1550 nm erbium glass lasers are primarily used for non-ablative dermal remodeling and induction of collagen synthesis to improve wrinkles, scars, and pore size [45–47]. Consequently, research on acne scars using lasers of this wavelength is quite active, and they are commonly utilized as the main lasers for acne scar treatment due to their noninvasive nature and short downtime. This wavelength can penetrate deep into the dermis and modulate sebaceous gland activity through heat coagulation, as shown in several studies demonstrating positive results in acne treatment [45, 48].

Several uncontrolled studies have been performed to evaluate the efficacy of the 1540 nm erbium glass laser for the treatment of acne. Angel and colleagues [49] treated 18 patients with face acne using 1540 nm erbium glass (3 ms, four pulses, 10 J/cm^2, cumulative fluence 40 J/cm^2). Four treatments were performed at 4-week intervals, and the results showed the mean reduction of 71%, 79%, and 73% at 6-, 12-, and 24-month follow-up, respectively [49]. Bogle and colleagues [48] reported 15 patients with inflammatory facial acne treated with four treatments at 2-week intervals using 1540 nm erbium:glass laser (active lesions treated with six pulses at 10 J/cm^2, entire face then treated with bursts of four pulses at 10 J/cm^2). At 6-month follow-up, mean investigator improvement assessment was 78%. A single retreatment 6 months after the initial course held clearance at 80% at 9-month follow-up [48]. Politi and colleagues [50] reported mild-to-moderate acne patients using 1540 erbium:glass laser with four to six treatment sessions at a 2-week interval. An acne lesion was initially manipulated upon contact by a vacuum cooling-assisted tip, followed by 3–4 stacked pulses to affected areas with the following parameters: 500–600 mJ, 4 mm spot size, and 2 Hz. Independent dermatologists rated improvement as moderate to significant in all patients [50]. In one study, improvement in both active acne and scars was evaluated after treatment with a 1540 nm erbium:glass fractional laser. Twenty patients with acne and scarring received entire face treatment with four sessions at 1-month interval [51]. Eighty percent of patients felt the improvement of the scars, and 85% of patients felt that their active acne had been improved. Pore size was evaluated as improved by 75%, and sebum secretion improved in 80% of cases [51].

The 1550 nm fractional erbium:glass fractional laser has also been studied and used in the treatment of active acne, particularly inflammatory acne. Moneib and colleagues [52] reported significant improvement in acne lesions after four treatments at 2-week intervals using a 1550 nm fractional erbium:glass laser (30–40 mJ, two passes of stamping mode, and one pass of continuous moving mode) on 24 acne patients. A significant reduction ($p < 0.0001$) in the mean count of lesions and in the size of sebaceous glands was observed after treatment. In particular, remission in papules and pustules was maintained for approximately 1 year after completion of sessions. The laser treatment was well tolerated by all patients without serious complications [52]. Liu and colleagues treated 45 acne patients with four sessions at monthly intervals with an 1550 nm erbium fractional laser and evaluated both the short-term and long-term clinical efficacy. Treatment parameters were 100–169 spot density, 15–30 mJ, one pass for sensitive skin, and two passes for general skin [53]. The results showed 72% reduction in mean lesion count at 6-month, 79% at 1-year, and 75% at 2-year follow-ups. Adverse effects were mild erythema and edema immediately posttreatment, which recovered after 1–2 days, in nearly all the patients, and transient acne flare-ups in two patients. After 2 years of follow-up, three patients said that their skin was a little sensitive. No other complications were reported.

1726 nm Laser

Sebum has an absorption coefficient higher than water at 1726 nm (1.8:1), and it may be a viable endogenous alternative to exogenous chromophores for sebaceous gland-selective photothermolysis. Sakamoto and colleagues successfully demonstrated that optical pulses with a wavelength of 1700–1720 nm could be used to destroy sebaceous glands selectively in ex vivo human facial skin samples [54].

Scopelliti and colleagues used Monte Carlo and finite element models to show the thermal damage on sebaceous glands and found that selective photothermolysis could be achieved with a 1726 nm laser energy and contact cooling [55]. In vivo human facial skin histologic examination results showed no signs of continuing inflammation in epidermis 5 days posttreatment during the biopsy, and damage to the sebaceous gland was observed across the length of the gland.

Goldberg and colleagues [56] conducted a single-center, open-label study on 17 mild-to-severe acne patients who received up to three facial laser sessions up to 7 weeks apart with the following parameters: delivered in an array of 3 × 3 laser beams with a total area = 68 mm^2, 10–60 J/cm^2 of fluence, 10–60 ms of pulse duration, 3.1 mm of spot size, and 5 °C of cooling temperature. All subjects tolerated the treatments well, and total number of inflammatory lesions was reduced by more than 52% within 1 month of treatment and improved further to 56% by the third month post-final treatment session. Long-term follow-ups showed progressive improvement 24 months posttreatment with a 97% reduction in inflammatory lesion count. Adverse effects occurred mildly and resolved entirely by the end of the study.

1726 nm Laser treatment can be a safe and effective treatment for acne of all severity. However, additional research is needed due to the small number and relatively narrow demographics of subjects of previous studies.

Light-Based Therapies

Blue Light

The *C. acnes* produces a large amount of coproporphyrin III and protoporphyrin IX (PpIX) within its cell [57, 58]. These porphyrins are photosensitized when light energy is absorbed in the spectrum of ultraviolet and blue light [57–59], producing a photodynamic reaction creating a singlet oxygen. Eventually, bacteria are destructed, indicating that acne can be successfully treated with phototherapy with blue visible light. Blue light may also exhibit anti-inflammatory effects [60].

Antoniou and colleagues [61] conducted a split-face study on 89 patients, by applying a photoconverter gel chromophore and then a multi-LED device with a wavelength from 415 to 446 nm, applied for 5 min at a distance of 5 cm (dose: 33–35 J/cm^2, irradiance: 110 and 150 W/cm^2) to one half of the face, and the other half of the face was used as a control group. Two weekly treatment sessions were performed for 6 weeks, and patients were followed up at 6 weeks after final treatment. There was a reduction of at least two degrees in the severity of acne according to the Investigator's Global Assessment (IGA) scale, which was demonstrated in 51.7% of patients at week 12, in the treated group. The number of inflammatory acne lesions dropped at least 40% in 81.6% of the hemifaces treated after 12 weeks. In the control group, with an untreated face, only 18% reached a reduction of 2 degrees in the acne scale [61]. Elman and colleagues [62] treated 46 acne patients with blue light. It was the split-face dose-response study, the full-face open trial, and the split-face, double-blind controlled study. Of these 46 patients, more than 80% of them showed a significant reduction of 59–67% of inflammatory acne lesions after eight treatments [62].

Gold and colleagues [63] performed Institutional Review Board (IRB)-approved randomized self-control study. For each patient (30 mild-to-moderate acne patients), two similar lesions, one of each side of the face, were chosen for treatment with either a blue-light LED handheld or sham device. Treatments were conducted twice daily in the clinic, and lesions were followed up till resolution. The results showed the effectiveness of using blue-light LED therapy on a daily basis for better improvement and faster resolution of inflammatory acne lesions [63].

There were several studies comparing blue light to another therapy. Gold and colleagues compared blue light to topical 1% clindamycin solution in the treatment of mild-to-moderate inflammatory acne [64]. Blue-light therapy reduced inflammatory acne vulgaris lesions by an average of 34%, as compared to 14% for topical 1% clindamycin solution [64]. Goldman and Boyce compared two sessions of blue light to blue-light PDT in 22 patients; results showed promise for this treatment in mild-to-moderate inflammatory acne vulgaris [65]. However, results in these two studies were not statistically analyzed [64, 65]. Kwon and colleagues [66] conducted a 20-week, randomized split-face study to compare 1450 nm diode laser (two passes of the stamp mode, spot size 6 mm, and 5–7 J/cm^2 of fluence) followed sequentially by blue light (450 nm, 3.5–7.0 mW/cm^2 of irradiance range) versus blue light alone in 24 patients with mild-to-moderate facial acne vulgaris. Patients received three consecutive sessions at 4-week intervals. Both combination and blue light sides demonstrated steady improvement of inflammatory acne lesions with 62.3% and 35.2% decreases at the 12-week follow-up visit compared with baseline, respectively. For noninflammatory lesions and seborrhea, only combination regimen demonstrated improvement. No severe adverse effect was observed on both sides [66].

The variable efficacy rates observed using blue-light treatment studies could be related to the varied spectral output of devices and overlap of the ultraviolet A (UV-A) range.

Red (± Blue) Light

Red light penetrates to the level of sebaceous glands in the dermis compared with 1–2 mm for light at 400–500 nm. Although *C. acnes* is inactivated with shorter wavelengths, red light (620–660 nm) seems to be more efficacious than blue light (400–500 nm) in the treatment of acne [67].

Li and colleagues [68] demonstrated anti-inflammatory effect of red LED light therapy using an in vitro model and obtained normalization of keratinization within the sebaceous glands by lowering the level of interleukin IL-α. They suggested that red LED light treatments can inhibit inflammation and normalize pilosebaceous duct hyperkeratinization [68].

Na and Suh [69] treated 28 mild-to-moderate acne patients with portable red light-emitting devices in this split-face randomized trial. Phototherapy was performed for 15 min (wavelength of 635–670 nm, irradiance of 6 mW, cumulative dose of 604.8 J/cm^2) twice a day for 8 weeks, and the percent improvement in noninflammatory and inflammatory lesion counts of the treated side was significant compared to the control side ($p < .005$) [69]. This study shows that phototherapy with red light alone is effective in acne.

The effectiveness of combination red and blue light therapy has been demonstrated in several studies. Papageorgiou and colleagues [70] reported that the simultaneous use of red and blue light was significantly more effective than blue light alone or 5% benzoyl peroxide. They proposed that phototherapy with mixed blue and red light, probably by combining antibacterial and anti-inflammatory action, is an effective means of treating acne vulgaris of mild-to-moderate severity, with no significant short-term adverse effects [70]. Kwon and colleagues [71] performed double-blinded, randomized, sham device-controlled study with combination blue and red LED devices for 35 mild-to-moderate acne patients. Twice-daily treatment of blue–red LED for 4 weeks significantly decreased both inflammatory and noninflammatory acne lesions by 77% and 54%, respectively, at 12 weeks. Sebum output reduction, attenuated inflammatory cell infiltrations, and a decreased size of the sebaceous gland were found only in the treatment group [71]. Combination blue and red light therapy was compared with 10% salicylic acid (SA) peel in adolescents [72]. The number of comedones, pustules, and papules also showed significant reduction after treatment in both groups. However, there was a significant difference between the number of pustules on phototherapy group compared to the SA group [72]. In a

12-week, randomized, evaluator-blinded study of patients with mild-to-moderate acne, 445 nm/630 nm light therapy was found to be more significantly effective, with 24.4% improvement in inflammatory acne lesions compared with 2.5% benzoyl peroxide lotion with 17.2% improvement [73]. Combination light therapy was also significantly effective in noninflammatory acne lesions compared with 2.5% benzoyl peroxide lotion (19.5% improvement vs. 6.3% improvement, respectively).

Intense Pulsed Light (IPL)

Intense pulsed light (IPL) delivers wide-spectrum, noncoherent visible light (green, yellow, and red) to near-infrared wavelengths. IPL therapy is widely used in a variety of dermatologic conditions, such as pigmentary disorders, vascular lesions, inflammatory conditions, acneiform eruption, premalignant lesions, and adnexal disease [74].

The action mechanism of IPL for acne treatment may be photoexcitation of porphyrins, synthesized and stored by *C. acnes*, to generate reactive oxygen species and photosensitivity [75, 76]. Sebaceous glands can be damaged by several mechanisms after IPL treatment, such as free oxygen radicals by photoactivation of porphyrins and destroying blood supply to the sebaceous gland by heat damage. This results in reducing the amount of sebum [77].

There were a few negative results for acne treatment with IPL. Chang and colleagues reported that IPL alone (530–750 nm filter, 7.5–8.0 J/cm^2 of fluence, three treatment sessions at 3-week intervals) was effective for acne red macules, irregular pigmentation, and skin tone [78]. However, there was no significant difference between IPL-treated and untreated sides of the face for mean papule plus pustule counts, 3 weeks after three sessions. Yeung and colleagues also showed no significant efficacy of IPL alone (530–750 nm filter, 7.0–9.0 J/cm^2 of fluence, four treatment sessions at 3-week intervals) or IPL combined with topical methyl aminolevulinic acid (MAL)-PDT for moderate inflammation in Chinese patients [79].

In contrast, more studies have demonstrated IPL efficacy in acne treatment, especially to inflammatory lesions [80–84]. This discrepancy may result from acne severity of patients or inaccurate targeting of the light source.

Seven patients with acne vulgaris alongside mild acne scarring were treated [80]. After four treatments spaced at 3-week intervals, patients assessed their improvement at 70%, whereas physician-assessed improvement was 75% [80]. In another study, 100 female inflammatory acne patients with Fitzpatrick skin types IV–VI were treated with IPL using a 530–1200 nm filter (7.0 J/cm^2 fluence with 3 ms of pulse width) once a week for a total duration of 6 weeks. Patient satisfaction scores revealed that approximately 80% of patients noticed good-to-excellent improvement, and approximately 11% of patients reported fair-to-good improvement [81]. Kawana and colleagues reported that IPL with dominant wavelengths of 400–700 nm had a satisfactory effect on acne vulgaris in Asians [82]. After five treatments, noninflammatory and inflammatory acne lesions were decreased to 12.9% and 11.7%, respectively.

Patidar and colleagues compared IPL at two different fluences in a split-face study with 45 Indians with inflammatory facial acne. Four treatments of IPL were delivered at 2-week intervals with normal fluence (35 J/cm^2) and subnormal fluence (20 J/cm^2). Both fluence treatments were effective (63.49% and 57.9% lesion count reduction, respectively), with no significant difference between the two [83].

IPL with a novel filter of dual-band spectral output (400–600 nm and 800–1200 nm) was used in one prospective study [85]. Five sessions of IPL treatment (first and second pulse fluences for the treatment were 9 and 6 J/cm^2, respectively; 3.5–4.0 ms of pulse width; 30–40 ms delay in a double-pulse mode) mode and the energy density of the first and second pulses at 4-week interval were administered to the subjects. Over 75% of subjects exhibited excellent or good response at 1 month posttreatment. The first band (400–600 nm) has an impact of photodynamic therapy on *C. acnes*, and the second band (800–1200 nm) can penetrate deeper into the skin and might directly target sebaceous glands [85].

Choi and colleagues compared the efficacy and safety of IPL and 585 nm PDL [84]. A split-face, single-blind, randomized controlled study was conducted with four treatment sessions at 2-week intervals. One half of the face was treated with 585 nm PDL (10 mm spot size, 40 ms pulse duration, 8–10 J/cm^2 fluence, and two passes in conjunction with cold air cooling). The other side was treated using IPL (530–750 nm filter, 7.5–8.3 J/cm^2 fluence, 2.5 ms pulse duration, triple light pulse with a 9.0 ms interval, and two passes). Both PDL and IPL were found to treat acne effectively, but PDL showed a more sustained effect.

There were a few studies using IPL with a pressure vacuum [86–88]. This vacuum serves to better target the pilosebaceous unit, thereby stretching the skin, elevating and everting the sebaceous gland, and allowing it to open up and empty its contents. Photopneumatic therapy is a safe and effective treatment for mild-to-moderate acne vulgaris. Lee and colleagues conducted four successive treatments at 2-week intervals on one side of the face with a combined photopneumatic device for 20 adults with mild-to-moderate facial acne vulgaris [86]. Significant lesion improvements and reduced numbers of acne lesions were observed on the treated side. Gold and Biron performed a study of 11 mild-to-moderate acne patients who received four treatments at 3-week intervals with photopneumatic therapy [87]. At 3 months, significant reductions in both inflammatory ($p = 0.0137$) and noninflammatory lesions ($p = .0383$) had occurred. In another study, four successive photopneumatic therapy was administered at 2-week intervals. Modest reduction in acne lesion counts and global clinical improvement were observed in the majority of patients [88]. In these three studies, no severe adverse effects occurred, with the most common adverse events encountered being mild pain and transient erythema.

Generally, IPL has been safely used even in dark skin types without severe adverse effects [81, 83].

Photodynamic Therapy (PDT)

PDT uses light in combination with a photosensitizer, typically applied topically, for treatment. It is hypothesized that PDT decreases the size and function of sebaceous glands, has anti-inflammatory effects, and downregulates the immune response, even decreasing inflammatory markers including TLR-2 and TLR-4 [89–91].

Three topical agents can be used as the photosensitizers in PDT: aminolevulinic acid (ALA), methyl aminolevulinate (MAL), and indocyanine green (ICG). ALA has the largest body of evidence, and 5% ALA is the most commonly used photosensitizer for conventional PDT for acne [92–94]. The largest randomized, single-blinded, self-controlled trial consisted of 180 Chinese patients and compared the efficacy of ALA at different concentrations (5, 10, 15, 20%) [95]. All groups had statistically significant reductions in inflammatory counts, with greater improvement at 24 weeks in the 15% and 20% groups. Treatment-related hyperpigmentation tended to occur earlier and longer at higher ALA strengths. Strength of the photosensitizer can lead to more treatment-related pain and adverse effects. The authors recommended the application of 10% and 15% ALA for 1.5 h with a red-light source as the preferred modality [95]. MAL is related to ALA, but is more lipophilic, and more preferentially localizes to diseased and inflamed skin [96]. Wiegell and colleague investigated the difference in response between MAL and ALA in a split-faced trial with 15 patients. There was a 59% reduction overall in acne lesions without a significant difference between the two photosensitizers. However, adverse effects, such as edema and PIH, were more severe on the ALA side than the MAL side in 80% of patients, possibly because ALA accumulates throughout normal and diseased skin, while MAL shows high selectivity for lesional skin [97]. Indocyanine green (ICG), a photosensitizing dye that can also be used as a photosensitizer, has shown improvement in acne, especially after multiple treatments [98–100].

Different light sources can be used including light-emitting diodes (LEDs), lasers, and

IPL. The wavelength selection of the light controls the penetration depth. Red light penetrates deeper into the dermis to target the sebaceous glands than blue light due to its longer wavelength. Red LED therapy was the most commonly described PDT light source in the literature [101]. Inflammatory acne reduction rate with red-light PDT was highly variable (from 28% to 94%) [102–104]. The total energy dose of red light could affect the results. One study showed that higher fluences of red light (35 vs. 25 J/cm^2) have greater rates of acne clearance [105]. Blue light as a light source was used in only a few small studies that investigated its use with MAL or ALA, showing a 66–71% reduction in acne lesions [106, 107]. IPL was the second most commonly used light source for PDT. In one randomized, split-face clinical trial, IPL was compared with red light for PDT light source, and MAL was used as a photosensitizer in 20 patients. With serial PDT sessions, both groups had a statistically significant decrease in inflammatory lesions from baseline [108]. Rojanamatin and Choawawanich reported beneficial effect of IPL alone (560–590 nm, 25–30 J/cm^2, three sessions at 3- to 4-week intervals) for inflammatory acne, although greater improvement was obtained with a combination of IPL and topical ALA-PDT [109]. PDL and long-pulse dye lasers (LPDLs) were the most frequently used laser in PDT [101]. The trials using PDL as the light source for PDT have shown inconsistent results [110–112]. PDT with PDL showed fewer adverse events than with red or blue light and less pain during treatment, which can be explained by gradual or even decreased overall photobleaching [101].

Conclusion

The use of lasers for acne treatment has shown significant efficacy on its own and can reduce the risk of acne recurrence by improving sebum production. Laser and light treatment for acne not only improves acne lesions but also induces collagen remodeling and neocollagenesis through heat delivery to the dermis, resulting in overall improvement in facial skin elasticity, pore size, and acne scar reduction. The choice of laser or light wavelength can be tailored to individual needs based on factors such as erythema, severity of acne, presence of acne scars, and availability of laser equipment at each clinic. Most acne laser and light treatments have minimal downtime and can be combined with other treatments such as scaling or broad-spectrum light therapy. Therefore, laser treatment for acne can be a suitable alternative for patients who have a poor response to oral or topical acne medications, as well as for patients who are pregnant, children, or with other internal medical conditions where drug therapy may be challenging.

Acknowledgments

Grant support: This study was not supported by any foundation.

Conflict of Interest Statement: The authors have no conflicts of interest or financial ties to disclose.

References

1. Yilmaz O, Senturk N, Yuksel EP, Aydin F, Ozden MG, Canturk T, et al. Evaluation of 532-nm KTP laser treatment efficacy on acne vulgaris with once and twice weekly applications. J Cosmet Laser Ther. 2011;13(6):303–7.
2. Baugh WP, Kucaba WD. Nonablative phototherapy for acne vulgaris using the KTP 532 nm laser. Dermatol Surg. 2005;31(10):1290–6.
3. Bhardwaj SS, Rohrer TE, Arndt K. Lasers and light therapy for acne vulgaris. Semin Cutan Med Surg. 2005;24(2):107–12.
4. Jung JY, Choi YS, Yoon MY, Min SU, Suh DH. Comparison of a pulsed dye laser and a combined 585/1,064-nm laser in the treatment of acne vulgaris. Dermatol Surg. 2009;35(8):1181–7.
5. Nouri K, Ballard CJ. Laser therapy for acne. Clin Dermatol. 2006;24(1):26–32.
6. Hamilton FL, Car J, Lyons C, Car M, Layton A, Majeed A. Laser and other light therapies for the treatment of acne vulgaris: systematic review. Br J Dermatol. 2009;160(6):1273–85.
7. Jih MH, Kimyai-Asadi A. Laser treatment of acne vulgaris. Semin Plast Surg. 2007;21(3):167–74.
8. Seaton ED, Charakida A, Mouser PE, Grace I, Clement RM, Chu AC. Pulsed-dye laser treatment for inflammatory acne vulgaris: randomised controlled trial. Lancet. 2003;362(9393):1347–52.
9. Orringer JS, Kang S, Hamilton T, Schumacher W, Cho S, Hammerberg C, et al. Treatment of acne

vulgaris with a pulsed dye laser: a randomized controlled trial. JAMA. 2004;291(23):2834–9.
10. Lekwuttikarn R, Tempark T, Chatproedprai S, Wananukul S. Randomized, controlled trial split-faced study of 595-nm pulsed dye laser in the treatment of acne vulgaris and acne erythema in adolescents and early adulthood. Int J Dermatol. 2017;56(8):884–8.
11. de Vries FMC, Meulendijks AM, Driessen RJB, van Dooren AA, Tjin EPM, van de Kerkhof PCM. The efficacy and safety of non-pharmacological therapies for the treatment of acne vulgaris: a systematic review and best-evidence synthesis. J Eur Acad Dermatol Venereol. 2018;32(7):1195–203.
12. Yang TH, Li CN, Huang YC. The efficacy of pulsed dye laser treatment for acne vulgaris: a systemic review and meta-analysis. Dermatol Surg. 2022;48(2):209–13.
13. Leheta TM. Role of the 585-nm pulsed dye laser in the treatment of acne in comparison with other topical therapeutic modalities. J Cosmet Laser Ther. 2009;11(2):118–24.
14. Yoon HJ, Lee DH, Kim SO, Park KC, Youn SW. Acne erythema improvement by long-pulsed 595-nm pulsed-dye laser treatment: a pilot study. J Dermatolog Treat. 2008;19(1):38–44.
15. Bae-Harboe YS, Graber EM. Easy as PIE (Postinflammatory Erythema). J Clin Aesthet Dermatol. 2013;6(9):46–7.
16. Alster TS, McMeekin TO. Improvement of facial acne scars by the 585 nm flashlamp-pumped pulsed dye laser. J Am Acad Dermatol. 1996;35(1):79–81.
17. Lekakh O, Mahoney AM, Novice K, Kamalpour J, Sadeghian A, Mondo D, et al. Treatment of acne vulgaris with salicylic acid chemical peel and pulsed dye laser: a split face, rater-blinded, randomized controlled trial. J Lasers Med Sci. 2015;6(4):167–70.
18. Glaich AS, Friedman PM, Jih MH, Goldberg LH. Treatment of inflammatory facial acne vulgaris with combination 595-nm pulsed-dye laser with dynamic-cooling-device and 1,450-nm diode laser. Lasers Surg Med. 2006;38(3):177–80.
19. Ibrahim SM, Farag A, Hegazy R, Mongy M, Shalaby S, Kamel MM. Combined low-dose Isotretinoin and pulsed dye laser versus standard-dose Isotretinoin in the treatment of inflammatory acne. Lasers Surg Med. 2021;53(5):603–9.
20. Gad SC, Sharp KL, Montgomery C, Payne JD, Goodrich GP. Evaluation of the toxicity of intravenous delivery of auroshell particles (gold-silica nanoshells). Int J Toxicol. 2012;31(6):584–94.
21. Paithankar DY, Sakamoto FH, Farinelli WA, Kositratna G, Blomgren RD, Meyer TJ, et al. Acne treatment based on selective photothermolysis of sebaceous follicles with topically delivered light-absorbing goLD microparticles. J Invest Dermatol. 2015;135(7):1727–34.
22. Fuchs CSK, Bay C, Adatto M, Lomholt H, Haedersdal M. Acne treatment with light absorbing gold microparticles and optical pulses: an open-label European multi-centered study in moderate to moderately severe acne vulgaris patients. Lasers Surg Med. 2019;51(8):686–93.
23. Park KY, Han HS, Hong JY, Seo SJ, Lee SJ. Gold nanoshell-mediated photothermal therapy for acne vulgaris. Dermatol Ther. 2020;33(1):e13189.
24. Suh DH, Park TJ, Jeong JY, Kim KE, Park JH, Lee SJ, et al. Photothermal therapy using gold nanoparticles for acne in Asian patients: a preliminary study. Dermatol Ther. 2021;34(3):e14918.
25. Goldberg DJ, Whitworth J. Laser skin resurfacing with the Q-switched Nd:YAG laser. Dermatol Surg. 1997;23(10):903–6; discussion 6–7.
26. Sumian CC, Pitre FB, Gauthier BE, Bouclier M, Mordon SR. Laser skin resurfacing using a frequency doubled Nd:YAG laser after topical application of an exogenous chromophore. Lasers Surg Med. 1999;25(1):43–50.
27. Friedman PM, Jih MH, Skover GR, Payonk GS, Kimyai-Asadi A, Geronemus RG. Treatment of atrophic facial acne scars with the 1064-nm Q-switched Nd:YAG laser: six-month follow-up study. Arch Dermatol. 2004;140(11):1337–41.
28. Jung JY, Hong JS, Ahn CH, Yoon JY, Kwon HH, Suh DH. Prospective randomized controlled clinical and histopathological study of acne vulgaris treated with dual mode of quasi-long pulse and Q-switched 1064-nm Nd:YAG laser assisted with a topically applied carbon suspension. J Am Acad Dermatol. 2012;66(4):626–33.
29. Monib KME, Hussein MS. Nd:YAG laser vs. IPL in inflammatory and noninflammatory acne lesion treatment. J Cosmet Dermatol. 2020;19(9):2325–32.
30. Chalermsuwiwattanakan N, Rojhirunsakool S, Kamanamool N, Kanokrungsee S, Udompataikul M. The comparative study of efficacy between 1064-nm long-pulsed Nd:YAG laser and 595-nm pulsed dye laser for the treatment of acne vulgaris. J Cosmet Dermatol. 2021;20(7):2108–15.
31. Yaghmai D, Garden JM, Bakus AD, Massa MC. Comparison of a 1,064 nm laser and a 1,320 nm laser for the nonablative treatment of acne scars. Dermatol Surg. 2005;31(8 Pt 1):903–9.
32. Bhatia AC, Dover JS, Arndt KA, Stewart B, Alam M. Patient satisfaction and reported long-term therapeutic efficacy associated with 1,320 nm Nd:YAG laser treatment of acne scarring and photoaging. Dermatol Surg. 2006;32(3):346–52.
33. Rogachefsky AS, Hussain M, Goldberg DJ. Atrophic and a mixed pattern of acne scars improved with a 1320-nm Nd:YAG laser. Dermatol Surg. 2003;29(9):904–8.
34. Deng H, Yuan DF, Yan CL, Ding XA. Fractional 1320 nm Nd:YAG laser in the treatment of acne vulgaris: a pilot study. Photodermatol Photoimmunol Photomed. 2009;25(5):278–9.
35. Orringer JS, Kang S, Maier L, Johnson TM, Sachs DL, Karimipour DJ, et al. A randomized, controlled, split-face clinical trial of 1320-nm Nd:YAG laser

therapy in the treatment of acne vulgaris. J Am Acad Dermatol. 2007;56(3):432–8.
36. Paithankar DY, Ross EV, Saleh BA, Blair MA, Graham BS. Acne treatment with a 1,450 nm wavelength laser and cryogen spray cooling. Lasers Surg Med. 2002;31(2):106–14.
37. Jih MH, Friedman PM, Goldberg LH, Robles M, Glaich AS, Kimyai-Asadi A. The 1450-nm diode laser for facial inflammatory acne vulgaris: dose-response and 12-month follow-up study. J Am Acad Dermatol. 2006;55(1):80–7.
38. Thiboutot D, Gollnick H, Bettoli V, Dreno B, Kang S, Leyden JJ, et al. New insights into the management of acne: an update from the Global Alliance to Improve Outcomes in Acne group. J Am Acad Dermatol. 2009;60(5 Suppl):S1–50.
39. Darne S, Hiscutt EL, Seukeran DC. Evaluation of the clinical efficacy of the 1,450 nm laser in acne vulgaris: a randomized split-face, investigator-blinded clinical trial. Br J Dermatol. 2011;165(6):1256–62.
40. Bernstein EF. A pilot investigation comparing low-energy, double pass 1,450 nm laser treatment of acne to conventional single-pass, high-energy treatment. Lasers Surg Med. 2007;39(2):193–8.
41. Uebelhoer NS, Bogle MA, Dover JS, Arndt KA, Rohrer TE. Comparison of stacked pulses versus double-pass treatments of facial acne with a 1,450-nm laser. Dermatol Surg. 2007;33(5):552–9.
42. Noborio R, Nishida E, Morita A. Clinical effect of low-energy double-pass 1450 nm laser treatment for acne in Asians. Photodermatol Photoimmunol Photomed. 2009;25(1):3–7.
43. Kwon HH, Choi SC, Jung JY, Bae YI, Park GH. Comparison of novel dual mode vs. conventional single pass of a 1450-nm diode laser in the treatment of acne vulgaris for Korean patients: a 20-week prospective, randomized, split-face study. J Cosmet Dermatol. 2018;17(6):1063–8.
44. Chua SH, Ang P, Khoo LS, Goh CL. Nonablative 1450-nm diode laser in the treatment of facial atrophic acne scars in type IV to V Asian skin: a prospective clinical study. Dermatol Surg. 2004;30(10):1287–91.
45. Lupton JR, Williams CM, Alster TS. Nonablative laser skin resurfacing using a 1540 nm erbium glass laser: a clinical and histologic analysis. Dermatol Surg. 2002;28(9):833–5.
46. Kim HJ, Kim TG, Kwon YS, Park JM, Lee JH. Comparison of a 1,550 nm erbium: glass fractional laser and a chemical reconstruction of skin scars (CROSS) method in the treatment of acne scars: a simultaneous split-face trial. Lasers Surg Med. 2009;41(8):545–9.
47. Solomon-Cohen E, Lapidoth M, Mimouni D, Akerman L, Slodownik D, Hodak E, et al. 1540-nm fractional erbium: glass laser is a safe and effective modality for nonablative facial rejuvenation. J Cosmet Dermatol. 2021;20(6):1679–83.
48. Bogle MA, Dover JS, Arndt KA, Mordon S. Evaluation of the 1,540-nm erbium:glass laser in the treatment of inflammatory facial acne. Dermatol Surg. 2007;33(7):810–7.
49. Angel S, Boineau D, Dahan S, Mordon S. Treatment of active acne with an Er:Glass (1.54 microm) laser: a 2-year follow-up study. J Cosmet Laser Ther. 2006;8(4):171–6.
50. Politi Y, Levi A, Enk CD, Lapidoth M. Integrated cooling-vacuum-assisted 1540-nm erbium:glass laser is effective in treating mild-to-moderate acne vulgaris. Lasers Med Sci. 2015;30(9):2389–93.
51. Isarria MJ, Cornejo P, Munoz E, Royo de la Torre J, Moraga JM. Evaluation of clinical improvement in acne scars and active acne in patients treated with the 1540-nm non-ablative fractional laser. J Drugs Dermatol. 2011;10(8):907–12.
52. Moneib H, Tawfik AA, Youssef SS, Fawzy MM. Randomized split-face controlled study to evaluate 1550-nm fractionated erbium glass laser for treatment of acne vulgaris—an image analysis evaluation. Dermatol Surg. 2014;40(11):1191–200.
53. Liu Y, Zeng W, Hu D, Jha S, Ge Q, Geng S, et al. The long-term effect of 1550 nm erbium:glass fractional laser in acne vulgaris. Lasers Med Sci. 2016;31(3):453–7.
54. Sakamoto FH, Doukas AG, Farinelli WA, Tannous Z, Shinn M, Benson S, et al. Selective photothermolysis to target sebaceous glands: theoretical estimation of parameters and preliminary results using a free electron laser. Lasers Surg Med. 2012;44(2):175–83.
55. Scopelliti MG, Kothare A, Karavitis M. A novel 1726-nm laser system for safe and effective treatment of acne vulgaris. Lasers Med Sci. 2022;37(9):3639–47.
56. Goldberg D, Kothare A, Doucette M, Kaur A, Ronan S, Fromowitz J, et al. Selective photothermolysis with a novel 1726 nm laser beam: a safe and effective solution for acne vulgaris. J Cosmet Dermatol. 2023;22(2):486–96.
57. Kjeldstad B, Johnsson A, Sandberg S. Influence of pH on porphyrin production in Propionibacterium acnes. Arch Dermatol Res. 1984;276(6):396–400.
58. Morton CA, Scholefield RD, Whitehurst C, Birch J. An open study to determine the efficacy of blue light in the treatment of mild to moderate acne. J Dermatolog Treat. 2005;16(4):219–23.
59. Goldberg DJ, Russell BA. Combination blue (415 nm) and red (633 nm) LED phototherapy in the treatment of mild to severe acne vulgaris. J Cosmet Laser Ther. 2006;8(2):71–5.
60. Shnitkind E, Yaping E, Geen S, Shalita AR, Lee WL. Anti-inflammatory properties of narrow-band blue light. J Drugs Dermatol. 2006;5(7):605–10.
61. Antoniou C, Dessinioti C, Sotiriadis D, Kalokasidis K, Kontochristopoulos G, Petridis A, et al. A multicenter, randomized, split-face clinical trial evaluating the efficacy and safety of chromophore gel-assisted blue light phototherapy for the treatment of acne. Int J Dermatol. 2016;55(12):1321–8.
62. Elman M, Slatkine M, Harth Y. The effective treatment of acne vulgaris by a high-intensity, narrow

band 405-420 nm light source. J Cosmet Laser Ther. 2003;5(2):111–7.
63. Gold MH, Sensing W, Biron JA. Clinical efficacy of home-use blue-light therapy for mild-to moderate acne. J Cosmet Laser Ther. 2011;13(6):308–14.
64. Gold MH, Rao J, Goldman MP, Bridges TM, Bradshaw VL, Boring MM, et al. A multicenter clinical evaluation of the treatment of mild to moderate inflammatory acne vulgaris of the face with visible blue light in comparison to topical 1% clindamycin antibiotic solution. J Drugs Dermatol. 2005;4(1):64–70.
65. Goldman MP, Boyce SM. A single-center study of aminolevulinic acid and 417 NM photodynamic therapy in the treatment of moderate to severe acne vulgaris. J Drugs Dermatol. 2003;2(4):393–6.
66. Kwon HH, Choi SC, Jung JY, Bae Y, Park GH. A novel combined light-based treatment of acne vulgaris with 1,450-nm diode laser and 450-nm blue light. Dermatol Surg. 2019;45(9):1147–54.
67. Kjeldstad B. Different photoinactivation mechanisms in Propionibacterium acnes for near-ultraviolet and visible light. Photochem Photobiol. 1987;46(3):363–6.
68. Li WH, Fassih A, Binner C, Parsa R, Southall MD. Low-level red LED light inhibits hyperkeratinization and inflammation induced by unsaturated fatty acid in an in vitro model mimicking acne. Lasers Surg Med. 2018;50(2):158–65.
69. Na JI, Suh DH. Red light phototherapy alone is effective for acne vulgaris: randomized, single-blinded clinical trial. Dermatol Surg. 2007;33(10):1228–33; discussion 33.
70. Papageorgiou P, Katsambas A, Chu A. Phototherapy with blue (415 nm) and red (660 nm) light in the treatment of acne vulgaris. Br J Dermatol. 2000;142(5):973–8.
71. Kwon HH, Lee JB, Yoon JY, Park SY, Ryu HH, Park BM, et al. The clinical and histological effect of home-use, combination blue-red LED phototherapy for mild-to-moderate acne vulgaris in Korean patients: a double-blind, randomized controlled trial. Br J Dermatol. 2013;168(5):1088–94.
72. Alba MN, Gerenutti M, Yoshida VM, Grotto D. Clinical comparison of salicylic acid peel and LED-laser phototherapy for the treatment of acne vulgaris in teenagers. J Cosmet Laser Ther. 2017;19(1):49–53.
73. Nestor MS, Swenson N, Macri A, Manway M, Paparone P. Efficacy and tolerability of a combined 445nm and 630nm over-the-counter light therapy mask with and without topical salicylic acid versus topical benzoyl peroxide for the treatment of mild-to-moderate acne vulgaris. J Clin Aesthet Dermatol. 2016;9(3):25–35.
74. Wat H, Wu DC, Rao J, Goldman MP. Application of intense pulsed light in the treatment of dermatologic disease: a systematic review. Dermatol Surg. 2014;40(4):359–77.
75. Handler MZ, Bloom BS, Goldberg DJ. Energy-based devices in treatment of acne vulgaris. Dermatol Surg. 2016;42(5):573–85.
76. Li MK, Liu C, Hsu JTS. The use of lasers and light devices in acne management: an update. Am J Clin Dermatol. 2021;22(6):785–800.
77. Barakat MT, Moftah NH, El Khayyat MA, Abdelhakim ZA. Significant reduction of inflammation and sebaceous glands size in acne vulgaris lesions after intense pulsed light treatment. Dermatol Ther. 2017;30(1) https://doi.org/10.1111/dth.12418.
78. Chang SE, Ahn SJ, Rhee DY, Choi JH, Moon KC, Suh HS, et al. Treatment of facial acne papules and pustules in Korean patients using an intense pulsed light device equipped with a 530- to 750-nm filter. Dermatol Surg. 2007;33(6):676–9.
79. Yeung CK, Shek SY, Bjerring P, Yu CS, Kono T, Chan HH. A comparative study of intense pulsed light alone and its combination with photodynamic therapy for the treatment of facial acne in Asian skin. Lasers Surg Med. 2007;39(1):1–6.
80. Myers P, Bowler P, Hills S. A retrospective study of the efficacy of intense pulsed light for the treatment of dermatologic disorders presenting to a cosmetic skin clinic. J Cosmet Dermatol. 2005;4(4):262–6.
81. Deshpande AJ. Efficacy and safety evaluation of high-density intense pulsed light in the treatment of grades II and IV acne vulgaris as monotherapy in dark-skinned women of child bearing age. J Clin Aesthet Dermatol. 2018;11(4):43–8.
82. Kawana S, Tachihara R, Kato T, Omi T. Effect of smooth pulsed light at 400 to 700 and 870 to 1,200 nm for acne vulgaris in Asian skin. Dermatol Surg. 2010;36(1):52–7.
83. Patidar MV, Deshmukh AR, Khedkar MY. Efficacy of intense pulsed light therapy in the treatment of facial acne vulgaris: comparison of two different fluences. Indian J Dermatol. 2016;61(5):545–9.
84. Choi YS, Suh HS, Yoon MY, Min SU, Lee DH, Suh DH. Intense pulsed light vs. pulsed-dye laser in the treatment of facial acne: a randomized split-face trial. J Eur Acad Dermatol Venereol. 2010;24(7):773–80.
85. Chen S, Wang Y, Ren J, Yue B, Lai G, Du J. Efficacy and safety of intense pulsed light in the treatment of inflammatory acne vulgaris with a novel filter. J Cosmet Laser Ther. 2019;21(6):323–7.
86. Lee EJ, Lim HK, Shin MK, Suh DH, Lee SJ, Kim NI. An open-label, split-face trial evaluating efficacy and safty of photopneumatic therapy for the treatment of acne. Ann Dermatol. 2012;24(3):280–6.
87. Gold MH, Biron J. Efficacy of a novel combination of pneumatic energy and broadband light for the treatment of acne. J Drugs Dermatol. 2008;7(7):639–42.
88. Wanitphakdeedecha R, Tanzi EL, Alster TS. Photopneumatic therapy for the treatment of acne. J Drugs Dermatol. 2009;8(3):239–41.
89. Hongcharu W, Taylor CR, Chang Y, Aghassi D, Suthamjariya K, Anderson RR. Topical ALA-photodynamic therapy for the treatment of acne vulgaris. J Invest Dermatol. 2000;115(2):183–92.

90. Stott B, Korbelik M. Activation of complement C3, C5, and C9 genes in tumors treated by photodynamic therapy. Cancer Immunol Immunother. 2007;56(5):649–58.
91. Jeong E, Hong JW, Min JA, Lee DW, Sohn MY, Lee WJ, et al. Topical ALA-photodynamic therapy for acne can induce apoptosis of sebocytes and downregulate their TLR-2 and TLR-4 expression. Ann Dermatol. 2011;23(1):23–32.
92. Asayama-Kosaka S, Akilov OE, Kawana S. Photodynamic therapy with 5% delta-aminolevulinic acid is safe and effective treatment of acne vulgaris in Japanese patients. Laser Ther. 2014;23(2):115–20.
93. Ma Y, Liu Y, Wang Q, Ren J, Xiang L. Prospective study of topical 5-aminolevulinic acid photodynamic therapy for the treatment of severe adolescent acne in Chinese patients. J Dermatol. 2015;42(5):504–7.
94. Ma L, Xiang LH, Yu B, Yin R, Chen L, Wu Y, et al. Low-dose topical 5-aminolevulinic acid photodynamic therapy in the treatment of different severity of acne vulgaris. Photodiagn Photodyn Ther. 2013;10(4):583–90.
95. Yin R, Hao F, Deng J, Yang XC, Yan H. Investigation of optimal aminolaevulinic acid concentration applied in topical aminolaevulinic acid-photodynamic therapy for treatment of moderate to severe acne: a pilot study in Chinese subjects. Br J Dermatol. 2010;163(5):1064–71.
96. Fritsch C, Homey B, Stahl W, Lehmann P, Ruzicka T, Sies H. Preferential relative porphyrin enrichment in solar keratoses upon topical application of delta-aminolevulinic acid methylester. Photochem Photobiol. 1998;68(2):218–21.
97. Wiegell SR, Wulf HC. Photodynamic therapy of acne vulgaris using 5-aminolevulinic acid versus methyl aminolevulinate. J Am Acad Dermatol. 2006;54(4):647–51.
98. Genina EA, Bashkatov AN, Simonenko GV, Odoevskaya OD, Tuchin VV, Altshuler GB. Low-intensity indocyanine-green laser phototherapy of acne vulgaris: pilot study. J Biomed Opt. 2004;9(4):828–34.
99. Kim BJ, Lee HG, Woo SM, Youn JI, Suh DH. Pilot study on photodynamic therapy for acne using indocyanine green and diode laser. J Dermatol. 2009;36(1):17–21.
100. Seo HM, Min HG, Kim HJ, Shin JH, Nam SH, Han KS, et al. Effects of repetitive photodynamic therapy using indocyanine green for acne vulgaris. Int J Dermatol. 2016;55(10):1157–63.
101. Boen M, Brownell J, Patel P, Tsoukas MM. The role of photodynamic therapy in acne: an evidence-based review. Am J Clin Dermatol. 2017;18(3):311–21.
102. Dessinioti C, Masouri S, Drakaki E, Katsambas A, Antoniou C. Short-contact, low-dose methyl aminolaevulinate photodynamic therapy for acne vulgaris. Br J Dermatol. 2016;175(1):215.
103. Calzavara-Pinton PG, Rossi MT, Aronson E, Sala R, Italian Group For Photodynamic T. A retrospective analysis of real-life practice of off-label photodynamic therapy using methyl aminolevulinate (MAL-PDT) in 20 Italian dermatology departments. Part 1: inflammatory and aesthetic indications. Photochem Photobiol Sci. 2013;12(1):148–57.
104. Pinto C, Schafer F, Orellana JJ, Gonzalez S, Hasson A. Efficacy of red light alone and methyl-aminolaevulinate-photodynamic therapy for the treatment of mild and moderate facial acne. Indian J Dermatol Venereol Leprol. 2013;79(1):77–82.
105. Bissonnette R, Maari C, Nigen S, Provost N, Bolduc C. Photodynamic therapy with methylaminolevulinate 80 mg/g without occlusion improves acne vulgaris. J Drugs Dermatol. 2010;9(11):1347–52.
106. Akaraphanth R, Kanjanawanitchkul W, Gritiyarangsan P. Efficacy of ALA-PDT vs. blue light in the treatment of acne. Photodermatol Photoimmunol Photomed. 2007;23(5):186–90.
107. Mavilia L, Malara G, Moretti G, Lo Re M, Puglisi Guerra A. Photodynamic therapy of acne using methyl aminolaevulinate diluted to 4% together with low doses of red light. Br J Dermatol. 2007;157(4):810–1.
108. Hong JS, Jung JY, Yoon JY, Suh DH. Acne treatment by methyl aminolevulinate photodynamic therapy with red light vs. intense pulsed light. Int J Dermatol. 2013;52(5):614–9.
109. Rojanamatin J, Choawawanich P. Treatment of inflammatory facial acne vulgaris with intense pulsed light and short contact of topical 5-aminolevulinic acid: a pilot study. Dermatol Surg. 2006;32(8):991–6; discussion 6–7.
110. Orringer JS, Sachs DL, Bailey E, Kang S, Hamilton T, Voorhees JJ. Photodynamic therapy for acne vulgaris: a randomized, controlled, split-face clinical trial of topical aminolevulinic acid and pulsed dye laser therapy. J Cosmet Dermatol. 2010;9(1):28–34.
111. Alexiades-Armenakas M. Long-pulsed dye laser-mediated photodynamic therapy combined with topical therapy for mild to severe comedonal, inflammatory, or cystic acne. J Drugs Dermatol. 2006;5(1):45–55.
112. Haedersdal M, Togsverd-Bo K, Wiegell SR, Wulf HC. Long-pulsed dye laser versus long-pulsed dye laser-assisted photodynamic therapy for acne vulgaris: a randomized controlled trial. J Am Acad Dermatol. 2008;58(3):387–94.

Laser-Assisted Drug Delivery

10

Pei-Ling Chi, Geun-Soo Lee,
and Patrick Po-Han Huang

Introduction

Topical medication is the mainstream treatment for most dermatologic diseases. Various modalities (e.g., occlusion therapy, iontophoresis, ultrasonophoresis, or intralesional injection) have been used by physicians to improve topical drugs' potency or transport active components more efficiently before initiating systemic therapy.

The primary barrier to topical medication or active ingredient absorption is the stratum corneum, which not only defends against environmental damage but also reduces the transcutaneous availability of applied medicine. Additionally, medications or active substances with a molecular weight greater than 500 kDa will be poorly absorbed, and the transcutaneous bioavailability was 1–5% of the topically applied medication dose [1–3].

In 2002, Rox Anderson found that erbium-yttrium aluminum garnet (Er:YAG) laser ablation of the stratum corneum substantially improved the effectiveness of topical anesthesia in their innovative trial about laser-assisted delivery of topical medication. Due to the pioneering insight of the fractionated laser idea by Rox Anderson in 2004, minimizing the damage to skin but keeping almost intact skin by delivering energy through fractional lasers became a giant leap in dermatology laser development. Based on the fractional photothermolysis concept, ablative fractional lasers (AFLs) were developed, including the carbon dioxide (CO_2) laser and the Er:YAG laser. The drilled holes allow the medications or active components to be easily absorbed and work on the targets, resulting in increased therapeutic results. The term "laser-assisted drug delivery (LADD)" refers to an idea that has altered conventional pharmacodynamic theory. Due to its controlled and selective destruction of the skin barrier, it may be an effective alternative for injectable or topical formulations of medications to increase penetration and absorption in treating cutaneous disorders [1, 2].

The predictability of LADD's efficacy and safety is always an issue of concern. While laser parameters influence tissue depth, future studies should focus on standardizing the applied medi-

P.-L. Chi · P. P.-H. Huang (✉)
Huang P. H. Dermatology and Aesthetics, Kaohsiung, Taiwan

G.-S. Lee
Dr. Woo and Hann's Skin and Laser Clinic, Seoul, South Korea

S. W. N. Cheng, C. L. Goh (eds.), *Updates on Lasers in Dermatology*, Updates in Clinical Dermatology, https://doi.org/10.1007/978-3-031-71155-8_10

cation concentration and its interaction with the laser system setting.

Different EBD and Medication Delivery Mechanisms

Many lasers have been used for LADD. The most common lasers studied in LADD are AFLs and, to a lesser degree, nonablative fractional lasers (NAFLs). Before fractional lasers were invented, LADD was performed by completely ablating the epidermis with greater local adverse effects; this is seldom performed nowadays. While both the CO_2 and Er:YAG lasers are equally effective at delivering therapeutic drugs through the stratum corneum, the CO_2 laser, with its deeper beam profile and coagulation zone (CZ), is theoretically preferred to the Er:YAG laser for more penetrating beam cutaneous medication delivery. In addition, a thin coagulation zone minimizes oozing and bleeding and may act as a reservoir for medication release into the tissue over time. Compared to other physical enhancement techniques (e.g., microneedling, microabrasion, nonablative laser), AFLs exhibit notable relative effectiveness [1, 2].

Whatever the type of energy-based device (EBD), the aim of fractional devices is the same (Fig. 10.1): to generate spatially dispersed columns of microthermal damage, referred to collectively as microscopic treatment zones (MTZs). The energy used to generate each column of MTZ causes thermal heating or ablation with minimal diffusion to surrounding tissue, preserving the epidermis integrity between the MTZs. Thus, fractional irradiation enables the laser beam to penetrate relatively deeply into the dermis while leaving the surrounding skin primarily intact.

All of the MTZ-inducing EBD opens channels for assisted drug delivery, while the absorption efficiency is affected by several factors: *application timing, drug properties and carrying vehicles, laser channel depth, laser density, and coagulation zone.*

Application Timing

Different modalities of MTZ-inducing EBD have different cutaneous channel formation effects and opening times. In Wang's observation through optical coherence tomography imaging, radiofre-

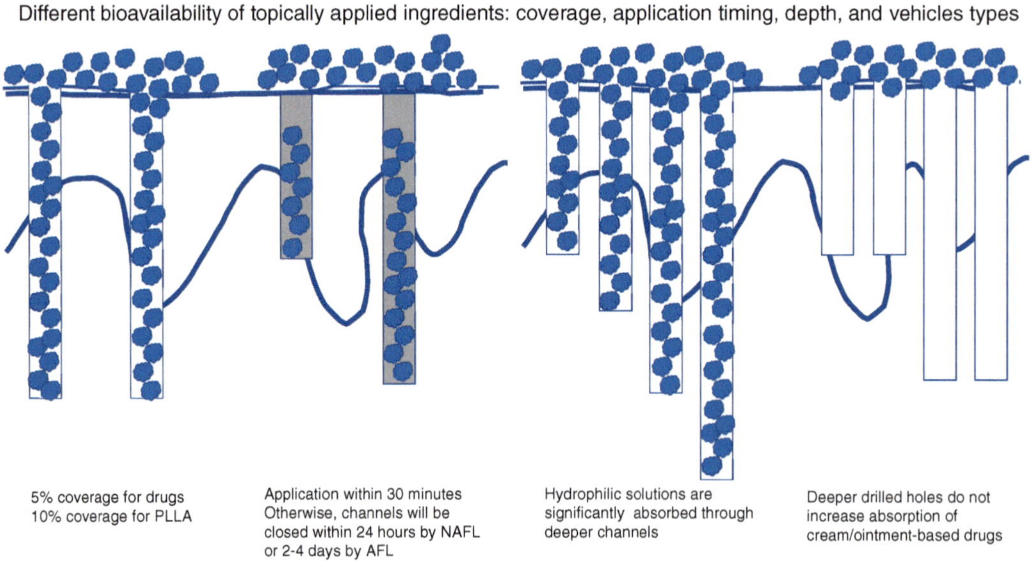

Fig. 10.1 LADD is affected by application timing and channel depth

quency microneedling demonstrated no cutaneous channels. Both low-energy, low-density, fractional 1927 nm thulium fiber and 1550 nm erbium fiber lasers produced transient channels, which close at 24 h. The thermomechanical fractional injury (TMFI) and the fractional ablative CO_2 laser produce open channels for 24 h. Regardless of the opening time for the channels, Haedersdal suggested that the best is to apply the drug for assisted delivery within 30 min.

Types of Drug Properties and Carrying Vehicles

It is easier for the lipophilic substances to cross an intact epidermis, but the laser-assisted delivery may enhance penetration of hydrophilic compounds. Besides, the vehicle types are also important. Liquid and gel formulations cross the channels drilled by AFL with greater affinity than creams or ointments [2].

Laser Channel Depth

Laser channel depth has been reported to be important for the topical delivery of hydrophilic molecules in Haedersdal's publication in 2016 [4]. Theoretically, deeper channels may result in higher drug penetration, especially for hydrophilic substances (e.g., methotrexate). The deeper channels accommodate a larger volume of drug solution, providing a larger contact surface and adding a reservoir for drug delivery. However, deeper channel depth does not necessarily increase absorption for hydrophobic/lipophilic substances (e.g., imiquimod, lidocaine). This may be due to the agent's diffusivity in the channel being less than or equal to that of adjacent skin layers [1, 3–6].

Laser Density

Laser density represents the width and number of microchannels generated per unit skin area. In vivo studies have demonstrated that some agents may increase cutaneous uptake if increasing channel density. Nevertheless, the methyl aminolevulinate (MAL) studies outlined no further increase in skin surface porphyrin fluorescence up to 5% laser density coverage [1–3, 5].

Coagulation Zone (CZ)

Coagulation zone dimensions depend on laser devices, pulse duration, energy, and stacking. Although the thicker CZ delays the initial delivery rate, they may maintain a reservoir for sustained release of the medication to surrounding tissue. The hydrophilic and low-molecular-weight drugs diffuse more easily through the CZ [1].

Laser-Generated Instant Pressure-Driven Microjet Drug Delivery

Without the thermal damage producing drug delivery route formation, laser-generated microjet-form drug delivery method was introduced recently. Using the characteristics that Er:YAG has a very high water absorption coefficient, Er:YAG laser is used to generate vapor bubbles. The laser energy is converted into pressure by sudden expansion of the vapor bubble, and the expanded chamber pushes the nozzle to inject drugs into the skin as a needleless microjet. Lee et al. [7] conducted a study using this needleless microjet device attached to Er:YAG laser and injected hyaluronic acid (HA) mixed with dye and poly-DL-lactic acid (PDLA) into the dermis.

Selected Common Indications for LADDs in Clinical Practices

Non-melanoma Skin Cancer

JAMA, European Dermatology, and other reviews recommended photodynamic therapy (PDT) combined with LADD for actinic keratosis (AK), actinic cheilitis, and cutaneous SCC in situ, using either MAL or aminolevulinic acid (ALA) as a photosensitizer [3, 8–11].

Actinic Keratosis (AK)

Togsverd-Bo K. et al. presented the first evidence that ablative fractional laser-assisted PDT (AFL-PDT) using fractional CO_2 laser is significantly more effective than conventional PDT in treating AK. The complete lesion response of grade II–III AK was 88% after AFL-PDT compared with 59% after PDT ($p = 0.02$); in grade I AK, 100% of lesions cleared after AFL-PDT compared with 80% after PDT ($p = 0.04$). The AFL-PDT group responded with significantly fewer new AK lesions and improved photoaging but more pain scores, erythema, crusting, and long-term pigmentary changes [12].

Ko D.-Y. et al. evaluated AFL-PDT (fractional Er:YAG laser used) in Asian facial AKs. The efficacy of AFL-PDT was most pronounced in treating Olsen grade III AKs (69.4% vs. 32.5%). In thin AKs, the complete response rate of AFL-PDT was 100%; AFL-PDT also showed a lower lesion recurrence rate than MAL-PDT (9.7% vs. 26.6%) and a higher long-term complete response rate (78.5% vs. 45.0%). Local adverse events were mild to moderate but higher in the AFL-PDT group. The author chose the fractional Er:YAG laser due to less thermal tissue damage, quicker wound healing, and fewer severe side effects of erythema, swelling, and postinflammatory hyperpigmentation (PIH) than the fractional CO_2 laser [13].

In a review of immunosuppressed organ transplant recipient patients with 542 AKs (Olsen grades I–III), complete response rate was 74% after ablative fractional laser-assisted daylight photodynamic therapy (AFL-dPDT; Er:YAG laser used at 2.3 mJ per pulse, 1.15 W, two stacks, 50 μs pulse duration, 2.4% density), compared with 46% after dPDT (daylight PDT) and 50% after cPDT (conventional PDT) at 3-month follow-up. AFL-dPDT has been associated with more pain and immediate skin reaction (e.g., erythema, crusting) compared with cPDT [14].

Bowen Disease, Squamous Cell Carcinoma In Situ (SCCIS), Actinic Cheilitis

A randomized trial demonstrated that Er:YAG AFL-MAL-PDT (550–600 μm ablation depth, level 1 coagulation, 22% treatment density, single pulse) was more effective than conventional MAL-PDT for lower extremity Bowen disease (BD) lesion in Asians with 3-month complete response rate of 93.8% vs. 73.1%. The recurrence rate was significantly lower for Er:YAG AFL-MAL-PDT than MAL-PDT (6.7% vs. 31.6%) at 12 months ($p = 0.022$). The efficacy of MAL-PDT was lower in Asians than in Caucasians, and more (two to four) treatment sessions and increased light doses would be required in Asians. However, a single session of Er:YAG AFL-MAL-PDT could be more effective than two sessions of conventional MAL-PDT in Asians [15].

The same group conducted another randomized controlled study with 5-year follow-up, with a sustained clearance rate of 84.7% of Er:YAG AFL-MAL-PDT vs. 44.7% of MAL-PDT, and the recurrence rate was 9.3% vs. 41.38% in the Er:YAG AFL-MAL-PDT vs. MAL-PDT group. Importantly, lesion size larger than 20 mm and previous treatment history were independent risk factors for unsuccessful treatment [16].

A small randomized, comparative trial on microinvasive squamous cell carcinoma (SCC) showed a 3-month complete response rate of 84.2% with Er:YAG AFL-MAL-PDT vs. 52.4% with MAL-PDT and a significantly lower recurrence rate in Er:YAG AFL-MAL-PDT (12.5%) than MAL-PDT (63.6%) at 12 months [17].

For actinic cheilitis, Choi et al. conducted a prospective randomized study, with a 3-month complete response rate of 92% vs. 59% in Er:YAG AFL-MAL-PDT group vs. MAL-PDT group; the differences in efficacy remained significant at the 12-month follow-up, and the recurrence rate was significantly lower for Er:YAG AFL-MAL-PDT (8%) than for MAL-PDT (50%) group at 12 months [18].

Basal Cell Carcinoma

Response of PDT in basal cell carcinoma (BCC) is influenced by tumor thickness, with reduced efficacy with increasing tumor thickness.

Whitaker et al. presented that combined CO_2 laser with MAL-PDT treatment at week 1, followed by repeated MAL-PDT at week 2, achieved 100% clearance at 18 months for 13 lesions of head and neck nodular BCC (nBCC); Shokrollahi et al. also reported 97.1% recurrence-free rate for 32-month follow-up with the same combination [19, 20].

A randomized, prospective, comparative study evaluated the efficacy of Er:YAG AFL-PDT and standard MAL-PDT in patients with thin nBCC (thickness $\leq$ 2 mm); the 3-month complete response rates were 84.2% with Er:YAG AFL-PDT vs. 50% with MAL-PDT ($p = 0.026$). The recurrence rate was significantly lower with Er:YAG AFL-PDT (6.3%) than with MAL-PDT (55.6%) at 12 months ($p = 0.006$) [21].

Another randomized study included facial nBCC with high-risk characters (diameter > 15 mm, tumors located in high-risk zones or on severely sun-damaged skin); the 3-month complete response rates were 100% in CO_2 AFL-PDT group (5% density, 80 mJ, 1000 μm ablation depth) vs. 88% in PDT group, and the recurrences tended to occur later and in lower numbers in CO_2 AFL-PDT group at 6, 9, and 12 months (6%, 19%, 19%) than PDT group (25%, 38%, 44%) [22].

Melasma

Fractional Er:YAG laser-assisted 4% HQ delivery had significantly improved Melasma Area and Severity Index (MASI) and Physician Global Assessment (PGA) compared with HQ alone, with 73.4% and 40%, respectively, for >50% improvement [23, 24].

Tawfic et al. and Mekawy et al. demonstrated that tranexamic acid (TXA) combined with low-power, low-density fractional CO_2 laser or TXA microinjection can significantly reduce melanin index (MI) and erythema index (EI), with no statistically significant difference in between [25, 26].

AFLs alone had successful reports in treating melasma with a significant reduction in MASI score [27–29]; electron microscopy analysis revealed a significant decrease in the number and size of melanocytes and also melanin granules in the surrounding keratinocytes [27]. However, postinflammatory hyperpigmentation and recurrence have been controversial issues in the past [28]. Combining AFL and topical TXA has a synergic effect in breaking the skin barrier for TXA absorption. The better absorption of TXA further avoids PIH [30].

Botsali et al. reported their study that performed Er:YAG AFL followed by topical 5% TXA cream application to Turkish women melasma patients. They concluded that laser-assisted delivery of TXA is an effective treatment strategy in melasma patients of Mediterranean descent [31]. 1927 nm Fractional thulium fiber laser has less water absorption than CO_2 and erbium:YAG lasers, so it can make controlled subablative tissue damage. According to the prospective pilot study of Wang et al., the combination of low-energy, low-density 1927 nm fractional thulium fiber laser and topical TXA improved clinical outcomes as well as skin radiance, texture, and tone [32].

Li et al. demonstrated more dyschromia improvements on the side of picosecond alexandrite laser and topical TXA combination therapy treated over laser monotherapy alone [33].

In addition to TXA, the first study to investigate using 1565 nm NAFL-assisted human umbilical cord mesenchymal stem cell-derived exosome (hUCMSC-Exos) delivery in the treatment of melasma was reported [34]. The combined 1565 nm NAFL and hUCMSC-Exos group achieved a significantly improved therapeutic effect and patient satisfaction ($p < 0.05$) toward promoting penetration compared with NAFL alone.

Vitiligo

In refractory, localized, stable non-segmental vitiligo, conventional treatment combined with various ablative methods has shown a good response.

In the past, ablative lasers followed by 5-FU or topical steroid application before NB-UVB therapy, dermabrasion combined with 5-FU, and microdermabrasion combined with pimecrolimus cream were reported to have better treatment response compared with topical medicine application [35–38]. However, dermabrasion or ablative laser resurfacing had difficulties in the depth control and wound care process. After fractional photothermolysis was introduced, it reduced the ablative laser side effects.

Shin et al. postulated that the CO_2 AFL induced various kinds of cytokines and growth factor secretion, which may act as mitogens for melanocytes, and the well-known matrix metalloproteinase-2 can enhance the migration of melanocytes from adjacent normal skin [37, 39].

Vasanop et al. conducted a randomized prospective study and demonstrated that combined CO_2 AFL, narrowband UVB (NB-UVB) phototherapy, and 0.05% clobetasol propionate produced significant improvement of vitiligo than the combination of NB-UVB and 0.05% clobetasol propionate in the recalcitrant area (dorsal hand) [40].

Hypertrophic and Keloid Scars

According to the most recent Cochrane systematic review and another review from Kelvin Truong et al., the treatment protocols and outcomes for hypertrophic and keloid scars were too varied to be combined for statistical analysis. This led to the low-certainty evidence of ablative fractional laser plus other treatments in scar management [41, 42]. Oosterhoff et al. outlined that the AFL (CO_2 and Er:YAG lasers) still yielded the most improvement across all scar characteristics [43].

Waibel et al. reported her outstanding findings in scar management in 2013 [44]. She found that CO_2 AFL followed by immediate topical application of triamcinolone acetonide suspension (10 or 20 mg/mL) at 2- to 3-month intervals resulted in an average overall improvement of 2.73/3.0. Another report focusing on the pediatric postburn hypertrophic scars also showed a mean reduction of 4.2 (range: 2.8–7) in Vancouver Scar Scale (VSS) after CO_2 AFL immediately followed by triamcinolone suspension 10 mg/mL and combined clobetasol gel application daily. Reduction of VSS by $\geq$4 points was observed in eight of ten cases, whereas PGA also revealed excellent response. The authors reported that the use of topical triamcinolone is painless and makes a more uniform distribution of the drug [45].

There were no statistically significant differences in VSS of the treated area between triamcinolone acetonide 10 mg/cm^3 intralesional injection and topical transparent film dressing occlusion after the Er:YAG AFL treatment in Park's publication in 2017 [46]. Waibel et al. also demonstrated the efficacy of CO_2 AFL-assisted delivery of 5-fluorouracil (50 mg/mL) and triamcinolone acetonide (20 mg/mL) and found no statistically significant difference in overall scar area reduction between the two modalities [47].

However, in a randomized clinical trial to compare fractional laser monotherapy and fractional laser-assisted topical clobetasol propionate 0.05% ointment delivery, Manuskiatti et al. from Thailand found that the application of topical corticosteroid provides a borderline significant improvement in scar flattening at 3-month follow-up but no long-term (longer than 3 months) synergistic effect to fractional laser monotherapy [48]. The main difference between Manuskiatti's research and the previous reports, which supported that corticosteroid plays a vital role in treating scars through LADD, is that topical clobetasol ointment is not hydrophilic, and the penetration and absorption might be limited and less than triamcinolone acetonide suspension that other reports had applied.

In treating scars and rejuvenating aging skin, it is always challenging to tell whether the effectiveness is mainly from AFL's thermal effects or added active ingredients' add-on effects. In addition, more and more industry-sponsored publications usually lack a control group with fractional laser alone. Therefore, further therapeutic trials are warranted to prove the safety and efficacy of LADD over fractional laser monotherapy.

Cosmetic Uses

Waibel et al. demonstrated that laser-assisted delivery of vitamins C and E and ferulic acid immediately postoperatively of fractional CO_2 laser could improve wound healing, with nonsignificant decreased edema and erythema; besides these agents being well tolerated, the upregulation of the basic fibroblast growth factor (bFGF) was also noted [49]. Another double-blind, prospective, randomized trial presented a significant reduction in both skin roughness and wrinkle depth in the group treated with vitamin C and growth factors than those treated with LADD followed by topical vitamin C alone; this study proved that LADD has a great potential to facilitate the absorption of exogenous macromolecules by the skin, with more direct intradermal delivery of growth factors [50].

Benzaquen et al. conducted a prospective, double-blinded, randomized split-face study on 20 patients to confirm the efficacy and safety of laser-assisted HA delivery (fractional CO_2 laser, spot size 300 μm, power 10 W, density 5%) in 2021 [51]. None of the skin remodeling parameters showed any statistically significant differences between the HA-treated and nontreated hemiface, despite the best improvement in skin radiance and greater improvement in skin texture and firmness being observed. There was no histologically approved evidence to support the effectiveness of HA in this study. Therefore, the gradually enhanced treatment effect at 1 month and 3 months may primarily originate from fractional CO_2 laser rather than the add-on effect from absorption of micronized, weakly cross-linked HA through laser-assisted delivery. The injectable form of HA is still the preferred option to offer more visible results in clinical practice.

Waibel et al. delivered poly-L-lactic acid (PLLA) through LADD to treat 19 patients with atrophic acne scars [52]. The PLLA was diluted with 6 mL of sterile saline and 2 mL of 1% lidocaine to evaluate the fractional CO_2 laser on the patient's skin and migration of the PLLA columns of the human cadaver cheek. The average overall improvement was 2.18 out of 3. On histologic examination, PLLA was visible within the upper dermis. Kim WJ from Korea reported a 21-year-old female with an atrophic, depressed, and hypopigmented scar on the nose treated with fractional CO_2 laser-assisted PLLA delivery [53]. PLLA was mixed with 3 mL sterile water and applied to the laser-treated area. After two laser treatment sessions, the hypopigmented atrophic and depressed scar color became similar to the existing skin color. In addition to the atrophic scar management, laser-assisted delivery of topical PLLA also improved the upper lip rhytids [54]. After three fractional CO_2 laser treatment sessions, the severity of upper lip wrinkles decreased by an average of 47%.

Cervantes et al. conducted a study on LADD utilizing various fillers as determined by histologic analysis. CO_2 AFL (eCO_2, 120 mm tip, 120 mJ), fractional radiofrequency microneedling (FRMN, Genius, 1.5 mm, 20 mJ/pin), and microneedling (2.0 mm) were applied to ex vivo human abdominoplasty skin samples. Immediately after PLLA, HA gel, calcium hydroxyapatite (CaHA), and black tissue marking dye were topically applied. Histology revealed that PLLA and black tissue marking dye were found within almost all channels in the papillary and upper to mid-dermis, while HA was also occasionally found. Because of their higher viscosity, CaHA particles were rarely found superficially within these channels. This study proved fractional CO_2 laser and PLLA to be the most effective combination for LADD in appropriate clinical indications. The authors mentioned that FRMN failed to show any significant channels for products to penetrate through and that further study investigating the timing of topical application in FRMN-assisted delivery is needed [55].

In regenerative medicine, LADD has also been used to deliver ambiguous active ingredients. Steven Cohen applied a topical nano-fat biocrème after using a 1550 nm erbium-doped and 1927 nm thulium NAFL [56]. To create a topical biocrème, harvested fat was processed into nano-fat and combined with a transdermal liposomal delivery vector. Histologically, the posttreatment postauricular skin specimens of two patients showed more elastin fibers and a slight increase in the thickness of the epidermis, even though the particles might be poorly absorbed through LADD due to early plugging with fibrin clots. In addition, compared to historical controls, patients' degrees of wrinkles, nasolabial fold depth, and texture all showed statistically significant improvements. According to the authors, the enhancement in the depth of nasolabial folds, the appearance of fine lines, and the general texture of the tissue were more substantial than those achieved with laser resurfacing alone. However, the long-term risks and benefits are not well known.

Kwon et al. evaluated the clinical efficacy of adipose tissue stem cell (ASC)-derived exosomes (ASCEs) as an adjuvant therapy after applying CO_2 AFL for acne scars through a 12-week prospective, double-blind, randomized, split-face trial. For rolling scars, the ASCE-treated side showed a significantly greater improvement than the control side; for ice pick and boxcar scars, a significant decrease in acne score was observed on both sides, but the ASCE-treated side had no significant difference from the other side. Overall, the ASCE treatment afforded more favorable responses, a shorter recovery time, and fewer side effects when combined with CO_2 AFL for acne scarring [57].

Ozog's team demonstrated that CO_2 AFL facilitated the transcutaneous penetration of botulinum toxin type A (BoNT-A) in 2015 [58]. In this randomized controlled trial for ten patients with lateral periorbital wrinkles, abobotulinumtoxinA (aboBoNTA) 100 units diluted in 0.1 mL of normal saline was applied within 60 s of the CO_2 AFL with the level of superficial dermis up to approximately 50 μm at non-overlapped but 100% coverage. On the treated side, there was a statistically significant difference in dynamic wrinkling between baseline and 1 week and baseline and 1 month. There was no statistically significant difference between the two groups regarding static wrinkles.

Manuskiatti et al. treated three patients of palmar hyperhidrosis with two CO_2 AFL treatments (with an average of 160–350 μm depth) on one palm administered with an average of 5% skin surface coverage at an interval of 2 weeks [59]. IncobotulinumtoxinA (incoBoNTA) solution at a concentration of 4 units/0.1 mL for 50 units was immediately applied at the laser-treated side. The authors found that the mean sweat production decreased 51.6% at 2 weeks after the first treatment and 88.5%, 67.8%, and 52.9% at 1, 2, and 3 months after the final treatment compared to the baseline. The second application of incobotulinumtoxinA significantly improved the absorption and efficacy in reducing palmar sweating. When 3 months had passed after treatment, the anhidrotic effects' duration had decreased. Agamia N et al. from Egypt published a comparative study on 30 patients with palmar hyperhidrosis [59]. In the groups treated with onabotulinumtoxinA (onaBoNTA) solution at a concentration of 2.5 units/0.1 mL over three sessions separated by 2 weeks, the efficacy of a total of 75 units of onaBoNTA application was found to be clinically equivalent to that of 50 units of injection. For each fractional laser session, 25 units of BoNTA were applied. Although LADD using botulinum toxin is effective and safe with less pain, it requires higher doses and frequent application to achieve optimal results [60].

Alopecia

Before considering the enhancement delivery of drugs for hair loss, Tosti et al. emphasized that physicians should consider the intended target and etiology of hair loss [61]. The CO_2 AFL, erbium:YAG AFL, and 1550 nm erbium:glass NAFL are promising treatment options for pattern hair loss (PHL) and alopecia areata (AA) [62, 63]. Fractional laser mono- and adjunctive therapy seem superior to any other therapy in total efficiency, but there were no statistical differences between them, according to a systematic review and meta-analysis [64]. Although the mechanisms are not fully understood, the microscopic injuries may induce a favorable wound-healing environment that promotes hair growth, and upregulation of the Wnt/B-catenin pathway has also been demonstrated; further topical treatment can potentiate the laser effect [61–63, 65].

The CO_2 AFL prolongs the duration of the anagen phase [65]. The erbium:YAG AFL can start the anagen phase significantly earlier and shorten the time period between the anagen and catagen phases in a murine model [66].

Lee W. et al. published the first report on laser-assisted delivery in the nude mouse skin and porcine skin model in 2014 [67]. Laser ablation at 6 and 10 mm depth enhanced drug accumulation in the skin. Minoxidil was two- to ninefold compared with the control, and diphencyprone (DPCP) was sixfold compared with the control.

In addition to the wound stimuli from laser therapy for male pattern hair loss (MPHL), Bertin ACJ added optimal dispersion of 2 mL of finasteride (0.05%) solution plus another 2 mL of a compounded solution of growth factors, including vascular endothelial growth factor, basic fibroblast growth factor, insulin-like growth factor, and copper peptide 1.2% on the scalp right after the treatment with 1550 nm erbium:glass NAFL [68]. Eight passes were performed at 7 mJ, 3–9% coverage, and 120 MTZ/cm2 density. All four patients showed increased hair regrowth and density 2 weeks after the final treatment. The authors believed that these cases may benefit from laser therapy and more optimal dispersion of growth factors and finasteride to the scalp. Yu AJ conducted another research on 30 male patients with moderate-to-severe MPHL. The patients in the combination group were treated with 1 mL of topical 5% minoxidil twice daily and six sessions of erbium:YAG AFL [69]. The combination group obtained a higher dermoscopy score than the patients receiving minoxidil alone ($p = 0.016$), but there was no difference between the two groups regarding the photography score ($p = 0.13$). Besides LADD by ABL and NABL improving alopecia, Lee YH et al. also confirmed that the FRMN enhanced the absorption of 5% topical minoxidil [70]. The combined therapy side had a higher degree of improvement in both hair count and hair thickness.

The application of ASC-conditioned medium (CM) with a microneedle roller once per week also showed efficacy in treating FPHL after 12 weeks of therapy. In this retrospective, observational study of outcomes in 27 patients with FPHL performed by Shin et al., the hair density increased from 105.4 to 122.7 hairs/cm^2 ($p < 0.001$). The hair thickness increased from 57.5 to 64.0 μm ($p < 0.001$). No serious side effects were observed in any patient [71].

A literature review was performed by Dabek RJ to evaluate the efficacy of fractional lasers and microneedling for AA [72]. There are not many studies or participants, but there is evidence that both triamcinolone acetonide at 20 mg/mL (0.1 mL dropped/cm^2) right after CO_2 AFL and triamcinolone acetonide at 10 mg/mL after microneedling are effective therapeutic approaches. Lario A et al. reported that the use of CO2 AFL and the application of intralesional methotrexate for two cases of refractory AA showed good hair regrowth response. They mentioned that the mean dose and frequency of drug application are still unknown and should be established in further studies [73].

In addition to laser-assisted drug delivery for AA, platelet-rich plasma (PRP) is a promising option for standard treatment, or it could serve as a supplemental therapy to enhance the effect of primary treatment. In both groups, total and terminal hair densities rose significantly during therapy compared to baseline. Throughout the study period, the mean total hair density rose considerably with high pulse energy (1.42 hair/cm^2) compared to low pulse energy (1.04 hair/cm^2) ($p = 0.023$; 4.89 hair/cm^2) [74].

Local Anesthesia

A randomized, controlled, split-face comparison study was performed by Yun et al.; they showed that topical anesthesia (EMLA cream) could be easily and painlessly enhanced by removing the stratum corneum with a low-fluence Er:YAG laser before application [75]. Baron et al. also demonstrated that a single, painless pulse of an Er:YAG laser increased the absorption of a lidocaine cream with enhanced penetration, consequently inducing anesthesia in just 5 min with two randomized trials [76]. However, Yun and Baron mentioned that laser-assisted topical anesthesia may not be adequate for laser resurfacing.

Meesters et al. designed a prospective, single-blinded, randomized study and found that superficial disruption of the epidermis by CO_2 AFL (2.5 mJ/microbeam, 5% density) pretreatment improved the efficacy of topically applied AHES (articaine hydrochloride 40 mg/mL + epinephrine 10 mg/mL solution), and the AHES gave superior anesthesia compared to EMLA cream. They believed that a liquid solution would more easily penetrate the ablation channels [77]. Meesters et al. further proved that both the CO_2 AFL and the Er:YAG AFL at very low energy settings are effective in AFL-assisted topical anesthesia, with no significant difference in visual analog scale (VAS) scores, and 15% density was more effective than 5% density [78].

Infantile Hemangioma

The use of timolol eye drops for superficial infantile hemangioma was reported in 2010 [79]. Since then, it has been widely used as one of the safe and effective alternatives to systemic use in treatment. Lin X. et al. used CO_2 AFL at 25–30 mJ/pulse, 5% density at 1-week intervals. Topical timolol maleate 0.5% under occlusion for 30 min was applied four to five times daily for an average treatment duration of 14.2 weeks. Eight out of the nine enrolled patients aged 1–6 months showed good (50–75% regression) to excellent (>75% regression) responses. Plasma timolol concentration was below the detected sensitivity limit [80].

Sun L et al. used Er:YAG AFL (11% coverage, depth: 80–110 μm) at 2-week intervals to assist the delivery of timolol for 24 weeks. 76.7% of the patients showed excellent regression, and 13.3% showed good regression, with no systemic adverse effects [81].

Laser Setting for Safety Concerns

Ablative lasers often maintain the potential risks for burning, scarring, and dyspigmentation. While the use of AFLs, particularly NAFLs, has significantly reduced these dangers, caution is still advised. The potential laser-induced risks are erythema, edema, blistering, scarring, and pigmentary changes with LADD, particularly at high fluences and high treatment densities. Therefore, the practitioner must consider how to achieve the desired results and the potential side effects associated with laser use as a whole. In addition, patients' skin type and skin character (e.g., hydration, age, anatomical region) may contribute to their tolerance to the treatment [1–3].

When AFLs are used in LADD, the laser parameters must be carefully calibrated to maximize efficacy while minimizing danger. Clinicians must be aware of the dangers associated with increased laser channel penetration. While deeper channels necessitate higher fluences, which also convey more heat, it raises the risk of local cutaneous adverse effects such as laser-induced discomfort, burns, scarring, prolonged downtime, and drug-induced local and systemic responses. Laser density and fluence are proportional to the size of the laser spots and the number of MTZ channels inside the treated area. Clinicians must recognize that increasing the density of laser channels results in increased thermal damage and, thus, an increased risk of burns and scarring. Because densities of more than 5% may not result in additional enhancement of cutaneous drug concentrations or therapeutic efficacy for specific medications, employing higher density settings may be problematic, in part because of increased adverse effects. While research has consistently shown that lower densities are more beneficial for LADD, this conclusion may vary per therapy [2, 3, 82].

Additionally, the size of the laser coagulation zone (CZ) may affect the efficacy and safety of LADD. The more significant CZs result in a more significant amount of heat damage being transferred to the skin, which raises the likelihood of undesirable consequences such as blistering and scarring; moreover, the existence of CZs may result in the persistent release of topically applied chemicals, raising the risk of local and systemic reactions [1, 2].

When administered through AFL, 5-FU and steroids have been related to an increase in local bacterial infections. As a result, prior to attempt-

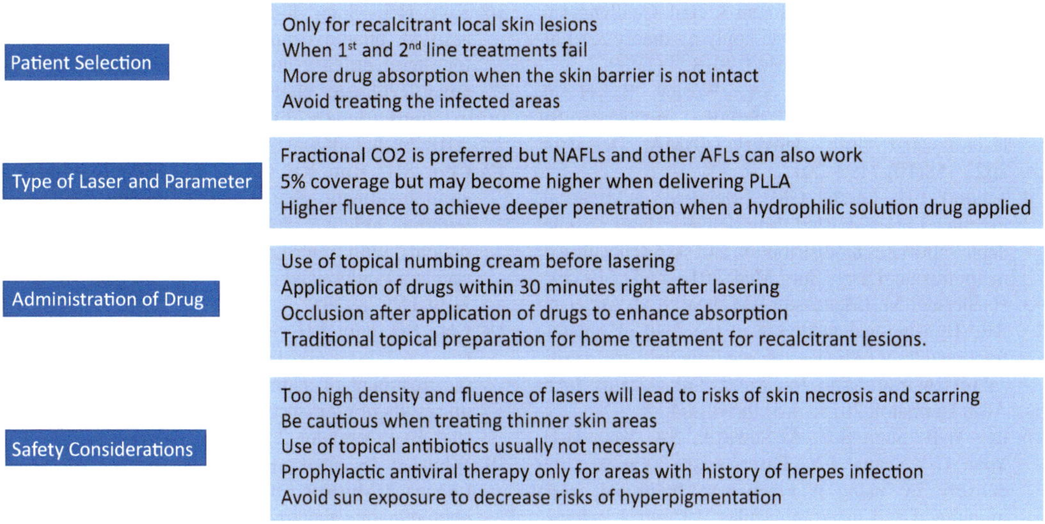

Fig. 10.2 Laser-assisted drug delivery: steps and concerns

ing LADD, strict pre- and post-procedural antiseptic care should be performed. Antibiotic or antifungal prophylaxis is not recommended except for impaired wound healing area; antiviral prophylaxis is recommended for the risk of herpes-infected area (Fig. 10.2) [2, 3].

Drugs to be Delivered and the Amplified Cutaneous Reactions

Although LADD enhances the dermal accumulation of topical drugs and chemicals used to treat several dermatological disorders, the amplified buildup of medication inside the dermis may exacerbate the medication's local reaction. Laser-assisted steroid administration has been shown to cause atrophy and hypopigmentation, while 5-FU administration has been shown to cause erythema, edema, and itch. As a result, it is necessary to be aware of known local adverse effects of topical medications and their potential induction by LADD; the risk of systemic absorption of the drugs following fractional ablative laser should be a concern when treating large skin areas, and the possibility of inducing systemic hypersensitivity also needs to be carefully considered [2, 3, 79].

With enhanced but physiologically normal therapeutic responses, transdermally delivered medicines may generate localized foreign-body or hypersensitive reactions. However, PLLA-induced granulomatous inflammation is important for healing atrophic scars.

The Future

LADD has emerged as a powerful tool to enhance drug delivery to and through the skin to achieve a fantastic clinical response to improve skin conditions. Ultrasound and other devices that can push the drug into the skin may help to enhance drug delivery efficacy. Practitioners should be familiar with the parameters of both drugs and lasers. However, classic pharmacodynamics has been significantly changed, but further investigations are warranted to establish an LADD version of the pharmacodynamic to accurately explain the efficacy and safety.

References

1. Wenande E, Anderson RR, Haedersdal M. Fundamentals of fractional laser-assisted drug delivery: an in-depth guide to experimental methodology and data interpretation. Adv Drug Deliv Rev. 2020;153:169–84.

2. Ibrahim O, Wenande E, Hogan S, et al. Challenges to laser-assisted drug delivery: applying theory to clinical practice. Lasers Surg Med. 2018;50(1):20–7.
3. Labadie JG, Ibrahim SA, Worley B, et al. Evidence-based clinical practice guidelines for laser-assisted drug delivery. JAMA Dermatol. 2022;158(10):1193–201.
4. Taudorf EH, Lerche CM, Erlendsson AM, et al. Fractional laser-assisted drug delivery: laser channel depth influences biodistribution and skin deposition of methotrexate. Lasers Surg Med. 2016;48(5):519–29.
5. Haedersdal M, Erlendsson AM, Paasch U, Anderson RR. Translational medicine in the field of ablative fractional laser (AFXL)-assisted drug delivery: a critical review from basics to current clinical status. J Am Acad Dermatol. 2016;74(5):981–1004.
6. Lee W-R, Shen S-C, Al-Suwayeh SA, Yang H-H, Yuan C-Y, Fang J-Y. Laser-assisted topical drug delivery by using a lowfluence fractional laser: imiquimod and macromolecules. J Control Release. 2011;153(3):240–8.
7. Lee J, Yi K, Kim H, et al. A novel needle-free microjet drug injector using Er:YAG laser: a completely new concept of transdermal drug delivery system. Clin Anat. 2022;35(5):682–5.
8. Zaleski-Larsen LA, Fabi SG. Laser-assisted drug delivery. Dermatol Surg. 2016;42(8):919–31.
9. Searle T, Ali FR, Al-Niaimi F. Lessons learned from the first decade of laser-assisted drug delivery. Dermatol Ther. 2021;11(1):93–104.
10. Paasch U, Grunewald S. Update on dermatologic laser therapy II—advances in photodynamic therapy using laser-assisted drug delivery. J Dtsch Dermatol Ges. 2020;18(12):1370–7.
11. Morton CA, Szeimies R-M, Basset-Seguin N, et al. European Dermatology Forum guidelines on topical photodynamic therapy 2019 part 1: treatment delivery and established indications—actinic keratoses, Bowen's disease, and basal cell carcinomas. J Eur Acad Dermatol Venereol. 2019;33(12):2225–38.
12. Togsverd-Bo K, Haak CS, Thaysen-Petersen D, et al. Intensified photodynamic therapy of actinic keratoses with fractional CO_2 laser: a randomized clinical trial. Br J Dermatol. 2012;166(6):1262–9.
13. Ko D-Y, Jeon S-Y, Kim K-H, Song K-H. Fractional erbium: YAG laser-assisted photodynamic therapy for facial actinic keratoses: a randomized, comparative, prospective study. J Eur Acad Dermatol Venereol. 2014;28(11):1529–39.
14. Togsverd-Bo K, Lei U, Erlendsson AM, Taudorf EH, et al. Combination of ablative fractional laser and daylight-mediated photodynamic therapy for actinic keratosis in organ transplant recipients—a randomized controlled trial. Br J Dermatol. 2015;172(2):467–74.
15. Ko DY, Kim KH, Song KH. A randomized trial comparing methyl aminolaevulinate photodynamic therapy with and without Er:YAG ablative fractional laser treatment in Asian patients with lower extremity Bowen disease: results from a 12-month follow-up. Br J Dermatol. 2014;170(1):165–72.
16. Kim H-J, Song K-H. Ablative fractional laser-assisted photodynamic therapy provides superior long-term efficacy compared with standard methyl aminolevulinate photodynamic therapy for lower extremity Bowen disease. J Am Acad Dermatol. 2018;79(5):860–8.
17. Choi SH, Kim KH, Song KH. Effect of methyl aminolevulinate photodynamic therapy with and without ablative fractional laser treatment in patients with microinvasive squamous cell carcinoma: a randomized clinical trial. JAMA Dermatol. 2017;153:289–95.
18. Choi SH, Kim KH, Song K-H. Efficacy of ablative fractional laser-assisted photodynamic therapy for the treatment of actinic cheilitis: 12-month follow-up results of a prospective, randomized, comparative trial. Br J Dermatol. 2015;173(1):184–91.
19. Whitaker IS, Shokrollahi K, James W, Mishra A, Lohana P, Murison MC. Combined CO(2) laser with photodynamic therapy for the treatment of nodular basal cell carcinomas. Ann Plast Surg. 2007;59:484–8.
20. Shokrollahi K, Javed M, Aeuyung K, et al. Combined carbon dioxide laser with photodynamic therapy for nodular and superficial basal cell carcinoma. Ann Plast Surg. 2014;73:552–8.
21. Choi SH, Kim KH, Song KH. Er:YAG ablative fractional laser-primed photodynamic therapy with methyl aminolevulinate as an alternative treatment option for patients with thin nodular basal cell carcinoma: 12-month follow-up results of a randomized, prospective, comparative trial. J Eur Acad Dermatol Venereol. 2016;30:783–8.
22. Haak CS, Togsverd-Bo K, Thaysen-Petersen D, et al. Fractional laser-mediated photodynamic therapy of high-risk basal cell carcinomas—a randomized clinical trial. Br J Dermatol. 2015;172(1):215–22.
23. Badawi AM, Osman MA. Fractional erbium-doped yttrium aluminum garnet laser-assisted drug delivery of hydroquinone in the treatment of melasma. Clin Cosmet Investig Dermatol. 2018;11:13–20.
24. Namazi N, Hesami A, Ketabi Y. The split-face comparison of the combined Er-YAG laser and hydroquinone 4% with hydroquinone 4% alone in the treatment of melasma in Iranian patients: a prospective, interventional case study. J Lasers Med Sci. 2020;11(1):70–3.
25. Tawfic SO, Abdel Hay RM, Abouelazm DI, Said ER. Tranexamic acid microinjection alone versus its combination with fractional carbon dioxide laser in melasma treatment: a dermoscopic evaluation. Dermatol Surg. 2022;48(5):556–61.
26. Mekawy KMM, Sadek A, Seddeik Abdel-Hameed AK. Micro-needling versus fractional carbon dioxide laser for delivery of tranexamic acid in the treatment of melasma: a split-face study. J Cosmet Dermatol. 2021;20(2):460–5.
27. El-Sinbawy ZG, Abdelnabi NM, Sarhan NE, Elgarhy LH. Clinical & ultrastructural evaluation of the effect of fractional CO_2 laser on facial melasma. Ultrastruct Pathol. 2019;43(4–5):135–44.

28. Lai D, Zhou S, Cheng S, Liu H, Cui Y. Laser therapy in the treatment of melasma: a systematic review and meta-analysis. Lasers Med Sci. 2022;37(4):2099–110.
29. Rokhsar CK, Fitzpatrick RE. The treatment of melasma with fractional photothermolysis: a pilot study. Dermatol Surg. 2005;31(12):1645–50.
30. Qu Y, Wang F, Liu J, Xia X. Clinical observation and dermoscopy evaluation of fractional CO_2 laser combined with topical tranexamic acid in melasma treatments. J Cosmet Dermatol. 2021;20(4):1110–6.
31. Botsali A, Esme P, Erbil H, et al. Comparison of fractional erbium:YAG laser assisted tranexamic acid delivery alone and in combination with oral tranexamic acid in melasma. Lasers Med Sci. 2022;37(7):2823–30.
32. Wang J, Christman M, Feng H, et al. Laser-assisted delivery of tranexamic acid for melasma: pilot study using a novel 1927 nm fractional thulium fiber laser. J Cosmet Dermatol. 2021;20(1):105–9.
33. Li Y, Yao C, Zhang H, et al. Efficacy and safety of 755 nm picosecond alexandrite laser with topical tranexamic acid versus laser monotherapy for melasma and facial rejuvenation: a multicenter, randomized, double blinded, split face study in Chinese patients. Lasers Med Sci. 2022;37(7):2879–87.
34. Wang T, Gao H, Wang D, Zhang C, Hu K, Zhang H, Lin J, Chen X. Stem cell-derived exosomes in the treatment of melasma and its percutaneous penetration. Lasers Surg Med. 2023;55(2):178–89.
35. Anbar TS, Westerhof W, Abdel-Rahman AT, et al. Effect of one session of ER:YAG laser ablation plus topical 5-fluorouracil on the outcome of short-term NB-UVB phototherapy in the treatment of non-segmental vitiligo: a left-right comparative study. Photodermatol Photoimmunol Photomed. 2008;24:322–9.
36. Farajzadeh S, Daraei Z, Esfandiarpour I, Hosseini SH. The efficacy of pimecrolimus 1% cream combined with microdermabrasion in the treatment of nonsegmental childhood vitiligo: a randomized placebo-controlled study. Pediatr Dermatol. 2009;26:286–91.
37. Doghaim NN, El-Tatawy RA, Ismail MA, et al. Study the effect of erbium:YAG laser plus topical 5-flurouracil in stable vitiligo resistant to NB-UVB phototherapy. J Cosmet Dermatol. 2020;19(1):122–30.
38. Li L, Wu Y, Li L, et al. Triple combination treatment with fractional CO_2 laser plus topical betamethasone solution and narrowband ultraviolet B for refractory vitiligo: a prospective, randomized half-body, comparative study. Dermatol Ther. 2015;28:131–4.
39. Shin J, Lee JS, Hann S-K, Oh SH. Combination treatment by 10600 nm ablative fractional carbon dioxide laser and narrowband ultraviolet B in refractory nonsegmental vitiligo: a prospective, randomized half-body comparative study. Br J Dermatol. 2012;166(3):658–61.
40. Vachiramon V, Chaiyabutr C, Rattanaumpawan P, et al. Effects of a preceding fractional carbon dioxide laser on the outcome of combined local narrowband ultraviolet B and topical steroids in patients with vitiligo in difficult-to-treat areas. Lasers Surg Med. 2016;48(2):197–202.
41. Leszczynski R, da Silva CA, Pinto ACPN, et al. Laser therapy for treating hypertrophic and keloid scars. Cochrane Database Syst Rev. 2022;9(9):CD011642.
42. Truong K, Prasidha I, et al. A systematic review of randomised controlled trials investigating laser assisted drug delivery for the treatment of keloid and hypertrophic scars. Lasers Med Sci. 2022;37(1):47–59.
43. Oosterhoff TCH, Beekman VK, van der List JP, Niessen FB. Laser treatment of specific scar characteristics in hypertrophic scars and keloid: a systematic review. J Plast Reconstr Aesthet Surg. 2021;74(1):48–64.
44. Waibel JS, Wulkan AJ, Shumaker PR. Treatment of hypertrophic scars using laser and laser assisted corticosteroid delivery. Lasers Surg Med. 2013;45(3):135–40.
45. Majid I, Imran S. Fractional carbon dioxide laser resurfacing in combination with potent topical corticosteroids for hypertrophic burn scars in the pediatric age group: an open label study. Dermatol Surg. 2018;44(8):1102–8.
46. Park JH, Chun JY, Lee JH. Laser-assisted topical corticosteroid delivery for the treatment of keloids. Lasers Med Sci. 2017;32:601–8.
47. Waibel JS, Wulkan AJ, Rudnick A, et al. Treatment of hypertrophic scars using laser-assisted corticosteroid versus laser-assisted 5-fluorouracil delivery. Dermatol Surg. 2019;45:423–30.
48. Manuskiatti W, Kaewkes A, Yan C, et al. Hypertrophic scar outcomes in fractional laser monotherapy versus fractional laser-assisted topical corticosteroid delivery: a randomized clinical trial. Acta Derm Venereol. 2021;101(3):adv00416.
49. Waibel JS, Mi QS, Ozog D, et al. Laser-assisted delivery of vitamin C, vitamin E, and ferulic acid formula serum decreases fractional laser postoperative recovery by increased beta fibroblast growth factor expression. Lasers Surg Med. 2016;48(3):238–44.
50. Machado BHB, Frame J, Zhang J, et al. Comparative study on the outcome of periorbital wrinkles treated with laser-assisted delivery of vitamin C or vitamin C plus growth factors: a randomized, double-blind, clinical trial. Aesthetic Plast Surg. 2021;45(3):1020–32.
51. Benzaquen M, Fongue J, Pauly V, et al. Laser-assisted hyaluronic acid delivery by fractional carbon dioxide laser in facial skin remodeling: a prospective randomized split-face study in France. Lasers Surg Med. 2021;53(9):1166–72.
52. Rkein A, Ozog D, Waibel JS. Treatment of atrophic scars with fractionated CO_2 laser facilitating delivery of topically applied poly-L-lactic acid. Dermatol Surg. 2014;40(6):624–31.
53. Kim WJ, Jung HR, Lee SJ, et al. Treatment of an atrophic scar with fractional carbon dioxide laser-assisted poly-L-lactic acid delivery. Med Lasers. 2021;10(3):181–4.
54. Ibrahim O, Ionta S, Depina J, et al. Safety of laser-assisted delivery of topical poly-L-lactic acid in

the treatment of upper lip rhytides. Dermatol Surg. 2019;45(7):968–74.
55. Cervantes J, Chang YF, Dover JS, et al. Laser-assisted and device-assisted filler delivery: a histologic evaluation. Dermatol Surg. 2023;49(9):865–70.
56. Cohen SR, Goodacre AK, Womack H, et al. Topical nanofat biocrème improves aesthetic outcomes of non-ablative fractionated laser treatment: a preliminary report. Aesthet Surg J. 2020;40(8):892–9.
57. Kwon HH, Yang SH, Lee J, et al. Combination treatment with human adipose tissue stem cell-derived exosomes and fractional CO_2 laser for acne scars: a 12-week prospective, double-blind, randomized, split-face study. Acta Derm Venereol. 2020;100(18):adv00310.
58. Mahmoud BH, Burnett C, Ozog D, et al. Prospective randomized controlled study to determine the effect of topical application of botulinum toxin a for crow's feet after treatment with ablative fractional CO_2 laser. Dermatol Surg. 2015;41:S75–81.
59. Junsuwan N, Manuskiatti W, Phothong W, et al. Fractional CO_2 laser-assisted botulinum toxin type A delivery for the treatment of primary palmar hyperhidrosis. Lasers Med Sci. 2021;36(1):233–6.
60. Agamia NF, Sobhy N, Abd-Elraouf A, et al. Fractional CO_2 laser for transcutaneous drug delivery of onabotulinumtoxinA in palmar hyperhidrosis. Dermatol Surg. 2021;47(5):678–83.
61. Alsalhi WA, Alalola AS, Randolph MJ, et al. Novel drug delivery approaches for the management of hair loss. Expert Opin Drug Deliv. 2020;17(3):287–95.
62. Perper M, Aldahan AS, Fayne RA, et al. Efficacy of fractional lasers in treating alopecia: a literature review. Lasers Med Sci. 2017;32(8):1919–25.
63. Dabek RJ, Austen WG Jr, Bojovic B. Laser-assisted hair regrowth: fractional laser modalities for the treatment of androgenic alopecia. Plast Reconstr Surg Glob Open. 2019;7(4):e2157.
64. Gao YL, Zhang Y, Zheng JC, et al. The efficacy and safety of fractional lasers for alopecia in mono and adjunctive therapy: a systematic review and meta-analysis. J Cosmet Dermatol. 2022;21(11):5500–8.
65. Bae JM, Jung HM, Goo B, et al. Hair regrowth through wound healing process after ablative fractional laser treatment in a murine model. Lasers Surg Med. 2015;47(5):433–40.
66. Ke J, Guan H, Li S, et al. Erbium: YAG laser treatment stimulates hair growth through upregulating Wnt 10b and beta-catenin expression in C57BL/6 mice. Int J Clin Exp Med. 2015;8(11):20883–9.
67. Lee W, Shen S, Aljuffali IA, et al. Erbium–yttrium–aluminum–garnet laser irradiation ameliorates skin permeation and follicular delivery of antialopecia drugs. J Pharm Sci. 2014;103(11):3542–52.
68. Bertin ACJ, Vilarinho A, Junqueira ALA. Fractional non-ablative laser-assisted drug delivery leads to improvement in male and female pattern hair loss. J Cosmet Laser Ther. 2018;20(7–8):391–4.
69. Mokhtari F, Zavare Z, Iraji F. Topical 5% minoxidil versus combined erbium YAG laser and topical 5% minoxidil in androgenetic alopecia: a randomized controlled trial. J Cosmet Dermatol. 2023;22(10):2737–43.
70. Yu AJ, Luo YJ, Xu XG, et al. A pilot split-scalp study of combined fractional radiofrequency microneedling and 5% topical minoxidil in treating male pattern hair loss. Clin Exp Dermatol. 2018;43(7):775–81.
71. Shin H, Ryu HH, Kwon O, et al. Clinical use of conditioned media of adipose tissue-derived stem cells in female pattern hair loss: a retrospective case series study. Int J Dermatol. 2015;54(6):730–5.
72. Dabek RJ, Roh DS, Ozdemir D, et al. Fractional laser-assisted hair regrowth and microneedling for the treatment of alopecia areata: a review. Cureus. 2019;11(6):e4943.
73. Lario A, Aguado-Garcia A, Andres-Lencina J, et al. Successful response to a combination of intralesional methotrexate and fractional CO_2 laser in refractory alopecia areata: case report. Skin Appendage Disord. 2022;8(6):486–91.
74. Hanthavichai S, Archavarungson N, Wongsuk T. A study to assess the efficacy of fractional carbon dioxide laser with topical platelet-rich plasma in the treatment of androgenetic alopecia. Lasers Med Sci. 2022;37(4):2279–86.
75. Yun PL, Tachihara R, Anderson RR. Efficacy of erbium:yttrium-aluminum-garnet laser-assisted delivery of topical anesthetic. J Am Acad Dermatol. 2002;47(4):542–7.
76. Baron ED, Harris L, Redpath WS, et al. Laser-assisted penetration of topical anesthetic in adults. Arch Dermatol. 2003;139(10):1288–90.
77. Meesters AA, Bakker MM, et al. Fractional CO_2 laser-assisted delivery of topical anesthetics: a randomised controlled pilot study. Lasers Surg Med. 2015;48(2):208–11.
78. Meesters AA, Nieboer MJ, et al. Parameters in fractional laser assisted delivery of topical anesthetics: role of laser type and laser settings. Lasers Surg Med. 2018;50(8):813–8.
79. Guo S, Ni N. Topical treatment for capillary hemangioma of the eyelid using β-blocker solution. Arch Ophthalmol. 2010;128(2):255–6.
80. Ma G, Wu P, Lin X. Fractional carbon dioxide laser-assisted drug delivery of topical timolol solution for the treatment of deep infantile hemangioma: a pilot study. Pediatr Dermatol. 2014;31(3):286–91.
81. Sun L, Wang C, Cao Y, et al. Fractional 2940-nm Er:YAG laser-assisted drug delivery of timolol maleate for the treatment of deep infantile hemangioma. J Dermatol Treat. 2021;32:1053–9.
82. Ng WHS, Smith SD. Laser-assisted drug delivery: a systematic review of safety and adverse events. Pharmaceutics. 2022;14(12):2738.

Lasers for Medical Dermatology Indications

11

Sophie Carrie Shan Cai and Sze Hon Chua

Conventional Ablative Laser (CO_2, Erbium:YAG)

Conventional ablative lasers utilise wavelengths that are well absorbed by water such as the 10,600 nm carbon dioxide (CO_2) laser and 2940 nm erbium:yttrium aluminium garnet (Er:YAG) laser. Their mode of action is purely photothermal, allowing destruction of diseased epidermis and, if required, progressive ablation down to diseased deeper skin layers. The ablation is necessarily followed by wound healing by secondary intention to achieve desired treatment outcomes.

Actinic Keratoses

Conventional ablative laser therapy has emerged as an attractive option for field-directed therapy of multifocal actinic keratoses (AKs). Several small randomised studies have demonstrated efficacy of 10,600 nm CO_2 laser and 2940 nm Er:YAG laser in treating actinic keratoses. A study of 27 patients with facial or scalp AKs showed significant 92% reduction in AKs with ablative CO_2 laser (5–6 W, superpulse mode, 1–2 passes) at 3 months post-treatment [1]. CO_2 laser ablation was also shown to be an effective treatment for multiple AKs in another randomised split-side comparative study, although photodynamic therapy appeared to be superior in AK reduction and overall satisfaction [2].

Er:YAG laser resurfacing (5.7–7.1 J/cm^2, 3 mm spot size, 8–15 Hz, 2–3 passes) [3] was used in another trial of 55 patients with multiple AKs on the scalp and/or the face, yielding significantly fewer recurrences at 3, 6 and 12 months post-treatment, compared to topical 5-fluorouracil treatment. More frequent side effects were reported, especially erythema and hypopigmentation [4].

Squamous Cell Carcinoma In Situ

CO_2 laser vaporisation demonstrated 86.3% clearance of intraepidermal squamous cell carcinoma in situ (SCCIS) in a large series of 44 patients (superpulse mode, 2 W/cm^2) after a single treatment session [5]. Recurrence occurred in 7.9% of these patients. 91% patients had solitary lesions mainly located on the lower limbs. Several passes were performed with the number determined intraoperatively according to the depth of the lesion with the aim to remove it in entirety. 11.3% of patients achieved clearance after more than one treatment (range 2–4 sessions), while 2.2% had no clinical resolution. 31.8% of patients sustained side effects including

S. C. S. Cai (✉) · S. H. Chua
National Skin Centre, Singapore, Singapore
e-mail: sophiecai@nsc.com.sg; shchua@nsc.com.sg

S. W. N. Cheng, C. L. Goh (eds.), *Updates on Lasers in Dermatology*, Updates in Clinical Dermatology, https://doi.org/10.1007/978-3-031-71155-8_11

minimal erythema, hypo- or hyperpigmentation with one patient developing a keloid scar.

Other smaller case series [6–9] have also reported success of CO_2 laser in treating SCCIS ranging from 80% to 100%, including on the digits where CO_2 laser provided excellent cosmesis and preservation of function. Ablative laser therapy may be preferred over standard surgical excision, which may result in scar contracture especially in the digit, leading to functional disability.

Several lesional characteristics may limit the success of ablative laser therapy in SCCIS clearance. These include tumour size and depth. Inadequate tumour control may result in thick or keratotic SCCIS. In a study of 13 SCCIS with their surrounding 3 mm margins treated with high-energy pulsed CO_2 laser (500 mJ, 2–4 W, 3 mm collimated handpiece), there was incomplete vaporisation in three of seven patients treated with three passes and in two of six patients treated with two passes [10]. Residual SCCIS was significantly thicker than that completely ablated on histological evaluation. Indeed, another case series of 16 patients with SCCIS on the legs treated with pulsed CO_2 laser showed that 12% developed recurrent lesions at 1-year follow-up [11]. On biopsy, these lesions revealed invasive SCC, which authors suggested were probably already present but undetected below the original laser treatment plane.

Thus, CO_2 laser ablation of SCCIS is likely suitable only for superficial SCCIS as thick keratotic SCCIS carries higher risks of residual tumour burden or recurrence with invasive SCC.

Cutaneous Human Papillomavirus (HPV) Warts

Ablative CO_2 laser has proven useful for the treatment of genital and non-genital verrucae [12–16]. Suggested settings include 9–15 W continuous mode for common warts, 4–6 W superpulse for flat warts and 8–15 W continuous mode for palmoplantar warts [16]. Across several studies, complete response rates were reported at 83–100% for Er:YAG laser and 59–100% for CO_2 laser [10]. No significant difference was found in efficacy or recurrence rates for laser therapy compared to conventional treatment modalities.

In the treatment of recalcitrant non-genital verrucae, variable response rates ranged from 30% to 80% [13]. A retrospective analysis of 200 patients with resistant verrucae treated with CO_2 laser vaporisation reported an overall cure rate of 64% at 12 months, with no difference between single and multiple warts and the duration or location of the wart [14]. However, ablative laser therapy carries significant morbidity risks of post-operative pain, infection and scarring. Special site considerations include the treatment of periungual verrucae, which may incur the risk of permanent onychodystrophy [15].

Operator safety considerations are important in the use of ablative laser treatment of cutaneous verrucae. Physicians and attending nursing personnel should wear effective protective masks to avoid inhalation of virus particles generated in the laser plume during vaporisation of verrucae.

Rhinophyma

Rhinophyma is a form of phymatous rosacea characterised by progressive sebaceous gland hypertrophy and fibrosis of the nasal skin leading to nodular distortion and significant disfigurement. Severe disease is suited for physical debulking and sculpting of the nose by physical treatment modalities such as the CO_2 ablative laser. A study of 124 patients with rhinophyma who were treated with CO_2 ablation (continuous mode to debulk larger rhinophymas followed by either resurfacing (20–40 W, 4–7 mm spot size) or continuous mode (10–20 W, defocused 2–3 mm beam) to reshape nasal contours) demonstrated good-to-excellent results in 118 patients with high satisfaction rates and long-term durable responses [17]. Side effects reported included pain with local anaesthetic injection, scarring and hypopigmentation (four patients) and open pores (two patients). A smaller retrospective study including patients with moderate and major rhinophyma treated with CO_2 ablation also showed excellent cosmetic outcomes, without major complications or recurrence at 1 year of follow-up [18]. As treatment of rhinophyma involves ablation of deeper skin tissues beneath the epidermis, significant operator skills are required. Meticulous wound management post-ablation is required to ensure good treatment outcomes.

Keloids and Hypertrophic Scars

Keloids and hypertrophic scars are forms of abnormal wound healing in which management remains challenging. Many treatment modalities have been applied including intralesional corticosteroid injection, surgery and laser therapy [19]. Debulking of earlobe keloids using CO_2 laser ablation was shown to be equally effective as cold steel surgery in a retrospective study of 16 patients with earlobe keloids, but recurrence of keloids at 2–18 weeks post-procedure occurred in both modalities [20]. Another prospective study of 28 patients with keloids on the trunk or limbs demonstrated that CO_2 laser vaporisation or excision (15 W, superpulse (for firm keloid) or continuous mode (for hard keloid), 0.1 mm point beam for excision or 1–3 mm point beam for vaporisation with low power 10 W), followed by intralesional triamcinolone acetonide 40 mg/mL 3–4 weeks apart for 6 months, was a useful treatment approach for keloid treatment [21]. Expectedly, CO_2 ablation alone was not sufficient in preventing recurrence as patients who were irregular with post-laser debulking intralesional corticosteroid demonstrated significantly higher recurrence at 6 and 12 months than those receiving regular intralesional corticosteroid. In general, ablative CO_2 laser debulking of keloids should be limited to areas of minimal wound tension such as the earlobe (suggested settings: 9–15 W continuous mode for large earlobe keloids; 4–7 W superpulse for smaller keloids) [16] and must be followed by regular intralesional corticosteroid injections and additionally the use of pressure ear clips to achieve better long-term treatment outcomes.

Hailey-Hailey Disease (HHD)

Hailey-Hailey disease (HHD) is a rare genetic disorder characterised by ruptured vesicles and blisters forming crusted painful erosions favouring the intertriginous areas especially the axillae and groin. Mutation in the Golgi-associated calcium transporter *ATP2C1* is responsible for the acantholysis. Laser therapy offers a safe, effective alternative treatment option for HHD besides medical and surgical therapy. One advantage of CO_2 laser ablation is that it allows large areas in HHD to be treated in a short period of time, with good aesthetic outcomes and acceptable side effects, compared to skin grafting or dermabrasion which is more invasive and associated with greater complications [22–28]. It is postulated that the ablation of the epidermal keratinocytes that express the molecular adhesion defect spares intact adnexa to regenerate normal epidermis [27] or that the dermal fibrosis generated contributes to better support of the diseased epidermis [28]. A systematic review identified a total of 23 HHD patients from case reports and case series who were treated with CO_2 laser ablation. At follow-up periods ranging from 4 to 144 months, 10 patients (43%) had no recurrence, 10 (43%) had greater than 50% improvement (with two patients showing recurrence at the periphery of treated area), 2 (8%) had less than 50% improvement and 1 (4%) patient had absence of improvement [23]. Suggested settings of CO_2 laser ablation: continuous, defocused mode 5–25 W, 1–9 mm spot size and 1–5 passes until normal vaporised reticular dermis were seen (yellowish tissue with pinpoint bleeding), with removal of char by moistened gauze after each pass [23]. Adverse events were minimal including pain, erythema and oedema, although long-term adverse effects such as dyspigmentation and scarring may occur with more aggressive laser settings.

Er:YAG laser ablation has also been used to treat HHD. Er:YAG is a more superficial laser than the CO_2 laser, causing minimal thermal injury or pain with better control of tissue ablation. However, it is unable to achieve haemostasis during treatment. Three patients with HHD were treated with Er:YAG laser (300–1000 mJ,

7.1–8.5 J/cm^2/pulse, 350 μs pulse width, 1.6–5 mm spot size, 5–10 Hz, overlap of 30% over large areas, 5 pulse series per lesion, end point punctate bleeding) [29] achieving complete remission in two patients, while the other patient had only partial remission with disease recurrence at the periphery [29, 30]. To prevent disease recurrence at the periphery of treated areas, some authors have suggested for laser treatment to extend beyond clinically visible disease [25].

In a case report, fractionated CO_2 laser was performed in a patient with long-standing HHD leading to remission in the right axilla and right groin, but symptomatic recurrences in the groin region required subsequent treatment using the Er:YAG laser [26]. Presumably, ablation of only the microthermal zones do leave behind areas of diseased epidermis leading to disease recurrences. Thus, conventional ablative lasers tend to be favoured over their fractionated counterparts as they offer superior treatment outcomes.

Fractional Ablative Laser

By using a scanning handpiece, the ablative laser may be converted from field or conventional ablation to fractional ablation. This modification employs the concept of fractional photothermolysis where microscopic thermal injury zones are surrounded by unaffected epidermis. Following fractional ablation, the normal skin surrounding the microscopic thermal injury zones enables rapid epidermal wound healing leading to less downtime and fewer adverse effects when compared to conventional laser ablation. Continued dermal tissue remodelling may lead to delayed improvements of deeper dermatological conditions. The microscopic thermal injury of fractional ablative lasers creates microscopic channels through the skin barrier. In fractional ablative laser-assisted drug delivery, this effect has been successfully capitalised to deliver drug molecules more effectively into the skin via the microscopic ablated channels, enhancing topical drug uptake and its efficacy.

Porokeratosis

CO_2 and Er:YAG ablative lasers have been successfully employed to treat porokeratosis of Mibelli, linear porokeratosis and disseminated superficial actinic porokeratosis (DSAP) [31–36]. Laser therapy side effects were minimal, including mild erythema, hyperpigmentation and moderate oedema. CO_2 laser vaporisation was successfully used to treat a large plaque of porokeratosis on the dorsal hand, fingers and web spaces with better cosmetic results and superior functionality than excision with split-thickness skin graft placement [33]. Recurrence of porokeratosis has been reported following CO_2 laser, and complete excision had to be performed thereafter [34]. Combination of CO_2 laser (superpulse 0.7 W, multiple passes applied to visible rims, with single pass to central area) and methyl aminolevulinate-photodynamic therapy (MAL-PDT) has been reported to improve but not completely clear DSAP lesions [37].

Actinic Keratoses (AKs)

In a randomised clinical trial of 15 patients with a total of 212 AKs on the face and scalp, fractional CO_2 laser-assisted methyl aminolevulinate photodynamic therapy (MAL-PDT) achieved significantly higher complete lesion response of AKs (88%) compared to MAL-PDT (59%) at 3-month follow-up, with fewer new AKs and improved photoaging effect [38]. However, fractional CO_2 laser-assisted PDT had more side effects of pain, erythema, crusting and pigmentary changes. Fractional CO_2 laser-assisted PDT (power 30 W, 140 MJ/pulse, 5.65 or 6.25 ms pulse duration, 5.2% or 5.3% density (first pass); 40 or 60 MJ/pulse, 1.32 or 2.06 ms pulse duration, 4.3% or 5.3% density (second pass)) also led to intensified PDT response for more effective clearance of acral recalcitrant AKs (73%) compared to laser alone (31%) in a randomised trial of ten organ transplant recipients with a total of 680 AKs [39]. Mild pigmentary changes were reported with no scarring.

Squamous Cell Carcinoma In Situ (SCCIS)

A study of 21 Asian patients with a total of 58 Bowen disease of the lower limbs demonstrated significantly increased efficacy of Er:YAG ablative fractional laser-assisted (550–600 μm ablation depth, level 1 coagulation, 22% density, single pulse) MAL-PDT (93.8%) than MAL-PDT alone (73.1%) with a lower recurrence rate (6.7% vs. 31.6%) at 12 months [40].

Keloids and Hypertrophic Scars

A recent Cochrane review evaluating randomised controlled trials of laser therapy used for treating hypertrophic and keloid scars stated unclear evidence whether fractional CO_2 laser improved hypertrophic and keloid scar severity compared with no treatment (very-low-certainty evidence) [41]. For instance, a randomised controlled split-lesion trial of 25 patients with scars from surgery or trauma yielded no significant difference between the treated and untreated side of the scar after three sessions of fractional CO_2 laser at 8-week intervals [42]. An earlier study of fractional CO_2 laser monotherapy treatment of keloids and hypertrophic scars also indicated mixed results as patient satisfaction was low even though Vancouver scar score was significantly reduced in the treatment group after 3 and 6 months, which was mainly attributed to increased scar pliability [43].

However, there appear to be promising results in combining fractional CO_2 laser and immediate laser-assisted drug delivery of topical triamcinolone acetonide for scar treatment [44]. Various studies have reported their combination use as safe and efficacious, with superiority compared to intralesional corticosteroid treatment alone [45, 46] and more significant reduction in keloid scar thickness compared to fractional CO_2 laser alone (power 20–25 W, stack 1–2, 300 ms, spacing 350 mm, 4 monthly sessions) [47].

Pulsed Dye Laser (PDL)

The pulsed dye laser (PDL) is a vascular-specific laser. It is postulated that its effectiveness in medical dermatology rests in its disruption of blood supply to lesional skin or the healing sequelae arising from microvascular destruction.

Basal Cell Carcinoma (BCC)

BCCs have vasculature that could serve as a chromophore target for vascular-selective laser such as the PDL. Compared to the 585 nm wavelength, the 595 nm wavelength penetrates deeper leading to coagulation depth of up to 2 mm, which enables the 595 nm PDL to treat BCCs more adequately within the upper 1–1.5 mm of skin [48].

The superiority of PDL (595 nm, 8 J/cm^2, pulse duration 0.5 ms, 10 mm spot size) compared to control sham treatment in treating superficial BCC was demonstrated in a randomised controlled study, with 78.6% (44/56) of cases showing histological clearance at 6-month follow-up after PDL [49]. Side effects included crusts and dyspigmentation. In a study of 29 patients with 39 biopsy-proven BCCs, one to four PDL sessions (595 nm, 15 J/cm^2, pulse duration 3 ms, 7 mm spot size) at 2–4-week intervals also achieved 75% (24/32) complete tumour resolution at a mean follow-up period of 11 months, with recurrence rate of 16% [50]. Nodular, infiltrative or mixed types of BCCs had higher risk of recurrence or non-response to treatment. Side effects reported were transient erythema, oedema and dusky purpura with no scarring. Another study of ten patients with 13 BCCs, which did not meet the criteria for Mohs micrographic surgery, used four combined PDL and Nd:YAG treatments at 2–4-week intervals but only attained 58% complete histologic clearance rate [51]. Superficial and nodular BCCs were the histologic types among complete responders, with 75% of tumours less than 1 cm in diameter showing complete response. Of note, all patients with residual tumours were receiving anticoagulation therapy, and the authors postulated that this inhibited laser-mediated intravascular coagulation leading to incomplete clearance of BCC.

Studies therefore suggest that the PDL is an effective and safe treatment option for BCCs, but its effectiveness is likely limited to smaller and more superficial BCCs.

Cutaneous Human Papillomavirus (HPV) Warts

As human papillomavirus infection stimulates epidermal hyperplasia and dermal neovascularisation, PDL may be useful in destroying cutaneous warts via laser-induced photocoagulation, targeting haemoglobin in their vasculature. The lack of bleeding and scarring is an advantage, but pre-laser paring of hyperkeratotic wart is required as PDL has limited penetration depth. A large retrospective study showed that 86% of the 209 patients with recalcitrant common or plantar warts attained complete or near-complete resolution of warts after an average of six treatment sessions with higher fluence levels (12.5–15 J/cm^2) [52]. However, another prospective randomised trial of 40 patients with verrucae assigned to monthly PDL (585 nm) for four treatment sessions or conventional treatment with cryotherapy or cantharidin did not find any increased efficacy for PDL (66% vs. 70%) [53]. Similar efficacy and relapse were seen between PDL (585 nm, 0.5 ms pulse duration, 8 J/cm^2, 7 mm spot size) and Nd:YAG laser (1064 nm, 20 ms pulse duration, 100 J/cm^2, 7 mm spot size) in a comparative study of treating plantar warts, although PDL appeared safer and less painful [54]. Overall, the variable wart clearance rates (20–95%) of PDL may be a result of different number and frequency of laser treatment sessions and applied fluences.

Keloids and Hypertrophic Scars

One of the earliest lasers used for scar remodelling is the PDL. It appears useful in treating vascular scars since it targets blood vessels with haemoglobin as the chromophore. The microvascular destruction causes resultant tissue hypoxia and neocollagenesis, with reduction in TGF-beta, collagen type III and fibroblast proliferation [55]. The efficacy of PDL for the treatment of keloids and hypertrophic scar has been evaluated in various studies and systematic reviews [41, 44, 56, 57]. Suggested settings for 595 nm PDL: 1.5 ms pulse duration, 7 mm spot size, 10 J/cm^2 fluence and dynamic cooling device duration 20 ms/delay 10 ms; for 585 nm PDL: 450 μs pulse duration, 7–10 mm spot size and 3.5–7.5 J/cm^2 (with lower fluence and 10 mm spot size in ethnic skin type) [57]. One case series demonstrated improvement in three patients with keloids post-shave excision 595 nm PDL treatment with no recurrence, and only hypopigmentation was noted in one patient [58]. A larger study of 26 patients with keloids treated with three sessions of 3–4 weekly 595 nm PDL found significant improvement in Vancouver scar scale (including improved pain, itch, pliability and erythema) and downregulation of connective tissue growth factor [59]. Similar improvements were reported in another study of 59 patients with keloids and hypertrophic postsurgical scars treated with 4–6 sessions of 585 nm PDL with 44 patients demonstrating moderate-to-excellent results, and only three patients were with minimal improvement at 6-month follow-up [60].

PDL treatment of keloids and hypertrophic scars is generally well tolerated with minor transient side effects. However, the variability in laser settings and outcome assessments has made comparison challenging, and a systematic review found only low or moderate evidence of improvement in scar erythema, volume and pliability with PDL treatment [56]. A more recent Cochrane review of laser therapy highlighted two randomised controlled trials suggesting greater improvement among PDL-treated scars compared with no treatment [41].

Long-Pulsed (LP) 1064 nm Nd:YAG

The chromophores for 1064 nm radiation are, in decreasing order, melanin, haemoglobin and water. The effectiveness of the long-pulsed 1064 nm Nd:YAG laser in medical dermatological conditions is based on its photothermal effects on target chromophores or, by extension, on tissues adjacent to the target chromophores.

Onychomycosis

Onychomycosis is a common chronic fungal infection of the nail, which remains challenging to treat. In view of the limited penetration and poor compliance to topical antifungal therapy as well as potential complications from systemic agents and surgical modalities, long-pulsed 1064 nm Nd:YAG has emerged as an alternative option for treatment. Varying clinical and mycological improvement rates have been demonstrated in largely uncontrolled studies (excellent mycological response or cure may range from 13% to 95%), with better efficacy in more severe cases and after extended Nd:YAG treatment [61–68]. Patients tolerated laser procedures well with no serious adverse event reported. The mechanism of long-pulsed Nd:YAG laser treatment of onychomycosis remains unclear, but laser irradiation has been shown to inhibit colony growth of *T. rubrum* and *T. mentagrophytes* and change their cellular ultrastructures [69]. Possibly, the photothermal heating effect leads to oxidative stress and cell apoptosis, contributing to a fungicidal effect [70]. The energy density and treatment durations have been described as the main factors affecting the efficacy of long-pulsed Nd:YAG laser (40–60 J/cm^2 depending on the nail plate thickness, 35 ms pulse duration, 4 mm spot size, 1 Hz, 6 weekly sessions) in treating onychomycosis [71].

Randomised controlled trials conducted have failed to demonstrate long-term efficacy of long-pulsed Nd:YAG laser as monotherapy to treat onychomycosis [72, 73]. There was no significant difference in mycologic clearance rates between the long-pulsed 1064 nm Nd:YAG laser group (17 patients) and control group (10 patients) in an early randomised trial, although the study had a small sample size of 27 patients with only two treatment sessions at fortnightly intervals [72]. A non-significant trend favouring greater proximal nail clearance in the laser group at 3 months was also not apparent by 12 months. Another small randomised trial of 20 patients evaluating short-pulsed 1064 nm Nd:YAG laser versus control group found that laser treatment was ineffective for mycologic remission or clinical improvement at 12 months [73]. A separate trial which compared long-pulsed Nd:YAG laser treatment to oral itraconazole also indicated no significant difference in their clinical efficacy at 12 months [71].

Given the incomplete clinical and mycological improvement, additional therapy is recommended to be combined with laser procedure to reduce recurrence, particularly for severe onychomycosis [66, 67]. A randomised clinical trial showed that 12 weeks of combined long-pulsed Nd:YAG laser with oral terbinafine treatment resulted in significantly greater and faster mycological and clinical clearance rates at 6 months than either treatment alone [74]. More recently, a clinical trial of 30 patients with onychomycosis also demonstrated best clinical results with combined long-pulsed Nd:YAG laser and itraconazole pulse therapy compared to pulse itraconazole alone, although there was no difference in mycological cure between the two groups [68]. In conjunction, another randomised clinical study of 60 patients found that combination treatment with long-pulsed Nd:YAG laser and topical amorolfine yielded better mycological cure rates (and clinical cure rates) than laser treatment alone at 65% (30%) versus 35% (10%), respectively [75].

While promising, more robust data for efficacy, optimal laser and combination regimen is needed before the long-pulsed Nd:YAG laser may find an established place in clinical practice to treat onychomycosis.

Cutaneous Human Papillomavirus (HPV) Warts

Lasers such as the long-pulsed Nd:YAG laser have greater depth of penetration compared to PDL, which has relatively shallow depth of penetration. The heat effect from long-pulsed Nd:YAG laser may induce coagulation of epidermal proteins and vasculature, stimulating a reactive inflammatory response to clear the wart. This laser hyperthermia effect has demonstrated wart clearance in verrucae on hands and plantar feet [76]. A randomised controlled trial of 150 patients with cutaneous warts comparing long-pulsed Nd:YAG laser (10 ms pulse duration, 160–360 J/cm^2, 2 mm spot size, or 45 ms pulse duration, 60–100 J/cm^2, 6 mm spot size, maximum four sessions at 3–4-week intervals) to cryotherapy demonstrated similar cure rates at 4-month (54.1% vs. 46.7%) and 6-month (59.5% vs. 57.3%) follow-up, respectively [77]. However, the study also indicated that long-pulsed Nd:YAG laser treatment may be more effective at treating relatively recalcitrant warts, leading to faster wart clearance, with milder adverse effects.

Hidradenitis Suppurativa

As hidradenitis suppurative (HS) is a chronic follicular occlusive disease, long-pulsed 1064 nm Nd:YAG laser is well placed as a hair epilation device to target the primary follicular pathogenesis of this disorder. It is safely used for hair removal, as it avoids burning the skin, especially for darker skin types. The long-pulsed 1064 nm Nd:YAG laser was shown to be effective in a randomised trial of 22 patients with stage II–III HS disease in reducing the severity of the inguinal, axillary and inframammary regions after a series of 3 monthly laser sessions [78]. Histologic examination of HS lesions after 2 monthly laser sessions showed that the mechanism of action of the long-pulsed Nd:YAG laser involved selective photothermolysis of the follicular unit and destruction of inflammatory lesions in the superficial to mid-dermis [79]. A multicentre, prospective, randomised intra-individual comparative trial of 36 patients also showed that the long-pulsed Nd:YAG laser hair removal (20 ms pulse duration, 45 J/cm^2 for skin types I–III and 35 ms pulse duration, 30 J/cm^2 for skin types IV–VI, 10–15 mm spot size, four sessions at 6-week intervals) was effective for reducing the number of HS inflammatory lesions at 1 month although the efficacy declined with time [80].

Q-Switched (QS) Nd:YAG

Xanthelasma

Xanthelasma palpebrarum is the most common cutaneous xanthoma arising on the eyelids, which may be associated with underlying hyperlipidaemia. While benign, these lesions can be disfiguring, prompting patients to seek treatment. Selective photothermolysis of lipid-rich tissue in vitro is feasible using 1064 nm laser light [81]. Fusade first showed the treatment of xanthelasma by 1064 nm Q-switched Nd:YAG laser in a prospective study of 11 patients with 38 xanthelasma where good or excellent results were achieved after a single treatment session for 26 of 38 lesions in eight patients with good rapid healing [82]. However, a larger study of 37 patients with 76 lesions who received two treatments with Q-switched Nd:YAG laser (6 J/cm^2 [1064 nm] or 2 J/cm^2 [532 nm], 4 mm spot size, 2–3 passes) failed to demonstrate similar results with majority of treated lesions showing no clearance [83]. A more recent retrospective study with 46 Asian patients with 103 lesions revealed that 93.2% of lesions treated with Q-switched Nd:YAG laser (7–10 J/cm^2 with increments of 0.5 J/cm^2 fluence at each subsequent treatment, 5 ns pulse width, 3–4 mm spot size, stacked pulses, 4–8-week intervals) had certain extent of clearance with all lesions achieving excellent-to-complete clearance after at least four treatment sessions [84]. Advantages of Q-switched Nd:YAG laser include avoidance of major scarring, atrophy or dyspigmentation, but it has been shown that with more passes or higher energy dose, higher risk of pigmentary changes and potential scarring could occur [85]. On the other hand, ultrapulse CO_2 ablative laser under local anaesthesia may also be used to treat xanthelasma palpebrarum with side effects of post-inflammatory hyperpigmentation, minimal scarring and about 20% recurrence rate [86]. A small retrospective study found that continuous CO_2 laser (five patients, continuous mode 3–5 W) was more efficacious than Q-switched Nd:YAG laser (12 patients) in the treatment of xanthelasma palpebrarum as it targets tissue water, allowing better haemostasis and thus being suitable for deep lesions [87]. However, erythema, hypopigmentation and hypertrophic scarring occurred in two patients in the CO_2 laser group compared to three patients with hypopigmentation and one with hyperpigmentation in the Nd:YAG laser group. Overall, Q-switched Nd:YAG laser offers a promising option, particularly for flat, superficial lesions, with its specific photoacoustic effect, yielding minimal thermal damage, better cosmetic outcomes and similar recurrence rate.

Conclusion

Lasers are gradually making inroads in medical dermatology, being used as effective monotherapy or serving as useful adjuncts to boost the efficacy of existing medical therapies (Table 11.1). In some dermatological conditions where previously only surgical options were recommended (e.g. SCCIS, BCCs), lasers now offer the dermatologist additional armamentarium where their clinical efficacy has been proven and where complications are fewer compared to surgery. It is appreciated that in some conditions, rather variable outcomes have been reported, making it difficult to advocate lasers as the primary modality of treatment. This variability in treatment responses could well be due to different laser treatment protocols such as laser parameters, technique and treatment schedules. When these variables are clarified by future studies, lasers will undoubtedly gain further prominence in the management of medical dermatological conditions.

Table 11.1 Lasers for medical dermatology indications

Medical dermatology indications	CO_2	Er:YAG	Fractional CO2	Fractional laser-assisted PDT	PDL	Fractional laser-assisted steroid delivery	LP Nd:YAG	QS Nd:YAG
Actinic keratosis	✓	✓	✓	✓				
Squamous cell carcinoma in-situ	✓	✓		✓				
Basal cell carcinoma					✓			
Hailey-Hailey disease	✓	✓	✓					
Porokeratosis	✓ +PDT	✓						
Cutaneous HPV warts	✓				✓		✓	
Onychomycosis							✓	
Rhinophyma	✓							
Hidradenitis suppurativa							✓	
Keloids and hypertrophic scars	✓				✓	✓		
Xanthelasma	✓							✓

References

1. Hantash BM, Stewart DB, Cooper ZA, et al. Facial resurfacing for nonmelanoma skin cancer prophylaxis. Arch Dermatol. 2006;142(8):976–82.
2. Scola N, Terras S, Georgas D, Othlinghaus N, Matip R, Pantelaki I, et al. A randomized, half-side comparative study of aminolaevulinate photodynamic therapy vs. CO_2 laser ablation in immunocompetent patients with multiple actinic keratoses. Br J Dermatol. 2012;167(6):1366–73.
3. Wollina U, Konrad H, Karamfilov T. Treatment of common warts and actinic keratoses by Er:YAG laser. J Cutan Laser Ther. 2001;3(2):63–6.
4. Ostertag JU, Quaedvlieg PJ, van der Geer S, et al. A clinical comparison and long-term follow-up of topical 5-fluorouracil versus laser resurfacing in the treatment of widespread actinic keratoses. Lasers Surg Med. 2006;38(8):731–9.
5. Covadonga Martínez-González M, del Pozo J, Paradela S, Fernández-Jorge B, Fernández-Torres R, Fonseca E. Bowen's disease treated by carbon dioxide laser. A series of 44 patients. J Dermatolog Treat. 2008;19(5):293–9.
6. Soleymani T, Abrouk M, Kelly KM. An analysis of laser therapy for the treatment of nonmelanoma skin cancer. Dermatol Surg. 2017;43(5):615–24.
7. Gordon KB, Garden JM, Robinson JK. Bowen's disease of the distal digit. Outcome of treatment with carbon dioxide laser vaporization. Dermatol Surg. 1996;22(8):723–8.
8. Tantikun N. Treatment of Bowen's disease of the digit with carbon dioxide laser. J Am Acad Dermatol. 2000;43(6):1080–3.
9. Vaïsse V, Clerici T, Fusade T. Bowen disease treated with scanned pulsed high energy CO2 laser. Follow-up of 6 cases. Ann Dermatol Venereol. 2001;128(11):1220–4.
10. Humphreys TR, Malhotra R, Scharf MJ, Marcus SM, Starkus L, Calegari K. Treatment of superficial basal cell carcinoma and squamous cell carcinoma in situ with a high-energy pulsed carbon dioxide laser. Arch Dermatol. 1998;134(10):1247–52.
11. Dave R, Monk B, Mahaffey P. Treatment of Bowen's disease with carbon dioxide laser. Lasers Surg Med. 2003;32(5):335.
12. Iranmanesh B, Khalili M, Zartab H, Amiri R, Aflatoonian M. Laser therapy in cutaneous and genital warts: a review article. Dermatol Ther. 2021;34(1):e14671.
13. Street ML, Roenigk RK. Recalcitrant periungual verrucae: the role of carbon dioxide laser vaporization. J Am Acad Dermatol. 1990;23(1):115–20.
14. Sloan K, Haberman H, Lynde CW. Carbon dioxide laser-treatment of resistant verrucae vulgaris: retrospective analysis. J Cutan Med Surg. 1998;2(3):142–5.
15. Logan RA, Zachary CB. Outcome of carbon dioxide laser therapy for persistent cutaneous viral warts. Br J Dermatol. 1989;121(1):99–105.
16. Krupa Shankar D, Chakravarthi M, Shilpakar R. Carbon dioxide laser guidelines. J Cutan Aesthet Surg. 2009;2(2):72–80.
17. Madan V, Ferguson JE, August PJ. Carbon dioxide laser treatment of rhinophyma: a review of 124 patients. Br J Dermatol. 2009;161(4):814–8.
18. Lim SW, Lim SW, Bekhor P. Rhinophyma: carbon dioxide laser with computerized scanner is still an outstanding treatment. Australas J Dermatol. 2009;50:289–93.
19. Wheeland RG. Clinical uses of lasers in dermatology. Lasers Surg Med. 1995;16:2–23.
20. Ang CC, Tay YK, Kwok C. Retrospective analysis of earlobe keloids treated with the carbon dioxide laser ablation or cold steel debulking surgery. J Cosmet Laser Ther. 2013;15(5):271–3.
21. Garg GA, Sao PP, Khopkar US. Effect of carbon dioxide laser ablation followed by intralesional steroids on keloids. J Cutan Aesthet Surg. 2011;4(1):2–6.
22. García-Zamora E, López-Estebaranz JL, Dradi GG, Álvarez-Fernández JG. Carbon dioxide laser treatment in Hailey-Hailey disease. Dermatol Surg. 2022;48(1):146–8.
23. Falto-Aizpurua LA, Griffith RD, Yazdani Abyaneh MA, Nouri K. Laser therapy for the treatment of Hailey-Hailey disease: a systematic review with focus on carbon dioxide laser resurfacing. J Eur Acad Dermatol Venereol. 2015;29(6):1045–52.
24. Salas-Marquez C, Boixeda de Miguel JP, Del Boz González J. Laser therapy for Hailey-Hailey disease: a series of 7 cases. Actas Dermosifiliogr. 2022;113(2):207–9.
25. Kruppa A, Korge B, Lasch J, Scharffetter-Kochanek K, Hunzelmann N. Successful treatment of Hailey-Hailey disease with a scanned carbon dioxide laser. Acta Derm Venereol. 2000;80:53–4.
26. Ortiz AE, Zachary CB. Laser therapy for Hailey-Hailey disease: review of the literature and a case report. Dermatol Rep. 2011;193(2):e28.
27. Don PC, Carney PS, Lynch WS, et al. Carbon dioxide laser ablation: a new approach to management of familial benign chronic pemphigus (Hailey-Hailey disease). J Dermatol Surg Oncol. 1987;13:1187–94.
28. Kartamaa M, Reitamo S. Familial benign chronic pemphigus (Hailey-Hailey disease). Treatment with carbon dioxide laser vaporization. Arch Dermatol. 1992;128:646–8.
29. Beier C, Kaufmann R. Efficacy of erbium:YAG laser ablation in Darier disease and Hailey-Hailey disease. Arch Dermatol. 1999;135(4):423–7.
30. Konrad H, Karamfilov T, Wollina U. Intracutaneous botulinum toxin A versus ablative therapy of Hailey-Hailey disease—a case report. J Cosmet Laser Ther. 2001;3:181–4.
31. Aird GA, Sitenga JL, Nguyen AH, Vaudreuil A, Huerter CJ. Light and laser treatment modalities for disseminated superficial actinic porokeratosis: a systematic review. Lasers Med Sci. 2017;32(4):945–52.

32. Barnett JH. Linear porokeratosis: treatment with the carbon dioxide laser. J Am Acad Dermatol. 1986;14(5 Pt 2):902–4.
33. Rabbin PE, Baldwin HE. Treatment of porokeratosis of Mibelli with CO2 laser vaporization versus surgical excision with split-thickness skin graft. A comparison. J Dermatol Surg Oncol. 1993;19(3):199–202.
34. McCullough TL, Lesher JL Jr. Porokeratosis of Mibelli: rapid recurrence of a large lesion after carbon dioxide laser treatment. Pediatr Dermatol. 1994;11(3):267–70.
35. Rosenblum J, Roenigk HH Jr. Erbium laser for the treatment of disseminated superficial actinic porokeratosis: a case report. Dermatol Surg. 2013;39(10):1543–5.
36. Aşkın Ö, Özkoca D, Uzunçakmak TK, Kutlubay Z. Verrucous porokeratosis treated with 2940 nm erbium:YAG laser. Dermatol Ther. 2022;35(4):e15342.
37. Kim HS, Baek JH, Park YM, Kim HO, Lee JY. Photodynamic therapy combined with CO_2 laser vaporization on disseminated superficial actinic porokeratosis: a report of 2 cases on the face. Ann Dermatol. 2011;23(Suppl 2):S211–3.
38. Togsverd-Bo K, Haak CS, Thaysen-Petersen D, Wulf HC, Anderson RR, Hædersdal M. Intensified photodynamic therapy of actinic keratoses with fractional CO_2 laser: a randomized clinical trial. Br J Dermatol. 2012;166(6):1262–9.
39. Helsing P, Togsverd-Bo K, Veierød MB, Mørk G, Haedersdal M. Intensified fractional CO_2 laser-assisted photodynamic therapy vs. laser alone for organ transplant recipients with multiple actinic keratoses and wart-like lesions: a randomized half-side comparative trial on dorsal hands. Br J Dermatol. 2013;169(5):1087–92.
40. Ko DY, Kim KH, Song KH. A randomized trial comparing methyl aminolaevulinate photodynamic therapy with and without Er:YAG ablative fractional laser treatment in Asian patients with lower extremity Bowen disease: results from a 12-month follow-up. Br J Dermatol. 2014;170(1):165–72.
41. Leszczynski R, da Silva CA, Pinto ACPN, Kuczynski U, da Silva EM. Laser therapy for treating hypertrophic and keloid scars. Cochrane Database Syst Rev. 2022;9(9):CD011642.
42. van Drooge AM, Vrijman C, van der Veen W, Wolkerstorfer A. A randomized controlled pilot study on ablative fractional CO_2 laser for consecutive patients presenting with various scar types. Dermatol Surg. 2015;41(3):371–7.
43. Azzam OA, Bassiouny DA, El-Hawary MS, El Maadawi ZM, Sobhi RM, El-Mesidy MS. Treatment of hypertrophic scars and keloids by fractional carbon dioxide laser: a clinical, histological, and immunohistochemical study. Lasers Med Sci. 2016;31(1):9–18.
44. Limmer EE, Glass DA 2nd. A review of current keloid management: mainstay monotherapies and emerging approaches. Dermatol Ther (Heidelb). 2020;10(5):931–48.
45. Kraeva E, Ho D, Jagdeo J. Successful treatment of keloid with fractionated carbon dioxide (CO_2) laser and laser-assisted drug delivery of triamcinolone acetonide ointment in an African-American man. J Drugs Dermatol. 2017;16(9):925–7.
46. Alexander S, Girisha BS, Sripathi H, Noronha TM, Alva AC. Efficacy of fractional CO_2 laser with intralesional steroid compared with intralesional steroid alone in the treatment of keloids and hypertrophic scars. J Cosmet Dermatol. 2019;18(6):1648–56.
47. El-Hamid El-Azhary EA, Abd Al-Salam FM, El-Hafiz HSA, Maghraby HM. Fractional carbon dioxide (CO_2) laser alone versus fractional CO_2 laser combined with triamcinolone acetonide or trichloroacetic acid in keloid treatment: a comparative clinical and radiological study. Dermatol Pract Concept. 2022;12(2):e2022072.
48. Pikkula BM, Chang DW, Nelson JS, Anvari B. Comparison of 585 and 595 nm laser-induced vascular response of normal in vivo human skin. Lasers Surg Med. 2005;36:117–23.
49. Karsai S, Friedl H, Buhck H, Jünger M, Podda M. The role of the 595-nm pulsed dye laser in treating superficial basal cell carcinoma: outcome of a double-blind randomized placebo-controlled trial. Br J Dermatol. 2015;172(3):677–83.
50. Minars M, Blyumin-Karasik M. Treatment of basal cell carcinomas with pulsed dye laser: a case series. J Skin Cancer. 2012;2023:286480.
51. Jalian HR, Avram MM, Stankiewicz KJ, Shofner JD, Tannous Z. Combined 585 nm pulsed-dye and 1,064 nm Nd:YAG lasers for the treatment of basal cell carcinoma. Lasers Surg Med. 2014;46(1):1–7.
52. Sparreboom EE, Luijks HG, Luiting-Welkenhuyzen HA, Willems PW, Groeneveld CP, Bovenschen HJ. Pulsed-dye laser treatment for recalcitrant viral warts: a retrospective case series of 227 patients. Br J Dermatol. 2014;171(5):1270–3.
53. Robson KJ, Cunningham NM, Kruzan KL, Patel DS, Kreiter CD, O'Donnell MJ, Arpey CJ. Pulsed-dye laser versus conventional therapy in the treatment of warts: a prospective randomized trial. J Am Acad Dermatol. 2000;43(2 Pt 1):275–80.
54. El-Mohamady A-S, Mearag I, El-Khalawany M, Elshahed A, Shokeir H, Mahmoud A. Pulsed dye laser versus Nd:YAG laser in the treatment of plantar warts: a comparative study. Lasers Med Sci. 2014;29(3):1111–6.
55. Kuo YR, Jeng SF, Wang FS, Chen TH, Huang HC, Chang PR, Yang KD. Flashlamp pulsed dye laser (PDL) suppression of keloid proliferation through down-regulation of TGF-beta1 expression and extracellular matrix expression. Lasers Surg Med. 2004;34(2):104–8.
56. Vrijman C, van Drooge AM, Limpens J, Bos JD, van der Veen JP, Spuls PI, Wolkerstorfer A. Laser and intense pulsed light therapy for the treatment of hypertrophic scars: a systematic review. Br J Dermatol. 2011;165(5):934–42.

57. Voraphol V, Patel SS, Nouri K. Lasers for scars. In: Nouri K, editor. Lasers in dermatology and medicine. Cham: Springer; 2018. p. 63–71.
58. Eke U, Diaz C, Abdullah A. Keloid scars in type VI skin successfully treated with combined surgery and pulsed dye laser therapy. Br J Dermatol. 2013;168(6):1360–2.
59. Yang Q, Ma Y, Zhu R, et al. The effect of flashlamp pulsed dye laser on the expression of connective tissue growth factor in keloids. Lasers Surg Med. 2012;44(5):377–83.
60. Cannarozzo G, Sannino M, Tamburi F, Morini C, Nistico SP. Flash-lamp pulsed-dye laser treatment of keloids: results of an observational study. Photomed Laser Surg. 2015;33(5):274–7.
61. Zhong S, Lin GT, Zhao JY. Efficacy of two-stage treatment of onychomycosis using a long-pulsed Nd:YAG 1064-nm laser. Evid Based Complement Alternat Med. 2019;16:3647519.
62. Piccolo D, Kostaki D, Del Duca E, Cannarozzo G, Sannino M, Nisticò S. Long-pulsed 1064-nm Nd:YAG laser for the treatment of onychomycosis. Photomed Laser Surg. 2017;35(4):213–6.
63. Okan G, Tarikci N, Gokdemir G. The effect of long-pulsed Nd:YAG laser for the treatment of onychomycosis. J Am Podiatr Med Assoc. 2017;107(1):54–9.
64. Waibel J, Wulkan AJ, Rudnick A. Prospective efficacy and safety evaluation of laser treatments with real-time temperature feedback for fungal onychomycosis. J Drugs Dermatol. 2013;12(11):1237.
65. Moon SH, Hur H, Oh YJ, Choi KH, Kim JE, Ko JY, Ro YS. Treatment of onychomycosis with a 1,064-nm long-pulsed Nd:YAG laser. J Cosmet Laser Ther. 2014;16(4):165–70.
66. Kim MS, Jung JY, Cho EB, Park EJ, Kim KH, Kim KJ. The effectiveness of 1,064-nm long-pulsed Nd:YAG laser in the treatment of severe onychomycosis. J Cosmet Laser Ther. 2016;18(6):317–22.
67. Li Y, Xu J, Zhao JY, Zhuo FL. Self-controlled study of onychomycosis treated with long-pulsed Nd:YAG 1064-nm laser combined with itraconazole. Chin Med J. 2016;129(16):1929–34.
68. Hamed Khater M, Khattab FM. Combined long-pulsed Nd-Yag laser and itraconazole versus itraconazole alone in the treatment of onychomycosis nails. J Dermatolog Treat. 2020;31(4):406–9.
69. Cao Y, Xu S, Kong W, Xu Y, Fang H. Clinical retrospective analysis of long-pulsed 1064-nm Nd:YAG laser in the treatment of onychomycosis and its effect on the ultrastructure of fungus pathogen. Lasers Med Sci. 2020;35(2):429–37.
70. Ortiz AE, Avram MM, Wanner MA. A review of lasers and light for the treatment of onychomycosis. Lasers Surg Med. 2014;46:117–24.
71. Liu C, Zhang L, Zeng HY, Bei H, Chen SP, Wu YX, Luo WX, Fang Q, Liu PM. The energy density and treatment times are the main factors that affect the efficacy of long-pulsed 1,064-nm Nd:YAG laser treatment for onychomycosis caused by Trichophyton rubrum. Dermatology. 2018;234(3–4):105–11.
72. Hollmig ST, Rahman Z, Henderson MT, Rotatori RM, Gladstone H, Tang JY. Lack of efficacy with 1064-nm neodymium:yttrium-aluminum-garnet laser for the treatment of onychomycosis: a randomized, controlled trial. J Am Acad Dermatol. 2014;70(5):911–7.
73. Karsai S, Jäger M, Oesterhelt A, Weiss C, Schneider SW, Jünger M, Raulin C. Treating onychomycosis with the short-pulsed 1064-nm-Nd:YAG laser: results of a prospective randomized controlled trial. J Eur Acad Dermatol Venereol. 2017;31(1):175–80.
74. Xu Y, Miao X, Zhou B, Luo D. Combined oral terbinafine and long-pulsed 1,064-nm Nd: YAG laser treatment is more effective for onychomycosis than either treatment alone. Dermatol Surg. 2014;40(11):1201–7.
75. Bunyaratavej S, Wanitphakdeedecha R, Ungaksornpairote C, Kobwanthanakun W, Chanyachailert P, Nokdhes YN, et al. Randomized controlled trial comparing long-pulsed 1064-nm neodymium: yttrium-aluminum-garnet laser alone, topical amorolfine nail lacquer alone, and a combination for nondermatophyte onychomycosis treatment. J Cosmet Dermatol. 2020;19(9):2333–8.
76. Pfau A, Abd-el-Raheem TA, Bäumler W, Hohenleutner U, Landthaler M. Nd:YAG laser hyperthermia in the treatment of recalcitrant verrucae vulgares (Regensburg's technique). Acta Derm Venereol. 1994;74(3):212–4.
77. Liu JJ, Li HT, Ren YY, Yang F, Cheng ZH, Xia TB, Liu JL, Cao XJ, Lu SC. Long-pulsed neodymium-doped yttrium-aluminum-garnet laser versus cryotherapy for the treatment of cutaneous warts: a randomized controlled trial. J Am Acad Dermatol. 2022;87(6):1328–35.
78. Tierney E, Mahmoud BH, Hexsel C, Ozog D, Hamzavi I. Randomized control trial for the treatment of hidradenitis suppurativa with a neodymium-doped yttrium aluminium garnet laser. Dermatol Surg. 2009;35(8):1188–98.
79. Xu LY, Wright DR, Mahmoud BH, Ozog DM, Mehregan DA, Hamzavi IH. Histopathologic study of hidradenitis suppurativa following long-pulsed 1064-nm Nd:YAG laser treatment. Arch Dermatol. 2011;147(1):21–8.
80. Naouri M, Maruani A, Lagrange S, Cogrel O, Servy A, Collet Vilette AM, et al. Treatment of hidradenitis suppurativa using a long-pulsed hair removal neodymium:yttrium-aluminium-garnet laser: a multicenter, prospective, randomized, intraindividual, comparative trial. J Am Acad Dermatol. 2021;84(1):203–5.
81. Anderson RR, Farinelli W, Laubach H, Manstein D, Yaroslavsky AN, Gubeli J 3rd, et al. Selective photothermolysis of lipid-rich tissues: a free electron laser study. Lasers Surg Med. 2006;38:913–9.
82. Fusade T. Treatment of xanthelasma palpebrarum by 1064-nm Q-switched Nd:YAG laser: a study of 11 cases. Br J Dermatol. 2008;158(1):84–7.
83. Karsai S, Schmitt L, Raulin C. Is Q-switched neodymium-doped yttrium aluminium garnet laser an effective approach to treat xanthelasma palpebrarum?

Results from a clinical study of 76 cases. Dermatol Surg. 2009;35:1962–9.
84. Heng JK, Chua SH, Goh CL, Cheng S, Tan V, Tan WP. Treatment of xanthelasma palpebrarum with a 1064-nm, Q-switched Nd:YAG laser. J Am Acad Dermatol. 2017;77(4):728–34.
85. Kaliyadan F, Dharmaratnam A. Q-switched Nd: YAG in the treatment of xanthelasma palpebrarum. J Cutan Aesthet Surg. 2010;3(2):127–8.
86. Pathania V, Chatterjee M. Ultrapulse carbon dioxide laser ablation of xanthelasma palpebrarum: a case series. J Cutan Aesthet Surg. 2015;8(1):46–9.
87. Konstantinou MP, Evangelou G, Hegazy S, Krasagakis K, Bulai-Livideanu C. Comparison of the efficacy and safety of continuous CO_2 laser and 1064 nm Q-switched Nd:YAG laser for the treatment of xanthelasma palpebrarum. Int J Dermatol. 2023;62(3):e120–2.

Intense Pulsed Light for Skin Rejuvenation

12

Nicole Marella G. Tan and Nancy Garcia-Tan

Introduction and Basic Physiology

Developed in the early 1990s by Dr. Mitchel Goldman, Dr. Richard Fitzpatrick, and Dr. Shimon Eckhouse, intense pulsed light (IPL) was initially used to treat telangiectasia of the lower extremities. Following Dr. Patrick Bitter's study on serial, full-face treatments with IPL in 2000, the method steadily gained popularity for nonablative photorejuvenation.

IPL is fundamentally different from lasers in that it uses polychromatic, noncollimated, incoherent light. Flashlamps produce short bursts of high-intensity broadband light with variable durations and fluences, and wavelengths ranging from 500 to 1400 nm. Emitted light can be absorbed by multiple chromophores in a single exposure, namely, melanin, oxyhemoglobin, deoxyhemoglobin, methemoglobin, and water. This polychromatic nature grants the system its versatility, presenting a wide range of therapeutic opportunities. Harnessing this versatility demands a more intensive learning period to ensure patient safety while delivering optimal results.

N. M. G. Tan (✉) · N. Garcia-Tan
MedDERM Asia Laser & Surgicentre, Manila, Philippines

Department of Internal Medicine, Section of Dermatology, Cardinal Santos Medical Center, Manila, Philippines
e-mail: ngtan1@alum.up.edu.ph

Device and Settings

Understanding the science behind the IPL devices is crucial to achieving therapeutic success. Similar to lasers, IPL utilizes the principle of selective photothermolysis, wherein specific wavelengths of light can selectively target chromophores while preserving surrounding tissue. Paying close attention to intended chromophore targets and energy-tissue interactions allows the provider to adjust parameters to optimize treatment (Table 12.1).

In addition to these parameters, treatment with IPL is directly influenced by the handpiece and cooling mechanisms. Most IPL handpieces deliver light through a large, flat, rectangular sapphire crystal, providing rapid coverage with fewer pulses, deeper penetration, and even distribution, expediting treatment. However, the large surface poses a challenge in treating areas with irregular curvature, such as around the nose. Newer models have spot adaptors to treat isolated areas. A simple, work-around method would be to use an opaque sheet with a manual cutout to decrease exposure from the device.

Cooling mechanisms permit the delivery of higher fluences while providing epidermal protection, significantly reducing discomfort and side effects. Most devices have continuous contact cooling integrated into the handpiece through circulation of chilled water around the IPL crystal, contributing to the weight of the handpiece.

S. W. N. Cheng, C. L. Goh (eds.), *Updates on Lasers in Dermatology*, Updates in Clinical Dermatology, https://doi.org/10.1007/978-3-031-71155-8_12

Table 12.1 Parameters of intense pulsed light

Parameter	Range of settings (device dependent)	Clinical correlation/unique to IPL
Wavelength	Polychromatic, noncollimated, incoherent light 400–1400 nm	Broadband light; able to treat multiple chromophores in a single exposure – 400–744 nm: melanin – 418 nm: oxyhemoglobin – 542 nm: deoxyhemoglobin – 577 nm: methemoglobin
Filters	Cutoff filters: block emission of wavelengths shorter than the set limit (e.g., 420, 515, 550, 560, 615, 645, 690, 695, 755, 800 nm)	Convenient "snap-on" or "slide-in" filters may be employed to block out undesired wavelengths and tailor IPL treatment for different skin types and indications
	Absorption filter (available on certain devices): absorbs given wavelengths, but allows emission of flanking wavelengths)	Suggested filter by skin type [1]: – FST I–III: 560 nm – FST IV–VI: 590 nm or longer Suggested filter by indication [2]: – Epidermal pigmentation/telangiectasia: 560 nm – Dermal lesions, enlarged pores, photoaged/wrinkled skin: 640 nm
Pulse duration	0.2–100 ms	Choice of pulse duration is determined by the size of the target chromophore and, consequently, its thermal relaxation time For example, thermal relaxation time of: – Melanosomes: 200–400 ns – Blood vessels: 4–10 ms
Multi-sequential pulsing	Single pulse Double pulse Triple pulse	Delivers the same total energy in successive smaller portions → provides more epidermal protection, permits successive heating of large vessels with adequate cooling of the epidermis [3]
Pulse delay	0–50 ms	In darker/tanned skin, longer pulse delay provides more epidermal protection Suggested pulse delay: – FST I–III: 10–12 ms – FST IV–VI: 20–40 ms [3]
Fluence	Up to 40 J/cm^2	Higher fluences may be used if the chromophore is located deep within the skin or has a limited light absorption capacity, keeping in mind that side effects are more likely to occur at higher fluences

Other internal cooling mechanisms include pulsed cryogen sprays or glass chambers. External cooling methods include ice packs, forced-air cooling, or cold ultrasound gel applied right before pulsing. Cold gel plays an additional role in decreasing the refractive index between air and skin, permitting deeper penetration and increased absorption.

Unique to IPL is the phenomenon of spectral shift. Given a set fluence, lengthening of the pulse duration causes a change in relative distribution of energy and decrease in power. The relative energy density emitted along the longer wavelength increases, while there is a relative decrease at the shorter wavelengths, as compared to the same fluence at a shorter pulse duration. Clinically, spectral shift enhances the effectiveness of IPL in treating deeper, darker lesions and larger blood vessels that respond well to longer wavelengths.

While self-evident to those with foundational knowledge on energy-based devices, fair warning must be given that not all IPL devices are created equally. Innumerable devices available in the market span a diverse price spectrum, indicative of disparities in quality, reliability, and safety. Settings for different IPL devices can greatly differ between brands and are not interchangeable.

Hence, it is difficult, if not frankly dangerous, to compare and copy treatment parameters across different devices. It is important to base your device settings according to the manufacturer's recommendations and adjust accordingly. Even when using the same device, it is advisable to use more conservative settings following recalibration.

Patient Considerations

Specific to photorejuvenation, candidates for IPL are those seeking treatment for concerns like diffuse redness, flushing, facial telangiectasia, solar lentigines, ephelides, irregular pigmentation, and fine wrinkling. When securing the patient's consent, pre-procedure discussions should include counseling on realistic expectations. Photorejuvenation with IPL is best observed after a series of treatments, developing gradual improvement with minimal to no downtime. Setting a patient's expectations to completion of at least three to five sessions at 3–4-week intervals is more realistic and provides leeway for more conservative settings in the first session. In doing so, the two most common IPL complications are reduced, namely, superficial burns and lack of results. It is now well observed that the more treatments a patient receives, the clearer, smoother, and healthier-appearing the skin was with progressive treatments. Patients looking for immediate, drastic improvements may be better suited to treatment with alternative options. It is strongly recommended that pre-procedure photos be taken regularly for monitoring improvement.

Patients with darker Fitzpatrick skin types (FSTs) V and VI are generally not suitable for IPL treatment. Those with naturally or artificially tanned skin have increased risk of adverse events with IPL and may be advised to postpone the procedure until they are no longer tanned. Tanning may be assessed by comparing the prospective treatment area to the inner forearm or inner upper arm as a baseline for untanned skin.

Patients will be provided with opaque eye protection, though they should be counseled that bright flashes of light may still be perceived due to the intensity of the flashlamp. Patients with photophobia or photosensitive epilepsy or those on photosensitizing medications may not be good candidates for the procedure. Patients who are pregnant or breastfeeding may be advised to postpone the treatment. Patients prone to recurrent herpes labialis may be treated with prophylactic antivirals (oral acyclovir, valacyclovir, or famciclovir) a day before treatment and continued for 2 weeks afterward [4].

Previously reserved for patients with fairer skin, IPL has proven to be equally effective, useful, and versatile in treating skin of color. For darker skin types, higher cutoff filters, such as 590 nm, are used for more epidermal protection. Complications can be greatly avoided with proper adjustment of treatment parameters—specifically, longer wavelengths, lower fluences, longer pulse durations, decreased repetition rate, prolonged delay between pulses, and adequate skin cooling throughout the entire procedure.

IPL for Photorejuvenation

At present, IPL is used for both corrective and adjunctive purposes. Corrective conditions include (1) noninvasive photorejuvenation, (2) treatment of vascular conditions, (3) acne, (4) scars, (5) hair reduction, (6) delay of skin aging, (7) fine wrinkle reduction, and (8) skin tightening. Adjunctive benefits include (1) early treatment of postsurgical scars, (2) post-procedure purpura, (3) post-laser erythema, and (4) post-inflammatory hyperpigmentation [5]. This chapter focuses primarily on IPL as a prominent modality in photorejuvenation, with brief explanations on its mechanisms of action for various target chromophores.

Skin aging, a sum total of intrinsic factors and photodamage, is characterized by wrinkles, pigmentary alterations, telangiectasias, skin thinning, and laxity. The polychromatic nature of IPL gives it its ability to treat these signs simultaneously. Acting on both pigmentary and vascular targets, irregular pigmentation and telangiectasia can be treated in a single session. While evident improvement occurs in areas with discrete lesions, patients also often remark that baseline skin tone and texture improve in comparison to pretreated skin. Later research showed its ability to stimulate neocollagenesis with dermal bulk heating, leading to improvements in skin texture, pore size, and fine wrinkles. This combined overall improvement was termed "photorejuvenation." While multiple treatments are recommended to see improvement, minimal adverse effects and negligible downtime give IPL a key advantage compared to other modalities like the CO_2, Er:YAG, and PDL. Various techniques have been developed to maximize improvement for various skin types and indications.

Benign Pigmentary Lesions

Solar Lentigines, Ephelides, Seborrheic Keratoses

Q-switched and picosecond lasers in the nano- and picosecond range effectively target individual melanosomes, which have a thermal relaxation time (TRT) of ~200–400 ns. IPL, which works in the millisecond range, instead hits clustered melanosomes, which have longer TRTs than solitary cells. This induces denaturation of melanin cap-containing cells, triggering epidermolysis of the basement membrane and accelerated basal keratinocyte differentiation [6]. Upward transfer and elimination of necrotic keratinocytes and melanosomes can be seen clinically as microcrust formation. As these microcrusts naturally flake off, smoother, less pigmented skin is visible underneath (Fig. 12.1).

The efficacy of IPL for pigment removal is dependent upon melanin density and distribution in the epidermis. It has greatest efficacy in treating superficial lesions like solar lentigines and ephelides [7–9]. Darker discrete lesions typically have significant improvement within the first two sessions, followed by lessening of background discoloration and lighter lesions with higher fluences in succeeding sessions [7]. A systematic review done in 2014 reported nine studies that used IPL for the treatment of solar lentigines and ephelides, with all studies uniformly reporting excellent efficacy after three to five treatments [1]. A study comparing its efficacy with a quality-switched alexandrite laser (QSAL) showed them to be equally effective for treatment of solar lentigines; however, the post-inflammatory pigmentation following treatment with QSAL may lead to IPL being preferred for patients with darker skin types [10].

On normal skin, a diffuse, slightly pinkish erythema may be observed as the endpoint. For benign pigmented lesions, transient, subtle darkening of lentigines and freckling is the targeted endpoint. Patients should be advised that dryness and microcrusting may occur over pigmented lesions. Microcrusts typically last for about 5–10 days on the face, 7–14 days on the chest, and longer on the extremities. Superficial, thin seborrheic keratoses may also be adequately treated with IPL, but thicker lesions may be better treated with other modalities.

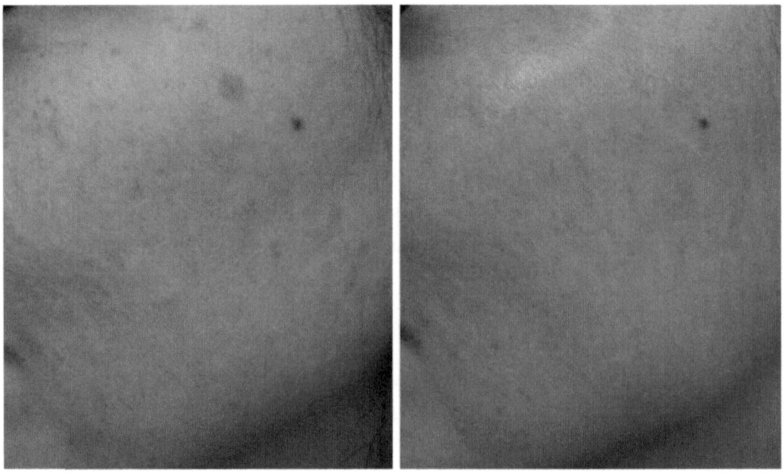

Fig. 12.1 34/F with improvement in ephelides, solar lentigines, and background melasma following three IPL treatments

Reflectance confocal microscopy studies suggest that while melanosomes are effectively extruded through microcrusts, active melanocytes are left behind [6]. Melanin-suppressive medications, such as hydroquinone, are recommended to be used in combination with IPL to maximize results.

Vascular Lesions

Facial Telangiectasia, Diffuse Erythema, Spider Angiomas, Small-Caliber Leg Veins

Pulsed dye lasers, the gold standard for vascular lesions, target hemoglobin to induce blood vessel damage, resulting in extensive purpura that may last up to 14 days. IPL is an alternative method of treatment of certain vascular conditions by photocoagulation of the vascular endothelium, leading to subsequent obliteration and fibrosis of blood vessels, significantly reducing side effects and downtime. Furthermore, IPL simultaneously acts on three vascular chromophores: oxyhemoglobin (predominant in reddish lesions) at 418 nm, deoxyhemoglobin (predominant in bluish lesions) at 542 nm, and methemoglobin at 577 nm.

Patients being treated for vascular lesions on the face may be positioned in a slight recline. Other practitioners also advocate the valsalva maneuver, armchair calisthenics, or gentle face heating with a blow-dryer to increase blood flow to the face [7]. Spot adaptors may be used to limit the spot size and isolate the pulse around the vessel. Pulse duration is set according to the vessel's diameter and should be shorter than the thermal relaxation time to avoid damage to surrounding tissues. Superficial blood vessels measuring 0.1–0.3 mm in diameter have TRTs of approximately 4–10 ms [11]. Efficacy of treatment depends heavily on blood vessel type and caliber; superficial blood vessels without feeding reticular veins, whether on the face or lower extremities, typically respond best to treatment. Telangiectasias near the nasal alae tend to be more recurrent [12].

Immediately after delivering a pulse, a transient color conversion from bright red to bluish-purple may be observed, signifying the conversion of oxyhemoglobin to deoxy- or methemoglobin. Some practitioners advocate performing a focal second pass with a slightly longer pulse duration, taking advantage of the spectral shift for better absorption by the converted chromophore [7]. Following the transient color change, the ideal endpoint is vasoconstriction with mild erythema and/or edema [12], leading to gradual control of redness (Fig. 12.2).While purpura may be achieved as an endpoint, most patients coming in

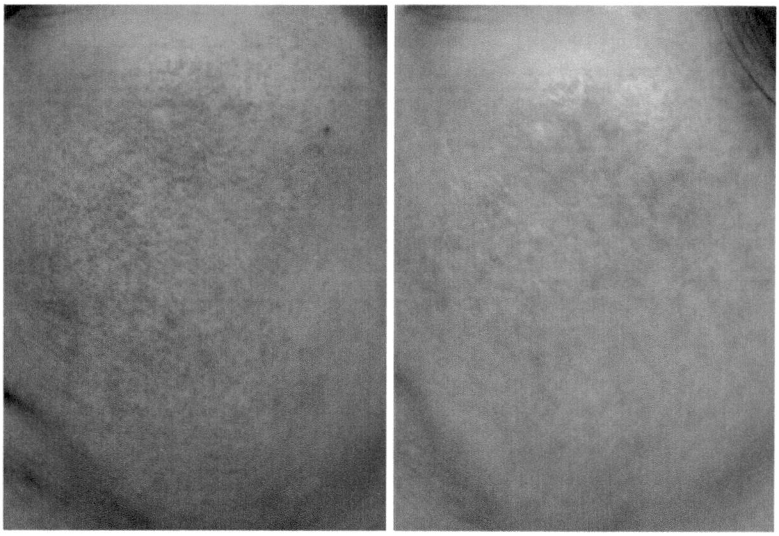

Fig. 12.2 40/F with stubborn facial redness, resistant to topical treatments. Diffuse facial erythema well controlled with quarterly IPL treatments

for aesthetic concerns would rather be treated to a sub-purpuric level.

In the largest study to date, 1000 patients (FST I–VI) with facial telangiectasia or other vascular marks were subjected to a mean of 2.16 IPL treatments. Majority of patients (89.70%) had a clearance of 75–100% [13].

Melasma

Epidermal, Dermal, Mixed Type

Melasma, a recognized photoaging disorder, presents with refractory hyperpigmentation and abnormal vascularization in genetically predisposed individuals. In comparison to laser modalities, IPL has the advantage of a broad wavelength spectrum that can simultaneously treat epidermal melasma, dermal melasma, as well as any vascular components that may be present. The millisecond duration causes greater diffusion of heat, reducing the risk of localized post-inflammatory hyperpigmentation. The large spot size allows for more homogenous treatment, reducing the risk of "polka-dot" treatment that can result from lasers with small round spot sizes [14].

On a molecular level, IPL has been found to attenuate tyrosinase activity and reduce the expression of melanogenic proteins, decreasing melanin production [15]. A study of 89 Chinese patients reported a decrease in melasma area and severity index (MASI) scores from 15.2 to 4.5, after undergoing four IPL treatments at 3-week intervals. On self-assessment, 70.8% of patients rated their improvement to be 50% or more. Subjects with epidermal melasma responded better than those with the mixed type [16].

A recent meta-analysis promotes short pulses of low fluence to achieve effective results without causing further darkening [17]. Combination treatments, such as with triple-combination cream (fluocinolone acetonide 0.01%, hydroquinone 4%, tretinoin 0.05%) or low-fluence Q-switched Nd:YAG or alexandrite lasers, deliver the best results [1, 17–20]. Treatments must be done at regular intervals to achieve control, owing to the recurrent nature of the condition.

Skin Texture, Pore Size, Fine Lines, and Skin Aging

Later discovered was IPL's ability to induce collagen synthesis in the long term. Studies suggest that cytokine inflammation and nonspecific dermal heating from the IPL exert a stimulatory effect on fibroblasts—treatment with low fluences induces fibroblast viability and pushes a significant percentage of fibroblasts into the synthesis stage of the cell cycle, as well as causes a fluence-dependent increase in the expression of procollagen (types I and III) [21]. Histopathologic analysis revealed that with repeated IPL treatments, both type 1 and type 3 collagen increased and appeared more organized. Elastic fibers decreased in content, but were more neatly arranged. Transelectron microscopy revealed increased fibroblast activity, with neater arrangement of collagen fibers within stroma [22]. Though less effective than ablative, water-targeted lasers, repeated treatment with IPL leads to clinical smoothening of overall skin texture, reduction in pore size, and mild skin tightening, especially evident around the periorbital and perioral areas [23].

While there is yet to be an established protocol, some clinicians believe that the use of a 570–690 nm cutoff filter better concentrates the fluence to deeper dermal structures, to better induce new collagen formation. Others believe that using wavelengths in the 900–1200 nm spectrum brings the IPL's target closer to that of water as in ablative lasers, triggering a cytokine reaction to stimulate neocollagenesis. Consensus among authors is that multiple treatment sessions are required for skin rejuvenation [24]. Severe rhytids or significant textural issues would best be addressed with combination treatments or more aggressive procedures.

Patients who have had repeated IPL sessions have been documented to have smoother, clearer, healthier-appearing skin than their chronological counterparts. Cumulative sessions can have a profound impact on skin health. Studies that explore its molecular effects have found that nearly 1300 genes relevant to cell division, tumor suppression, and cell and organism longevity were "functionally rejuvenated" following IPL

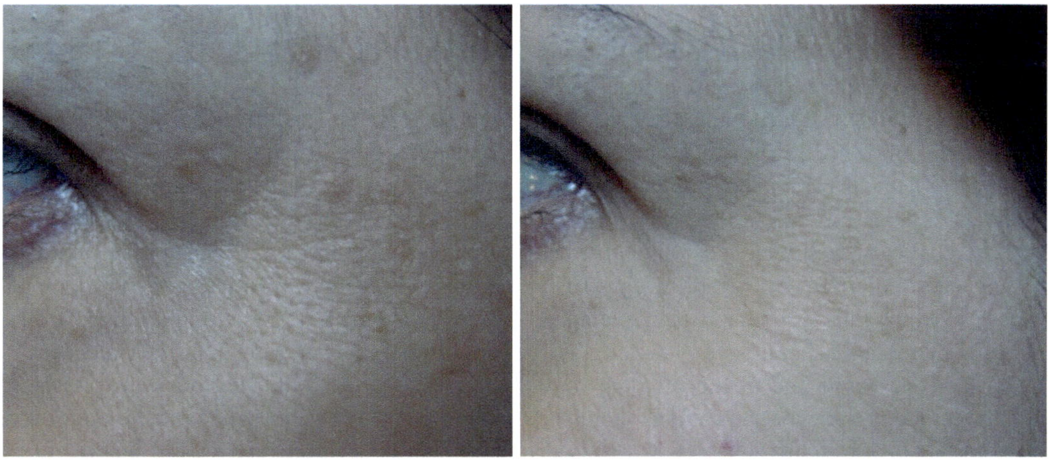

Fig. 12.3 61/F with visible improvement of fine lines and overall texture around the periorbital area following five IPL treatments

treatments, with a gene expression and immune profile resembling young skin [25]. Clinically, this was observed in a retrospective analysis of 2534 patients, with patients who received a minimum of three IPL treatments over a 12-year period for any of the following concerns: wrinkles, vascular skin concerns, pigmented skin concerns, and worsening skin texture. The total effective rate of IPL on reversing skin aging and photodamage was found to be between 88.24% and 96.45% [2]. While further studies are warranted, IPL treatments have been found to be capable of delaying, or even reversing, skin aging (Fig. 12.3).

Other Indications and Possible Future Directions of IPL

IPL is well known for treating vascular conditions such as rosacea and as an adjuvant treatment for stubborn hemangiomas and port-wine stains. Its improvement of the vascular, pigmented, and atrophic changes in poikiloderma of Civatte is well documented. Acne vulgaris and post-inflammatory erythema from acne likewise respond well to IPL treatment, which can be combined with photodynamic therapy. It is also commonly used as a hair reduction modality in patients with fairer skin. Most recently, it was FDA approved in 2021 as a treatment for dry eye disease due to meibomian gland dysfunction. Multiple small case series and anecdotal reports also exist on its use as treatment in other conditions, such as Becker nevus, actinic keratoses, porokeratosis, and hidradenitis suppurativa, among many others.

Following evidence of IPL's prowess in restoring gene expression of younger skin [25] and recognition of its ability to delaying skin aging in vivo, future directions may see benefits in skin cancer prevention. To date, there is early anecdotal evidence for reduced nonmelanoma skin cancer incidence in patients receiving regular pulsed light treatments. Many practitioners advocate for its use in the treatment of early postsurgical scars, possibly extending its effects to expedition of wound healing. Systemic rejuvenation is another possible future field, but the effects of IPL on the blood reached through the cutaneous vascular plexus have yet to be explored.

Treatment Protocol

Pretreatment

It is imperative that the clinician take a detailed history and perform a thorough physical exam, paying particular attention to genotypic and phenotypic ethnicity and density of target chromophore. Photorejuvenation with IPL may be done on any skin type and any anatomic area, provided that high vigilance is exercised and appropriate settings are used. Close attention to light-tissue interactions and keen clinical judgment are critical, and this allows the experienced practitioner to adjust treatment parameters optimally as the treatment progresses.

IPL is typically well tolerated without the use of any anesthesia. However, topical anesthesia may be used for patients with low pain tolerance, use of higher fluences, and longer wavelengths.

All persons within the treatment room must don proper protective eyewear. Patients should be provided with disposable adhesive eye pads or blackout goggles. Practitioners and assistants commonly wear goggles tinted with green or brown; however, these may hinder visibility. Newer flash sensor goggles darken only during a flash of light, allowing practitioners to appreciate transient graying or subtle erythema of the skin that would be very difficult to catch otherwise.

The treatment area should be properly cleansed to clear away any make-up or topical products which may interfere with light transmission. Patients undergoing the procedure for hair reduction should have the hair shaved before treatment.

After cleansing, cold gel is applied onto the treatment area as a thin and even layer. Cold gel cools the skin temperature, protecting the epidermis and reducing the patient's perceived pain, as well as enhances the optical transmission of light, delivering energy effectively into the target area. It plays a crucial role in optimizing treatment outcomes.

Performing a test spot was previously encouraged prior to proceeding with full treatment. However, as IPL often results in delayed tissue reactions, performing a test spot on the same day of treatment may lead to a false sense of security. Additionally, different anatomic areas may respond differently, especially as target density varies from location to location. Experienced clinicians, attuned to their devices and familiar with expected energy-tissue interactions, can often assess for potential complications after a few initial pulses in each area.

Procedure Proper and Device Settings

As seen in Table 12.1, treatment with IPL can be challenging due to the numerous parameters involved, making it a steep learning curve. Choice of filter depends primarily on the skin type and target/s, aiming for correct penetration depth and optimal absorption by the target chromophore. Patients should be advised that energy will be most absorbed by areas with the heaviest density of chromophores, clinically translating to more perceived heat or pain. Experienced practitioners adjust settings throughout treatment to achieve desired endpoints while ensuring patient safety and comfort. Typically, more exuberant erythema responses correlate to better clinical improvement [11]. However, care must be exercised as overly aggressive parameters may lead to adverse effects.

There is no prescribed sequence for treating specific areas, and order may vary depending on practitioner preference and patient's needs. Clinicians may prefer to treat the forehead first and work down, start from the chin and work up, or start from the cheeks and work around. Areas over bone, such as the forehead and bony prominence of the lower jaw, and areas with thinner skin such as the neck, may be more sensitive to higher fluences. Energy may be adjusted so that it is 1–2 J/cm^2 less than the rest of the face [2]. The forehead often has less chromophore density and is preferred by some clinicians as to assess initial energy-tissue interactions and patient's tolerance of pulses. However, caution should be exercised as a burn in this area would be very evident. Efficiency is a major consideration when treating multiple areas of the body; clinicians may choose an order that minimizes the time needed for setup and transitions between areas. Hair-bearing areas, such as the eyebrows, hairline, and beard area in men, should be avoided if hair reduction is not desired.

The number of passes performed is also dependent on the clinician's preference and technique. Some clinicians prefer a single pass with minimal overlap (10%) using higher energy, while others prefer multiple passes with lower energy, orienting the sapphire-crystal in different directions with each pass. The serial, full-face, two-step technique developed by Dr. Patrick Bitter is a combination of the two. The first step is to perform two passes over the entire face using conservative parameters, typically with fluences less than 10 J, to produce overall clearing of irregular pigmentation and smoother texture. This stimulates neocollagenesis, producing favorable gene expression changes in keratinocytes and dermal fibroblasts. Performing two passes at low fluences avoids the complications of uneven striping and superficial burns. The second step uses smaller spot sizes and higher fluences to target discrete lesions that would be unlikely to resolve at lower fluences—telangiectasias, areas of erythema, stubborn pigmented lesions, fine wrinkles, and scars. Typical full-face treatments garner about 240–400 pulses per session. When done correctly, this technique can lead to reproducible and better overall improvement. In addition, it greatly increases procedure safety and patient comfort. The same technique can be applied to any other anatomic location, most commonly, the neck, décolletage, and dorsal hands.

In delivering each pulse, it is imperative to keep the handpiece parallel to the skin surface. Excessive elevation or pressure may lead to nonuniform treatment or burns, as beam divergence changes effective fluence of the pulse. Keeping the cooled sapphire-crystal in close proximity to the skin provides adequate contact cooling to the epidermis. Other practitioners advocate additional external icing before, during, and after the procedure. Difficult-to-treat areas such as the alar groove may require additional cooling gel to ensure adequate contact or use of a spot adaptor.

The first treatment session generally begins with more conservative settings, while targets are at their most dense. Treatment intensity can be gradually increased with subsequent sessions as the target chromophores become more subtle and the patient develops more tolerance to the procedure. Similar to other energy-based procedures, the face can tolerate more aggressive settings than the neck and chest, while extremities require the gentlest settings. Fluences may be feathered from the lower face down to the clavicle for a more pleasing result. Recording pulse counts on each area of the face helps to build more consistent and reproducible results, especially for beginners, who may not realize that they are applying more pulses to the side of their handedness.

In all techniques, the most crucial component of successful treatment is a keen eye and constant vigilance. It is imperative that the clinician look and listen attentively to ensure that treatment is proceeding appropriately. Communication and live feedback from the patient will help to avoid most complications. If there is prolonged graying, intense erythema, imminent blistering or edema, or excessive pain at any point, the procedure should be stopped. Full treatment can proceed if the patient is tolerating the treatment well and the skin reacts as expected.

Posttreatment

Once the cooling gel is removed from the skin surface, application of a cooled moisturizer or anti-redness cream can provide immediate comfort. Patients should be counseled that skin may feel slightly drier after the procedure and to apply a simple moisturizer as needed. For milder treatments, patients can immediately walk out of the clinic with only very faint erythema as evidence of the procedure. Use of make-up can be permitted immediately after treatment. More aggressive treatments require immediate and liberal posttreatment chilling. Some practitioners advise a minimum of 10–15 min every waking hour for the first 24–48 h to decrease discomfort, redness, edema, and risk of PIH.

Patients treated for pigmented lesions should be advised that a fine, superficial microcrust may form over the next few days, which will slough off naturally in less than a week. Simple moisturizers may be applied. Those treated for vascular conditions should be counseled to avoid strenuous activities for 3 days after the procedure to minimize recanalization of coagulated vessels. Patients should be advised to avoid direct sun exposure.

Complications

In the hands of trained medical providers, side effects following IPL treatment are typically transient and easily managed. The most commonly reported adverse effects are mild discomfort, erythema, edema, and desquamating microcrusts. These typically resolve within 48 h, occasionally lasting up to 1 week, and respond well to conservative management such as post-treatment cooling and emollients.

However, inappropriate device settings or improper technique may lead to excess thermal energy, causing exuberant reactions and complications such as blistering, persistent purpura, leukotrichia, scarring, keloid formation, undesired hair reduction or hair growth, and risk of infections. Icing, compression, and focal application of topical corticosteroids immediately after treatment may help minimize subsequent complications. Hyperpigmentation and hypopigmentation to varying degrees may also occur. "Zebra striping" (Fig. 12.4) occurs due to skipped segments and uneven treatment and can be avoided with appropriate spacing and passes. Rarer complications like traumatic tattoos have also been reported.

Extra vigilance must be taken when treating darker skin types. It may be prudent to avoid treating near or over tattoos, as the long pulse duration can lead to prolonged heating of the exogenous pigmented and unwanted thermal damage to tissues. Balancing efficacy with safety of IPL treatments lies most heavily on an experienced clinician and appropriate device settings.

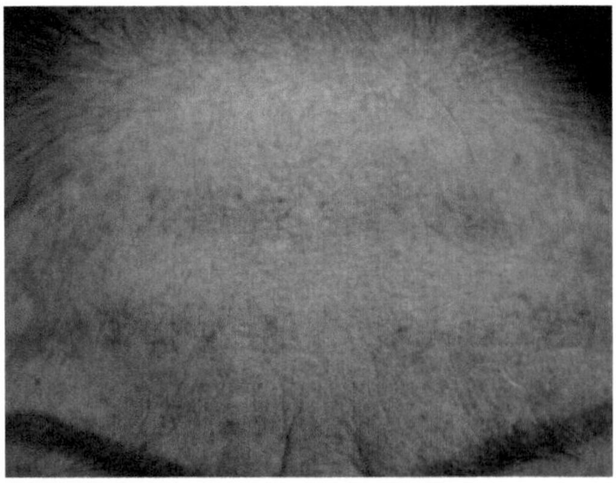

Fig. 12.4 "Zebra striping" that developed within 1 h after treatment

Conclusion

Intense pulsed light has solidified its role in the realm of photorejuvenation, following over three decades of constantly improving technology and track record of favorable results. Its capacity to target multiple chromophores and adaptability for various skin types and conditions make it exceptionally versatile and remarkably effective, positioning it as a fundamental tool for addressing a myriad of dermatological conditions.

As the demand for noninvasive cosmetic procedures continues to surge, IPL will remain a cornerstone in the landscape of modern aesthetic procedures for photorejuvenation. However, given its extensive range of settings, it is best entrusted to an experienced dermatologist or practitioner with deep understanding of its complexities to ensure optimal effectiveness and safety.

References

1. Wat H, Wu DC, Rao J, Goldman MP. Application of intense pulsed light in the treatment of dermatologic disease: a systematic review. Dermatol Surg. 2014;40(4):359–77.
2. Ping C, Xueliang D, Yongxuan L, Lin D, Bilai L, Shaoming L, Gold MH. A retrospective study on the clinical efficacy of the intense pulsed light source for photodamage and skin rejuvenation. J Cosmet Laser Ther. 2016;18(4):217–24.
3. Almukhtar R, Carr E, Goldman M. Intense pulsed light: the early years. Dermatol Rev. 2021;2(2):50–9.
4. Gilbert S, McBurney E. Use of valacyclovir for herpes simplex virus-1 (HSV-1) prophylaxis after facial resurfacing: a randomized clinical trial of dosing regimens. Dermatol Surg. 2000;26(1):50–4.
5. Bitter P. Broad band light and skin rejuvenation. Facial Plastic Surg Clin. 2020;28(1):29–36.
6. Yamashita T, Negishi K, Hariya T, Kunizawa N, Ikuta K, Yanai M, Wakamatsu S. Intense pulsed light therapy for superficial pigmented lesions evaluated by reflectance-mode confocal microscopy and optical coherence tomography. J Investig Dermatol. 2006;126(10):2281–6.
7. Brauer J, Dover KJ, Watchmaker J, Gwinn C. Treatment of skin with intense pulsed light sources.

Procedures in Cosmetic Dermatology: Lasers, Lights, and Energy Devices-E-Book. 2022;20:72–84.
8. Bjerring P, Christiansen K. Intense pulsed light source for treatment of small melanocytic nevi and solar lentigines. J Cutan Laser Ther. 2000;2(4):177–81.
9. Kawada A, Asai M, Kameyama H, Sangen Y, Aragane Y, Tezuka T, Iwakiri K. Videomicroscopic and histopathological investigation of intense pulsed light therapy for solar lentigines. J Dermatol Sci. 2002;29(2):91–6.
10. Wang CC, Sue YM, Yang CH, Chen CK. A comparison of Q-switched alexandrite laser and intense pulsed light for the treatment of freckles and lentigines in Asian persons: a randomized, physician-blinded, split-face comparative trial. J Am Acad Dermatol. 2006;54(5):804–10.
11. Lipp MB, Angra K, Wu DC, Goldman MP. Intense pulsed light: a methodical approach to understanding cllinical endpoints. J Drugs Dermatol. 2021;20(2):203–7.
12. Kalil CL, Reinehr CP, de Mattos Milman L. Intense pulsed light: review of clinical indications. Surg Cosmet Dermatol. 2017;9(1):9–17.
13. Clementoni MT, Gilardino P, Muti GF, Signorini M, Pistorale A, Morselli PG, Cavina C. Intense pulsed light treatment of 1,000 consecutive patients with facial vascular marks. Aesthet Plast Surg. 2006;30:226–32.
14. Zaleski L, Fabi S, Goldman MP. Treatment of melasma and the use of intense pulsed light: a review. J Drugs Dermatol. 2012;11(11):1316–20.
15. Kim J, Lee J, Choi H. Intense pulsed light attenuates UV-induced hyperimmune response and pigmentation in human skin cells. Int J Mol Sci. 2021;22:3173.
16. Li YH, Chen JZ, Wei HC, Wu Y, Liu M, Xu YY, Dong GH, Chen HD. Efficacy and safety of intense pulsed light in treatment of melasma in Chinese patients. Dermatol Surg. 2008;34(5):693–701.
17. Yi J, Hong T, Zeng H, Li P, Li P, Wang S, Chen J, Li P, Zhou J. A meta-analysis-based assessment of intense pulsed light for treatment of melasma. Aesthet Plast Surg. 2020;44:947–52.
18. Goldman MP, Gold MH, Palm MD, Colon LE, Preston N, Johnson LA, Gottschalk RW. Sequential treatment with triple combination cream and intense pulsed light is more efficacious than sequential treatment with an inactive (control) cream and intense pulsed light in patients with moderate to severe melasma. Dermatologic surgery. 2011;37(2):224–33.
19. Vachiramon V, Sirithanabadeekul P, Sahawatwong S. Low-fluence Q-switched Nd: YAG 1064-nm laser and intense pulsed light for the treatment of melasma. J Eur Acad Dermatol Venereol. 2015;29(7):1339–46.
20. Figueiredo Souza L, Trancoso SS. Single-session intense pulsed light combined with stable fixed-dose triple combination topical therapy for the treatment of refractory melasma. Dermatol Ther. 2012;25(5):477–80.
21. Cao Y, Huo R, Feng Y, Li Q, Wang F. Effects of intense pulsed light on the biological properties and ultrastructure of skin dermal fibroblasts: potential roles in photoaging. Photomed Laser Surg. 2011;29(5):327–32.
22. Feng Y, Zhao J, Gold MH. Skin rejuvenation in Asian skin: the analysis of clinical effects and basic mechanisms of intense pulsed light. J Drugs Dermatol. 2008;7(3):273–9.
23. González-Rodríguez AJ, Lorente-Gual R. Current indications and new applications of intense pulsed light. Actas Dermo Sifiliográficas. 2015;106(5):350–64.
24. Sales AF, Pandolfo IL, de Almeida Cruz M, Parisi JR, Garcia LA, Martignago CC, Renno AC, Vassão PG. Intense pulsed light on skin rejuvenation: a systematic review. Arch Dermatol Res. 2022;314(9):823–38.
25. Chang AL, Bitter PH Jr, Qu K, Lin M, Rapicavoli NA, Chang HY. Rejuvenation of gene expression pattern of aged human skin by broadband light treatment: a pilot study. J Investig Dermatol. 2013;133(2):394–402.

Complications from Dermatological Lasers

13

Nancy Garcia-Tan

Introduction

Advances in laser technology in dermatology more than four decades ago brought to the fore new armamentarium to manage skin conditions for which treatment was previously unavailable or unsatisfactory. Selective damage to cutaneous cells from selective absorption of optical radiation gave rise to devices that have become essential in dermatologic practice, such as the treatment of vascular and pigmented lesions.

With continued advancement and innovation, numerous devices have been developed, each one categorized according to the type of technology used (i.e., laser, light, radiofrequency, ultrasound); the target involved (i.e., pigment, tattoo, hair, vessels, fat); or the indication intended (i.e., skin tightening, resurfacing, liposculpting). With this came the challenge of determining optimum treatment protocols to avoid complications. While certain adverse reactions are unique to the individual technology, certain side effects and complications may be common given that they all involve the delivery of energy in defined areas of the skin that almost always involves the introduction or evacuation of heat [1].

N. Garcia-Tan (✉)
Department of Internal Medicine, Section of Dermatology, Cardinal Santos Medical Center, Manila, Philippines

MedDERM Asia Laser & Surgicentre, Manila, Philippines

Side effects and complications that may occur with the use of these devices in general, and those more specific to each category, are discussed. Equally important are management strategies to avoid complications and mitigate its sequelae.

Prevention

The prevention of complications begins with the initial consultation. It is important to first identify the chief concern of the patient, as the perception of the practitioner may differ from that of the patient. However, the doctor should say "no" when the procedure being requested will cause harm or not be beneficial to the patient. Simply put—what the doctor wants may not be what the patient wants; conversely, what the patient wants may not be what he or she needs.

Second, it is imperative that the correct diagnosis be established and prior treatments be known. One has to distinguish the initial problem from complications that may have occurred secondary to past procedures, e.g., melasma vs. post-inflammatory hyperpigmentation (PIH) secondary to previous laser treatments or products used. Knowledge of past treatments also gives the clinician a gauge of the patient's response or adverse effects that may have occurred.

History taking should include past health and surgeries done as these may have altered anatomical areas or impact the choice of procedures to

S. W. N. Cheng, C. L. Goh (eds.), *Updates on Lasers in Dermatology*, Updates in Clinical Dermatology, https://doi.org/10.1007/978-3-031-71155-8_13

be performed (e.g., pacemakers and metal implants may be affected by electromagnetic devices or radiofrequency). Underlying medical conditions and medications may predispose to infection or affect healing (e.g., immunocompromised states, intake of corticosteroids), and some supplements or maintenance drugs such as blood thinners may contribute to troublesome bleeding or bruising. Allergies particularly to analgesics, antibiotics, antivirals, or anti-inflammatory agents should be taken note of as these may be needed pre- or post-procedure. Health habits, occupation, hobbies, and activities including cigarette smoking, alcohol intake, and sun exposure may affect postoperative care, treatment timeline, and outcome.

With complete knowledge of the above, the physician should then weigh whether the patient is suitable for the treatment contemplated. Patient selection implies having the right patient for the right procedure. Aside from an informed consent, pre- and posttreatment photographs are a must especially for cosmetic procedures.

Complications may occur secondary to physician error or poor patient compliance but may also be due to device malfunction. Regular preventive maintenance is mandatory; beam alignment, handpiece, and tips should be checked prior to each use. It would be important to note that devices that have been recently serviced may have a different output than before servicing. It is thus important to be knowledgeable about expected reactions and clinical endpoints rather than to memorize device settings and be able to promptly identify when there is something amiss with the reaction of the skin.

Managing Expectations

Failure to manage expectations for each and every procedure contemplated results in an unhappy patient, with a negative effect on the doctor-patient relationship. The patient needs to know the degree of improvement that may be achieved, the side effects and potential complications that may occur, the presence of pain and downtime, the number of sessions needed, the costs involved, and what cannot be achieved with a particular procedure as patients often get confused as to which procedure achieves which result.

Even in the most experienced hands, adverse reactions may happen. Such adverse effects are usually better received by patients when they have been informed beforehand, not when the side effect has already occurred. Discussing potential complications makes the patient aware of inherent risks. An *informed* consent is thus obtained, not simply a signature on a form. Patient complaints are less likely to occur in these conditions, averting malpractice suits.

General Side Effects

When used appropriately, side effects from laser-, light-, and energy-based devices are usually mild and transient, and may even be the expected or the desired clinical endpoint (Table 13.1). On the other end of the spectrum are serious complications that may be permanent.

Erythema

Erythema is likely to occur after almost any laser-, light-, or energy-based device procedure. While most laser technologies can deliver energy selectively, some heat is likely to dissipate in and around the treated areas. Erythema is usually mild and transient and fades within 24 h. In most cases, ice packs on the area will suffice with no need for further treatment. Intense or prolonged erythema which lasts for more than 3–7 days may however lead to PIH, particularly in darker skin types (Figs. 13.1 and 13.2). In such instances, mild topical corticosteroids may be needed to avoid discomfort and subsequent hyperpigmentation; sun protection is advised post-procedure.

Edema

Edema is usually accompanied by erythema (Fig. 13.3) and fades within 24 h except in the

Table 13.1 Side effects/complications of lasers and energy-based devices

Side effect/complication	Management
A. General side effects	
Erythema	Cold packs, topical corticosteroids, sun protection
Edema	Cold packs, topical or oral corticosteroids
Purpura	Cold packs, sun protection
Hyperpigmentation	Depigmenting creams, sun protection
Hypopigmentation	Narrowband UVB/excimer laser/fractional lasers
Burns	Cold packs, topical corticosteroids, sun protection
Blisters, crusting	Cold compress, topical or oral antibiotics
Urticaria	Topical corticosteroid, oral antihistamines
Allergic reactions	Topical or oral corticosteroid, oral antihistamines
Infection (bacterial, viral, yeast)	Topical or oral antibiotics, antiviral prophylaxis for HSV, topical or oral anti-yeast agents
Scarring	Topical/intralesional corticosteroids, PDL for hypertrophic scars; fractional lasers for hypertrophic/atrophic scars, sun protection
Pain	Topical/local anesthetic, cooling methods
B. Laser hair removal	
Perifollicular erythema and edema	Cold packs, topical corticosteroids, oral antihistamine
Paradoxical hypertrichosis	Continue laser treatment of areas involved
C. Laser resurfacing	
Acne and milia formation	Regular acne medication
Line of demarcation	Prevent by feathering on the periphery of treated areas
D. Cryolipolysis	
Bruising and tenderness	Cold packs, oral analgesic
Numbness, paresthesia	No treatment
Paradoxical hypertrophy	No treatment
E. Intense pulsed light	
Footprinting	Prevent by slight overlap
F. Pigment lasers	
Erythema, crusting, PIH	As above
Purpura/pinpoint bleeding	As above
G. Vascular lasers	
Purpura	As above
H. RF, US, HIFEM	
Temporary/prolonged nerve damage	No treatment

periorbital area where it may last longer. Cold compresses and a short course of oral or topical corticosteroids may be needed if edema is significant.

Purpura

Purpura is an expected side effect of pulsed dye lasers (PDL) and usually fades in 7–10 days. This may also occur after treatment with 1064 nm Q-switched neodymium:yttrium aluminum garnet (QS Nd:YAG) lasers (Fig. 13.4). The use of longer pulse widths, lower fluences, and skin cooling lessens this side effect. In patients with darker skin, purpura may lead to PIH once the bruising subsides. Ice packs may be applied immediately posttreatment, followed by sun avoidance and use of depigmenting agents if PIH sets in.

Dyspigmentation

Post-inflammatory hyperpigmentation is a relatively common side effect occurring more fre-

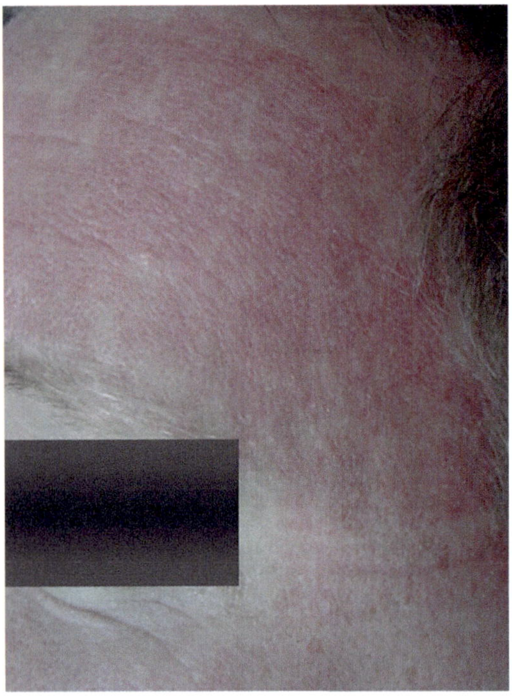

Fig. 13.1 Erythema on Fitzpatrick skin type I; usually fades within 24 h

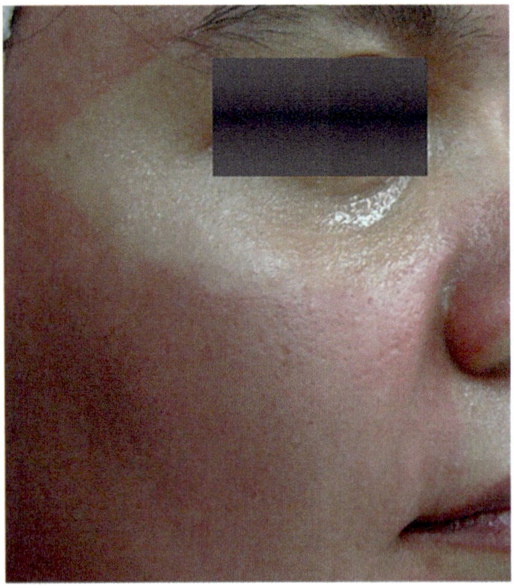

Fig. 13.2 Erythema on Fitzpatrick skin type V has higher risk for PIH

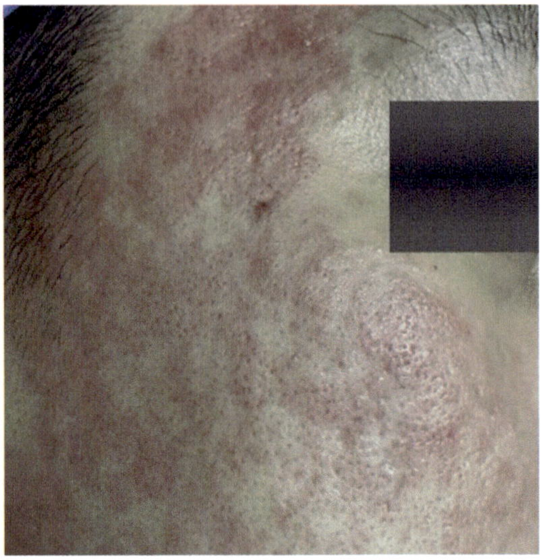

Fig. 13.3 Edema and erythema following fractional bipolar radiofrequency treatment for acne scars

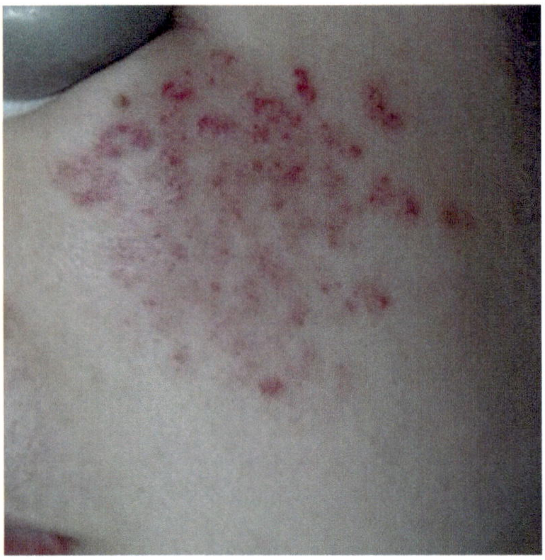

Fig. 13.4 Purpura following 1064 nm QS Nd:YAG laser treatment for Hori's nevus

quently in darker skinned patients. Common causes include the use of high fluences and inadequate cooling during treatment, but may also result from the use of excessive cryogen cooling (Fig. 13.5) or following marked erythema or purpura. Aside from the Fitzpatrick skin type, other factors that may contribute to its development include tanning prior to treatment, degree of dermo-epidermal junction (DEJ) disruption, and degree of inflammation at the DEJ [2]. PIH usually dissolves slowly over time; strict sun protection and depigmenting creams may be used in conjunction.

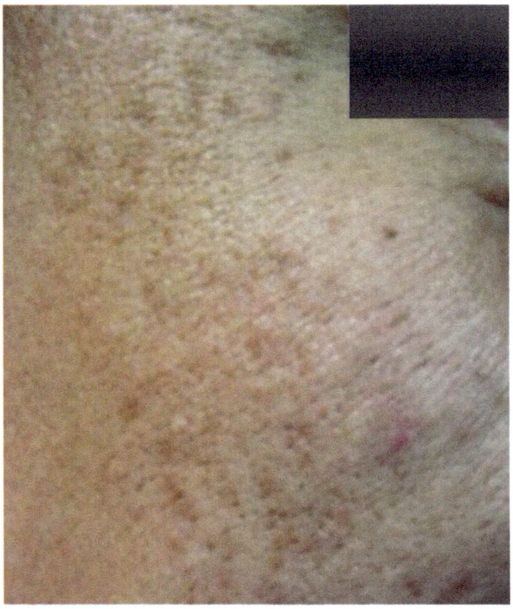

Fig. 13.5 PIH from cryogen cooling from a diode laser

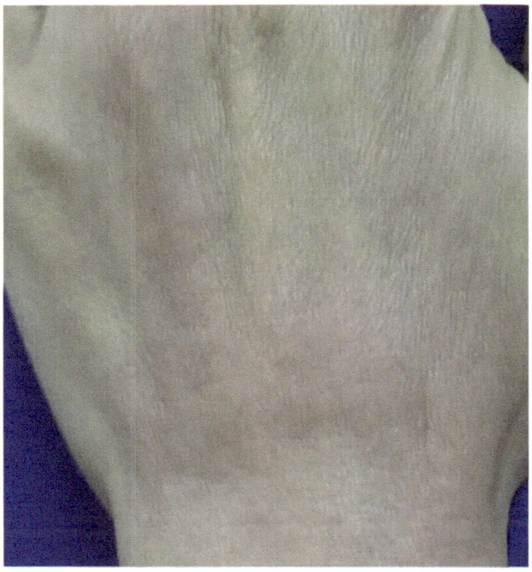

Fig. 13.6 Wheals following fractional skin resurfacing using thermomechanical ablation device on the dorsum of hand

Hypopigmentation is less common than PIH. It may be transient or permanent and difficult to treat. Narrowband UVB phototherapy, excimer laser, and fractional lasers have been tried with varying results [3].

Burns

Burns can result from the use of excessive fluences, long-pulse durations, pulse stacking, overlapping, or inadequate cooling. Blisters, crusting, PIH, and scarring may be the unwanted sequelae. The risk of burns is higher when using continuous beams versus pulsed or fractionated beams [4].

Urticaria

Wheals may occur following laser procedures (Fig. 13.6). These mostly represent a form of physical urticaria [3] and usually fade spontaneously with no further treatment required. If marked pruritus occurs, short-term topical corticosteroids and/or oral antihistamines may be given.

Allergic Reactions

Allergic reactions may result from the use of anesthetics, antibiotics, anti-inflammatory drugs, and other agents such as antiseptics, adhesives, or latex. These include type I hypersensitivity reactions such as urticaria, anaphylaxis, or angioedema or type IV delayed hypersensitivity reactions such as contact dermatitis [5] which may be secondary to the active ingredient itself or the vehicle used (Fig. 13.7). Short-course oral or topical corticosteroids and antihistamines help relieve related symptoms.

Infections

The risk of infection increases with the disruption of the epidermal barrier and is highest with ablative resurfacing procedures. Pain is a useful diagnostic sign, accompanied by patchy erythema, erosions, and superficial crusting, usually occurring 48 h post-ablation [6]. Infection may lead to scarring which can be permanent and thus should be treated promptly. Infection may be secondary to bacteria, virus, or yeast. Bacterial infections are usually due to *Staphylococcus aureus*, while viral infections are commonly a

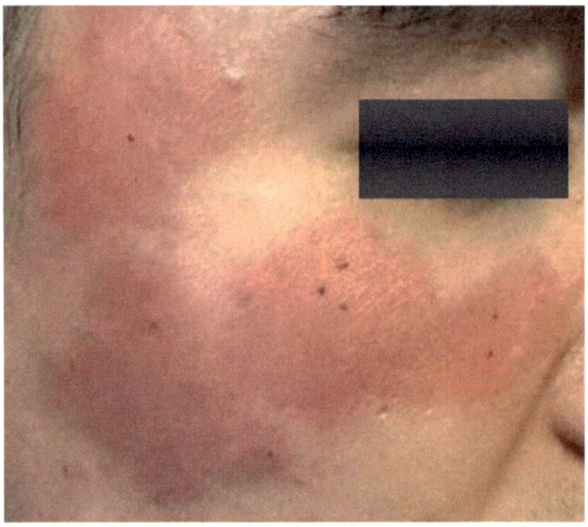

Fig. 13.7 Contact dermatitis to antibiotic-steroid cream applied s/p CO_2 laser for wart removal

reactivation of herpes simplex virus (HSV) infection. Antiviral prophylaxis may be warranted for those with a positive history of HSV infection. Yeast infections are rare and are commonly due to *Candida* species.

Scarring

Scarring is the most feared laser complication. Risk factors include using high fluences, pulse stacking, excessive overlap, high repetition rate, and inadequate cooling. It may also result from crusting, blistering, and infection. Caution should be exercised when resurfacing the neck as this area is more prone to scarring, likely due to a thinner dermis and lower concentration of pilosebaceous units [7]. Treatment for hypertrophic scars includes topical or intralesional corticosteroids and silicone gel sheets. Ironically, fractional lasers which may induce scarring in itself are also used in the treatment of hypertrophic and atrophic scars.

Pain

Pain may be minimized by the skin cooling and topical and local anesthesia but with careful attention to the total area involved. Application of local anesthetics over extensive areas may result in systemic absorption and consequent adverse reactions. Maximum dose of plain lidocaine is 4.5 mg/kg (not to exceed 300 mg). Symptoms of lidocaine toxicity include circumoral numbness, tongue paresthesia, dizziness, tinnitus, blurred vision, restlessness, muscle twitches, and seizures [8].

Eye Complications

Eye complications that have been reported with the use of laser- and energy-based devices include cataracts, iritis, iris atrophy, pupillary distortion, uveitis, photophobia, posterior synechiae, and visual field defects. It is important to note that some of the cases reported occurred despite the use of protective eyewear. This may be due to incorrect goggles used, improper positioning, or heat accumulation on corneal metal eye shields during periocular CO_2 resurfacing procedures [9].

Complications from Laser Plume

Laser plume produced during laser resurfacing or hair removal has been shown to contain particulate tissue debris, vapors, and smoke that have been reported to be carcinogenic, as well as being a teratogen. This presents as a health hazard to all those exposed including the operators and their assistants [10]. Use of appropriate surgical masks and smoke evacuators with appropriate filters are advised when performing these procedures.

Complications Related to Specific Indications

Aside from general side effects, certain complications are seen more commonly with specific devices or in relation to specific indications (Table 13.1).

Laser Hair Removal (LHR)

LHR has gained popularity in the past decade driven by patient demand. Though a relatively safe procedure when performed by trained practitioners, the incidence of side effects has increased in the past decade particularly with nonmedical personnel performing these procedures. In a review of liability claims due to a cutaneous laser surgery device from 2012 to 2020 in the United States, out of 69 cases, the most common litigated was LHR (64%), with 49 cases (71%) involving nonphysician operators [11]. Data gathered were consistent with an earlier study that reviewed cases from 1985 to 2012, which showed LHR as the most litigated procedure with a substantial subset of cases due to nonphysician operators [12].

Lasers and light devices used for hair reduction include ruby laser (694 nm), alexandrite laser (755 nm), diode laser (810 nm), Nd:YAG laser (1064 nm), and intense pulse light (IPL) or broadband light (BBL) (500–1200 nm) [13]. The target chromophore in laser hair removal is melanin located in the hair shaft and the hair bulb. Light energy absorbed by the target chromophore is converted to intense heat energy that diffuses into and destroys the hair follicle. The stem cells located in the hair bulge do not contain melanin but are destroyed by thermal damage through the diffusion of heat energy; damage to these cells prevents future hair regrowth [10].

The skin type and history of recent tanning from sun exposure play a role in the incidence of laser hair removal complications. In patients with dark or tanned skin, melanin in the epidermis competes with melanin in the hair follicle. Absorption of photons in the epidermis leads to thermal injury. The most common complications with LHR include folliculitis, erythema, perifollicular edema, pain, crusting, and purpura. More severe complications include thermal burns, permanent scarring, blisters, pigmentary changes (hyper- and hypopigmentation), and eye complications.

Perifollicular erythema and edema (Fig. 13.8) are desired endpoints in LHR and generally fade in a few hours. Some patients may experience accompanying pruritus, which is usually relieved by mild topical corticosteroid creams applied for a few days posttreatment and oral antihistamine.

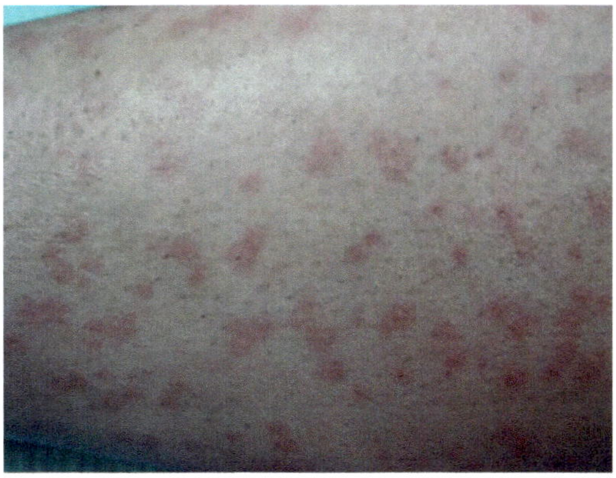

Fig. 13.8 Perifollicular erythema and edema after LHR on the legs using 1064 nm Nd:YAG laser

Patients with darker skin types are more at risk for pigmentary changes and scarring, due to their greater epidermal melanin content. Use of longer wavelengths, longer pulse durations, efficient cooling, and conservative fluence can help minimize these complications. For patients with darker skin, the Nd:YAG laser has been shown to be effective with less side effects [14].

Paradoxical hypertrichosis (PH) has been reported in about 4% of patients undergoing hair removal with IPL or lasers on the face; it is exceedingly rare in non-facial areas. The pathogenesis is unclear, but it is thought to be secondary to subtherapeutic thermal injury, which induces terminal hairs from vellus hairs. Continued treatment in areas where PH has occurred has been the management approach [15].

Devices designed for home use have recently gained popularity due to their lower cost and convenience. Safety concerns and complications have arisen because of the shift from professionally done LHR in the clinics to unsupervised use by inexperienced users (Fig. 13.9). These devices based on light or laser technology emit lower fluences compared to in-office devices. Despite FDA regulatory measures, accidental injury to the skin and the eyes of the user and those nearby continues to pose a concern [14].

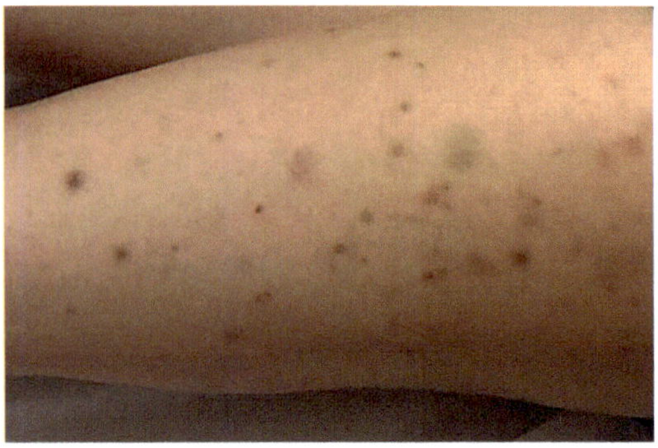

Fig. 13.9 Papular eruption and PIH following hair removal using a home device

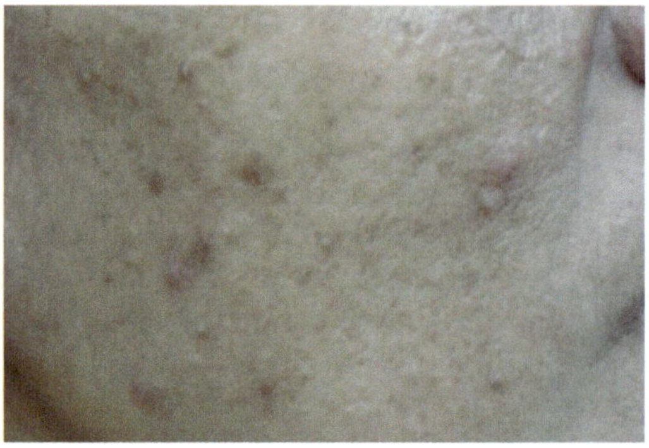

Fig. 13.10 Acne and milia formation following fractional CO_2 treatment

Laser Resurfacing

Ablative laser resurfacing uses high-energy, carbon dioxide (CO_2) and erbium-doped yttrium aluminum garnet (Er:YAG) devices in the treatment of photodamaged skin and scars. Complete ablation of the epidermis and upper papillary dermis results in oozing, copious serous discharge, and crusting, with reepithelialization occurring within an average of 8.5 days for CO_2 laser-resurfaced skin and 5.5 days for Er:YAG laser-treated skin [16].

The prolonged recovery and potential side effects which include infections (viral, bacterial, fungal), prolonged erythema, permanent scarring, ectropion, and post-inflammatory hypo- or hyperpigmentation have made ablative resurfacing less favored as a treatment modality. Other complications include acne and milia formation, contact dermatitis, pruritus, reactivation of herpes simplex virus (HSV) infection, and hypopigmented line of demarcation particularly above the angle of the mandible.

PIH is a common complication especially for darker skin types; hence, there should be a shift to non-ablative or fractional resurfacing for this segment of patients, since even with these modalities, PIH cannot be totally avoidable. Postoperative care for optimum healing, sun avoidance, and use of sunscreens are of utmost importance. Hypertrophic scars may be treated with corticosteroids or PDL. Line of demarcation is best avoided by feathering the laser beam in the peripheral borders of areas being treated.

Fractional photothermolysis generates microthermal treatment zones in the dermis which are columns of thermally denatured skin with controlled width and depth. This concept has revolutionized laser resurfacing, with shortened recovery period and decreased incidence of serious complications such as infections and scarring that occur more frequently with ablative resurfacing. Erythema immediately posttreatment is an expected side effect and usually subsides in 1–3 days. Acneiform eruptions and milia formation (Fig. 13.10) have been reported though incidence is lower compared to ablative mode and responds favorably to regular acne medication.

Carbon Dioxide Laser for Removal of Benign Cutaneous Growths

CO_2 lasers have been used extensively in dermatologic surgery to treat benign cutaneous lesions including warts, seborrheic keratosis, actinic keratosis, acrochordon, melanocytic nevi, sebaceous hyperplasia, syringoma, xanthelasma, rhinophyma, and angiofibroma. Parameter setting depends on the specific device used and type and depth of lesion. Immediate side effects include pain, erythema, edema, and crusting. Delayed side effects include infection, pigmentary changes, and scarring (Fig. 13.11).

Pain is averted with the use of topical or locally infiltrated anesthesia. Erythema and edema usually disappear after a few hours, but topical corticosteroids may be used if persistent.

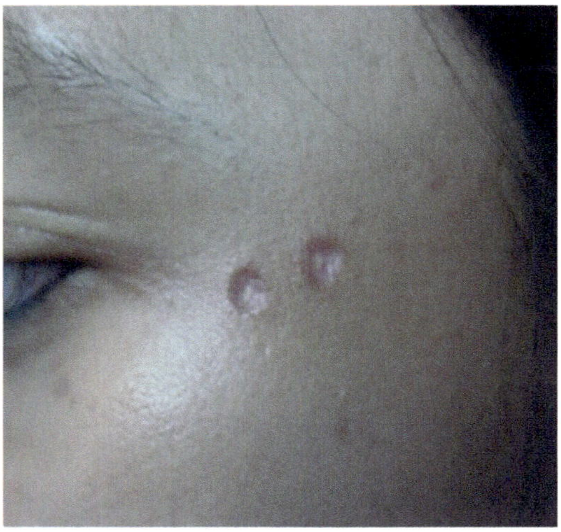

Fig. 13.11 Depressed scars following laser removal of warts

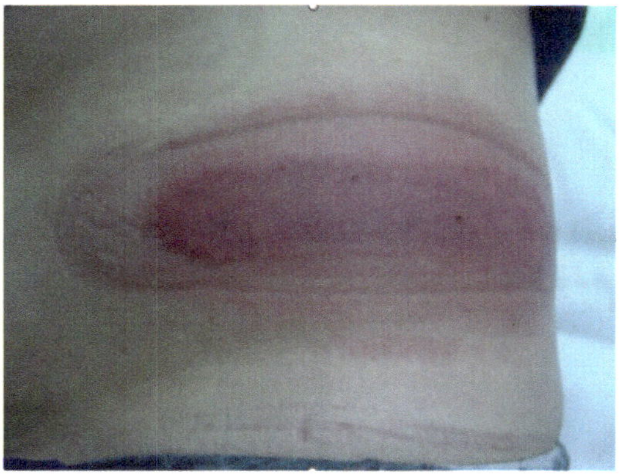

Fig. 13.12 Erythema, edema, bruising after cryolipolysis on the trunk

Infection is rare, but topical antibiotics may help prevent its occurrence. Sun avoidance and use of sunscreens help prevent PIH. As with any device, scarring is best prevented with proper training with the specific device and correct parameter settings.

Cryolipolysis

Cryolipolysis involves the application of freezing temperatures to induce adipocyte apoptosis. Erythema, edema, bruising (Fig. 13.12), tenderness, numbness, and paresthesia may occur immediately after a few days of treatment. Less common side effects include dysesthesia which may present as tingling, burning, or increased sensitivity over the treated area; delayed or persistent severe pain; PIH; and contour irregularities.

Though rare, patients should be informed about the risk of paradoxical hypertrophy, which presents as well-demarcated hyperplasia of subcutaneous fat. This complication may develop months after treatment and does not resolve spontaneously. The exact mechanism is unknown, but it is hypothesized that subapoptotic injury due to inadequate contact with the cooling applicator stimulates adipocyte growth [17].

Complications Related to Specific Devices

Intense Pulsed Light

IPL utilizes high-intensity light sources to treat a wide range of dermatological conditions which include photoaging, pigmented lesions, vascular lesions, and photoepilation. IPL treatments are relatively safe for patients with lighter skin types, but should be used with caution in those with darker skin types, tanned skin, or recent sunburn. The most common side effects of IPL include erythema, pain, edema, crusting, and pigmentary changes (Fig. 13.13). Slight overlap between pulses avoids skipped areas, which may leave a footprint of dyspigmentation in contrast to adjacent treated areas (Fig. 13.14). Use by untrained personnel and inappropriate settings can lead to more serious complications such as superficial burns and scarring due to nonspecific thermal damage. Reactivation of HSV has also been reported; prophylaxis with antivirals may be needed for patients with past history of infection.

Pigment Lasers

Laser and light devices have been used to treat pigmentary conditions such as ephelides, lentigines, nevus of Ota, Hori's nevus, melasma, PIH, and melasma. Most frequently used devices are

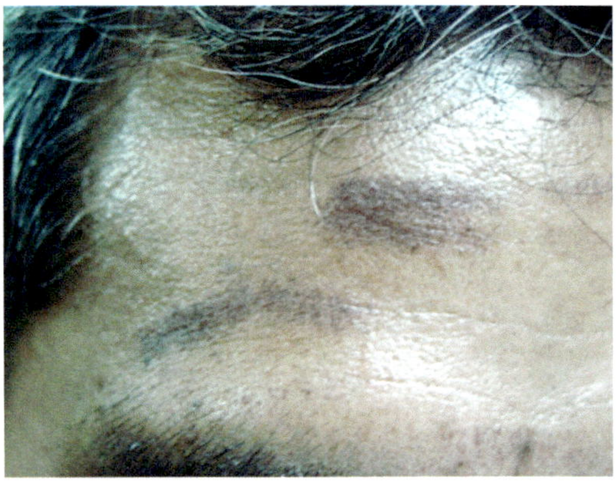

Fig. 13.13 Linear crusting and PIH on the forehead following IPL treatment

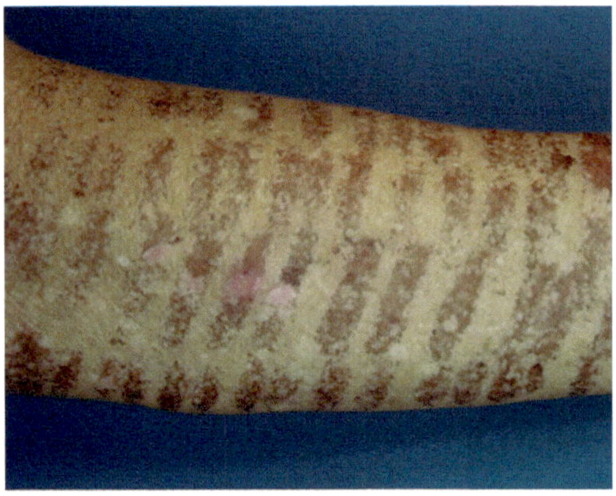

Fig. 13.14 Crusting, PIH, and foot printing on the forearm following IPL treatment

1064 nm QS Nd:YAG, 532 nm QS Nd:YAG, 532 nm potassium titanyl phosphate (KTP) laser, 755 nm QS alexandrite laser, and IPL. Complications from the use of these devices include pain, erythema, edema, petechiae, blistering, crusting, and dyspigmentation (Figs. 13.15 and 13.16).

The risk for PIH (Fig. 13.17) is greater for patients with darker skin types and tanned skin. Care should therefore be taken in patient selection and treatment timelines. Mild topical steroids may be used right after the procedure to alleviate erythema, which may lead to PIH. Sun avoidance and use of sunscreens are important reminders post-procedure. Use of depigmenting

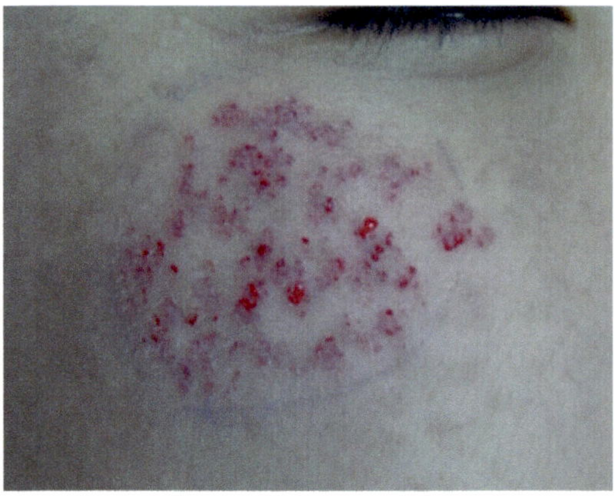

Fig. 13.15 Petechiae, pinpoint bleeding following 1064 nm QS Nd:YAG laser treatment for Hori's nevus

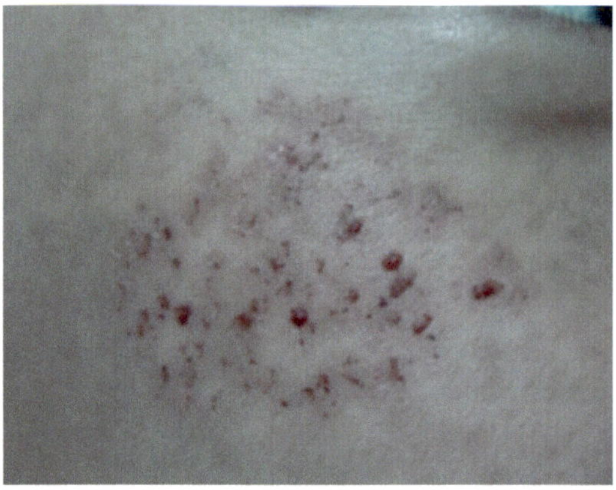

Fig. 13.16 Crusting following 1064 nm QS Nd:YAG laser treatment for Hori's nevus

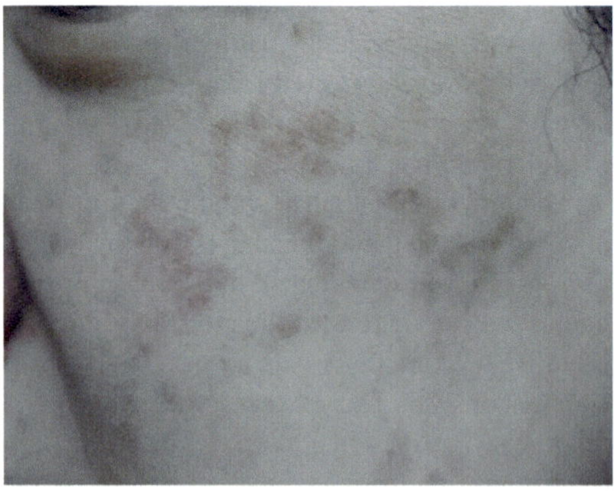

Fig. 13.17 PIH following 532 nm QS Nd:YAG laser treatment for ephelides

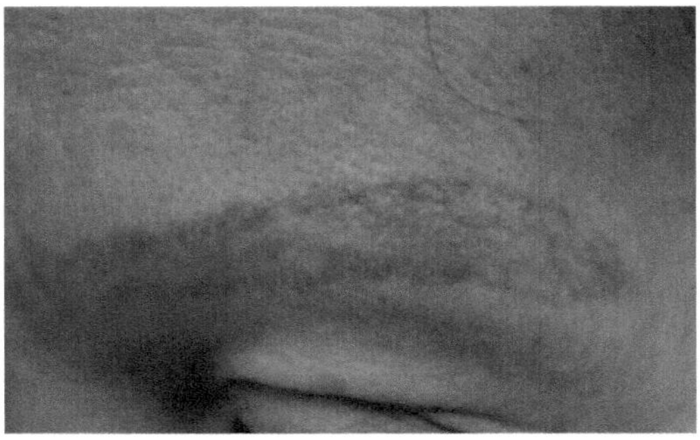

Fig. 13.18 Paradoxical darkening of eyebrow tattoo following 1064 nm QS Nd:YAG laser treatment

agents such as hydroquinone—alone or in triple combination with steroids and retinoic acid—and other products containing niacinamide, arbutin, and kojic acid may be used to treat PIH. Ironically, lasers have also been used to treat PIH that resulted from laser treatments of pigmentary conditions.

Paradoxical darkening of tattoos treated with QS Nd:YAG laser (Fig. 13.18) is believed to be due to the reduction of metallic compounds such as ferric oxide to ferrous oxide or titanium to titanium oxide. Continued treatment with Nd:YAG laser has been shown to eventually lighten the pigment. It would be prudent to do a test spot when removing cosmetic tattoos especially over the eyebrows as it may be difficult to treat this complication.

Vascular Lasers

Pulsed dye lasers (585, 595 nm), KTP lasers (532 nm), and longer wavelength lasers such as alexandrite lasers (755 nm), diode lasers (800–900 nm), millisecond Nd:YAG lasers (1064 nm), and IPL have been used to treat vascular lesions.

Purpura and bruising (Fig. 13.19a) are immediate side effects and usually fade in 7–10 days. Appearance of gray or pale white discoloration of the epidermis is a sign of dermal damage secondary to inappropriately high radiant exposures. Blister formation and subsequent crusting may occur following this sign,

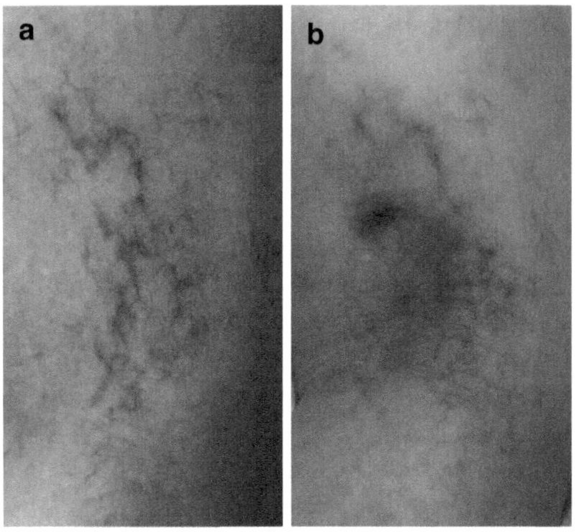

Fig. 13.19 (**a**) Purpura, bruising, and (**b**) subsequent PIH after 1064 nm long-pulsed Nd:YAG treatment for leg veins

which appears only for a few seconds. Other complications include dyspigmentation (hypo- or hyperpigmentation) (Fig. 13.19b), textural changes, and scarring. Skin cooling, lower energy densities, longer pulse durations, and avoidance of pulse stacking help decrease these complications.

Radiofrequency (RF), Ultrasound, and High-Intensity Focused Electromagnetic (HIFEM) Devices

RF devices including monopolar RF for skin tightening, RF microneedling for rejuvenation, and scar treatment can interfere with cardiac pacemakers, hence the importance of eliciting this history during the first consultation as this may have lethal outcomes. It is also important to know if the patient has dental metal implants or hip/knee replacements or other implantable devices. Use of HIFEM over these areas should be avoided. Temporary or prolonged nerve damage may also occur following the use of these devices. When treating the face or submental area, it is advised to avoid the temporal and marginal mandibular branches of the temporal nerve [18].

Conclusion

Even in the most experienced hands, adverse reactions may occur with the use of lasers and energy-based devices. Thorough history taking, careful patient selection, management of patient expectations, and discussion of potential complications are imperative in preventing problems postoperatively. Certain side effects are expected and may be the desired endpoint for certain procedures and hence must be differentiated from complications.

Informed consent, pre- and posttreatment photographs, and clear postoperative instructions are needed for each procedure, each and every time they are performed, even if the patient has undergone the same procedure in the past.

As technology evolves and indications for these tools increase, so will the number of complications, particularly with usage extending beyond physicians to technicians and aestheticians. It is imperative that practitioners are fully aware of the spectrum of adverse reactions and how these can be minimized to avoid negative outcomes.

References

1. Alam M, Warycha M. Complications of lasers and light treatments. Dermatol Ther. 2011;24(6):571–80.
2. Chan NPY, Ho SGY, Yeung CK, Shek SYN, Chan HH. The use of non-ablative fractional resurfacing in Asian acne scar patients. Lasers Surg Med. 2010;42(10):870–5.
3. Al-Niaimi F. Laser and energy-based devices' complications in dermatology. J Cosmet Laser Ther. 2016;18(1):25–30.
4. Prohaska J, Hohman MH. Laser complications. In: StatPearls. Treasure Island: StatPearls Publishing; 2023.
5. Rachidi S, Goldberg DJ. Complications and legal considerations of laser, light, and energy-based treatments. Proc Cosmet Dermatol. 2022;221–7.
6. Cavallini M, Molinari P. Managing errors and complications in aesthetic medicine. Officina Editoriale Oltrarno; 2016.
7. Metelitsa AI, Alster TS. Fractionated laser skin resurfacing treatment complications: a review. Dermatol Surg. 2010;36(3):299–306.
8. Torp KD, Metheny E, Simon LV. Lidocaine toxicity. StatPearls; 2022.
9. Van Gemert MJ, Bloemen PR, Wang WY, Van der Geld CW, Nuijts RM, Hortoglu H, Wolkerstorfer A, de Bruin DM, van Leeuwen TG, Neumann HM, Jager MJ. Periocular CO_2 laser resurfacing: severe ocular complications from multiple unintentional laser impacts on the protective metal eye shields. Lasers Surg Med. 2018;50(10):980–6.
10. Thomas MM, Houreld NN. The "in's and outs" of laser hair removal: a mini review. J Cosmet Laser Ther. 2019;21(6):316–22.
11. Khalifian S, Vazirnia A, Mohan GC, Thompson KV, Jalian HR, Avram MM. Causes of injury and litigation in cutaneous laser surgery: an update from 2012 to 2020. Dermatol Surg. 2022;48(3):315–9.
12. Jalian HR, Jalian CA, Avram MM. Common causes of injury and legal action in laser surgery. JAMA Dermatol. 2013;149(2):188–93.
13. Vaidya T, Hohman MH, Kumar D. Laser hair removal. StatPearls; 2022.
14. Gan SD, Graber EM. Laser hair removal: a review. Dermatol Surg. 2013;39(6):823–38.
15. Snast I, Kaftory R, Lapidoth M, Levi A. Paradoxical hypertrichosis associated with laser and light therapy for hair removal: a systematic review and meta-analysis. Am J Clin Dermatol. 2021;22(5):615–24.
16. AlNomair N, Nazarian R, Marmur E. Complications in lasers, lights, and radiofrequency devices. Facial Plast Surg. 2012;28(03):340–6.
17. Hedayati B, Juhász M, Chu S, Mesinkovska NA. Adverse events associated with cryolipolysis: a systematic review of the literature. Dermatol Surg. 2020;46:S8–13.
18. Hitchcock TM, Dobke MK. Review of the safety profile of microfocused ultrasound with visualization. J Cosmet Dermatol. 2014;13:329–35.

Index

S. W. N. Cheng, C. L. Goh (eds.), *Updates on Lasers in Dermatology*, Updates in Clinical Dermatology, https://doi.org/10.1007/978-3-031-71155-8

GPSR Compliance

The European Union's (EU) General Product Safety Regulation (GPSR) is a set of rules that requires consumer products to be safe and our obligations to ensure this.

If you have any concerns about our products, you can contact us on ProductSafety@springernature.com

In case Publisher is established outside the EU, the EU authorized representative is:

Springer Nature Customer Service Center GmbH
Europaplatz 3
69115 Heidelberg, Germany

Batch number: 10732809

Printed by Printforce, the Netherlands